Kate Cole-Adams is a journalist and writer. Her novel *Walking to the Moon* is also published by Text.

ANAESTHESIA

THE GIFT OF OBLIVION AND
THE MYSTERY OF CONSCIOUSNESS

KATE COLE-ADAMS

TEXT PUBLISHING MELBOURNE AUSTRALIA

textpublishing.com.au

The Text Publishing Company
Swann House
22 William Street
Melbourne Victoria 3000
Australia

The Text Publishing Company (UK) Ltd
130 Wood Street
London, EC2V 6DL
United Kingdom

First published in 2017 by The Text Publishing Company

Index by Karen Gillen
Cover design by Sandy Cull
Cover photograph by Milles Studio/Stocksy
Page design by Jess Horrocks
Typeset in Granjon 12/16.75 by J&M Typesetting

Printed in Australia by Griffin Press, an Accredited ISO AS/NZS 14001:2004 Environmental Management System printer.

National Library of Australia Cataloguing-in-Publication entry
Creator: Cole-Adams, Kate, author.
Title: Anaesthesia : the gift of oblivion and the mystery of consciousness / by Kate Cole-Adams.
ISBN: 9781925498202 (paperback)
ISBN: 9781925410525 (ebook)
Subjects: Anesthesia—Australia.
 Anesthesia—Popular works.
 Anesthetics—Physiological effect.

This book is printed on paper certified against the Forest Stewardship Council® Standards. Griffin Press holds FSC chain-of-custody certification SGS-COC-005088. FSC promotes environmentally responsible, socially beneficial and economically viable management of the world's forests.

This project has been assisted by the Australian Government through the Australia Council, its arts funding and advisory body.

For Pete, Finn and Frannie
With love and gratitude

Contents

Into the blue

I am in a smallish, whitish room in a hospital in Brisbane. It is night. On the wall opposite my bed I can dimly make out a crucifix with its limp passenger. Beneath it float wide blank windows through which I watch the synapses of city light: a web of tiny illuminations and extinctions that seem, when I loosen my gaze, almost to form patterns; as if they are about to make sense. I am surprised at how calm I feel.

In the weeks leading up to this moment I have set my affairs in order. Made a will, written letters for the children, waxed my legs. Said my farewells at the airport and boarded the flight from Melbourne with my mother. July 2010.

Some months before this, after decades of resistance, I gave in at last to the inevitability of major surgery. My capitulation was sudden and took place in a different wing of this same hospital, where I had come to consult a respected spinal surgeon. The surgeon had a quiet, almost diffident, manner and a moustache that put me in mind of a doleful Groucho. I am not sure what made my mind up, the moustache or the way his finger traced my wayward spine quite gently on the X-ray before him. But just as he began to tell me that I would not be a candidate for the type of non-invasive surgery we had been talking about, I realised with a small thud of certainty that, not only was I going to have this surgery—invasive though it might be—I was going to come back to Brisbane and he was going to do it.

In the aftermath of my decision, I was buoyed in a backwash of something like relief; a giving up of hope and its attendant efforts, a yielding to forces beyond my will. But when I lay awake at night, disquiet rose around me. It was not just the surgery that was worrying me—the cutting and drilling, the inevitable risk—it was that in some blank corner of myself I felt that I would not wake up afterwards. I knew logically, and during the day could convince myself, that for an otherwise healthy forty-eight-year-old, the likelihood of calamity was low. But at night, there in my bed in Melbourne, the conviction multiplied inside me that even if everything went according to plan, the me who woke after surgery would not be the same in some essential way as the me who had been wheeled into the operating theatre beforehand. I developed a dread of the moment when the anaesthetic drugs would take effect and I would cease to be. I pictured myself in a stark, poorly lit room with two doors, one in, one out, neither of which I could open from within. Otherwise the room was empty. No windows, no furniture. In this darkness—which I now realise had the same sinuous quality as the shadows beneath my childhood bed—I would be trapped alone. Perhaps forever. At least until such time as someone else chose to release, not me but some other, ostensibly similar, version of me who would slip soundlessly into the life that had once been mine.

Shortly after making my decision I rang a separate Brisbane medical practice. I asked to speak to the doctor whose job it would be to render me unconscious and keep me that way during the long operation. Halting, almost apologetic, I explained to the receptionist that I had spent some years researching the process known as anaesthesia, and that I was now rather nervous about what was going to happen to me. 'I think I know too much,' I said.

'Oh dear,' said the receptionist. 'That's not good.'

o

This book explores perhaps the most brilliant and baffling gift of modern medicine: the disappearing act that enables doctors and dentists to carry out surgery and other procedures that would otherwise be impossibly, often fatally, painful.

Anaesthesia. The term was appropriated from the Greek by New England physician and poet Oliver Wendell Holmes in 1846 to describe the effect of the drug ether following its first successful public demonstration in surgery. *Anaesthetise*: to render insensible.

These days there are other sorts of anaesthetics that can numb a tooth or a torso simply (or unsimply) by switching off the nerves in the relevant part of the body. But the most widespread and intriguing application of this curious craft is what is now known as general anaesthesia. In general anaesthesia it is not the nerve endings that are switched off, it is your brain—or at least parts of it. These, it seems, include the connections that somehow enable the operation of our sense of self, or (loosely) consciousness, as well as the parts of the brain responsible for processing messages from the nerves telling us that we are in pain: the neurological equivalent of shooting the messenger. Which is, of course, a good thing.

More than a good thing. I would not have boarded that plane to Brisbane had it been otherwise. And I don't assume my fears were greater than those of anyone else in my predicament. But it was also true that for the previous decade I had been deeply preoccupied with a question or series of questions, often nebulous and contradictory, that amounted to this: what really happens to us when we are anaesthetised?

By this I mean not what happens to the pinging, crackling apparatus of our nerves and spinal cords and brains, but what happens to *us*—to the person who is me or the person who is you—as doctors go about the messy business of slicing and delving within us? And, fused somehow to this, another odd and stubborn question: can whatever happens (or doesn't happen) while we are under anaesthesia continue to affect us in our waking lives? Can it change the way we feel or think or behave in the minutes, months and even years after surgery? Finally I wondered—a niggling, almost soundless irritation largely obscured by the first two questions—why did I care?

o

Not so long ago, if you were unlucky enough to need surgery and strong enough to withstand it, you would be tied down and cut open, usually conscious and probably screaming. Poppy. Hemlock. Hemp. Over the centuries healers tried every imaginable way of preventing or deadening pain: pressing on arteries, pinching nerves, soaking sponges in narcotic herbs for patients to breathe through. Some practitioners favoured a blow to the jaw; others rubbed stinging nettles on one part of the body to distract from another. Alcohol. Opium. Hypnosis. Prayer. Until the mid-1800s, surgery was almost always an agonising last resort. Most of today's routine operations were impossible, and even when they weren't, many patients chose death in preference. 'Suffering so great as I underwent cannot be expressed in words,' wrote one survivor. 'The particular pangs are now forgotten; but the blank whirlwind of emotion, the horror of great darkness and the sense of desertion by God and man...I can never forget.'

In the end a patient's best hope was often simply speed. A Napoleonic surgeon called Langeback claimed he could amputate a shoulder 'in the time it took to take a pinch of snuff'. The brutality of their trade made some surgeons wretched and others hard-hearted, but even amid the burgeoning humanism of the Enlightenment, pain was considered so integral to life that few could imagine surgery without it. 'To avoid pain, in surgical operations, is a chimera,' said the French surgeon Velpeau in 1839. 'Knife and pain, in operative surgery, are two words which never suggest themselves the one without the other...and it is necessary to admit the connection.'

Surgical anaesthesia brought the gift of oblivion.

Yet 170-odd years after a Boston dentist named William Morton gave the first successful public demonstration—removing a lump from the jaw of twenty-year-old Gilbert Abbott—we still don't understand fully how anaesthetics work. Each day specialist doctors known as anaesthetists (or, in America, anesthesiologists) put hundreds of thousands of people like you and me into chemical comas to enable other doctors to enter and alter our insides. Then they bring us back again. It is mind-blowing. But quite how this daily extinction happens and un-happens remains uncertain. Researchers know that a general anaesthetic acts on the central nervous system—reacting with the slick membranes of the nerve cells in the brain to hijack responses such as sight, touch and awareness. They have nominated areas and processes they know are important: the microscopic channels through which neurons blast their chemical relays; the electrical circuits that pulse and groove between different regions of the brain. But they still can't agree on just what it is that happens in those areas, or which of the things that happen matter the most, or why they sometimes happen differently with different anaesthetics, or even on the manner—a sunset? an eclipse?—in which the human brain segues from conscious to *not*.

Nor, as it turns out, can anaesthetists ultimately measure what it is they do.

For as long as doctors have been sending people under, they have been trying to fathom how deep they have sent them. In the early days, this meant relying on signals from the body; later, on calculations based on the blood concentration of the various gases used. More recently brain monitors have come on the market that translate the brain's electrical activity into a numeric scale—a de facto consciousness meter. For all that, however, doctors still have no way of knowing for sure how deeply an individual patient is anaesthetised— or even if that person is unconscious at all.

o

I am not an anaesthetist, or a surgeon, or even a doctor. I am, however, one of the hundreds of millions of humans alive today who have undergone a general anaesthetic. It is an experience now so common as to be mundane. These days there are gases and vapours and chemical infusions. Drugs to knock you out, to wake you up, to make you lie still in between; drugs to take away pain. There are machines to measure your heart rate, blood pressure, oxygen level, brainwaves; machines to breathe for you when you cannot. Anaesthesia has become a remarkably safe endeavour: less an event than a short and unremarkable hiatus. The fact that this hiatus has been possible for fewer than two of the two thousand or so centuries of human history; the fact that only since then have we been able to routinely undergo such violent bodily assaults and survive; the fact that anaesthetics themselves are potent and sometimes unpredictable drugs—all this seems to have been largely forgotten. *An-es-thee-zha*. Most of us can barely pronounce it. Yet it has allowed the body's defences to be breached in ways previously unimaginable except during warfare or other catastrophe. Through the use of powerful poisons, it has enabled entry into the secret cavities of the chest and the belly and the brain. It has freed surgeons to saw like carpenters through the bony fortress of the ribs. It has made it possible for a doctor to hold in her hand a steadily beating heart. It is a powerful gift. But what exactly is it?

..

Part of the difficulty in talking about anaesthesia—not how to do it, but what it actually does—is that any discussion veers almost immediately onto the *mystery of consciousness*. And despite a renewed focus in recent decades, scientists cannot yet even agree on the terms of that debate, let alone settle it.

Is consciousness one state or many? Can it be wholly explained in terms of specific brain regions and processes, or is it something more? Is it even a mystery? Or just an unsolved puzzle? And in either case, can any single explanation account for a spectrum of experience that includes both sentience (what it feels like to *be*—sound, sensation, colour) and self-awareness (what it feels like to be *me*—the subjective certainty of my own existence)? Not to mention the mechanisms by which information and attention wash in and out of these inexact, internal realms. In all this, unconsciousness remains the mute twin. Anaesthetists point out that you don't have to know how an engine works to drive a car. But stray off the bitumen, and it is surprising how quickly pharmacology and neurology give way to philosophy: *If a scalpel cuts into an unconscious body, can it still cause pain?* And then ethics: *If, under anaesthesia, you feel pain but forget it almost in the moment, does it matter?*

o

Sitting in my window seat en route to that small room in Brisbane, I was doing my best not to think about any of it. Until this point in my life, I had had three general anaesthetics—all short, and all, to my knowledge, uneventful: minor surgery. I had a composite memory of lying on my back on a trolley: the porous white ceiling tiles that have colonised hospitals the world over; the masked figures in caps and faded pyjamas; the jokes, the clatter; the sweet, dark swoop. And then, immediately it seemed, waking. Abruptly, and unrefreshed. As if the two parts of my life had been spliced together, and where there should have been something, there was now nothing, a blank. Perhaps it was this absence that worried me—the eviscerated, unaccounted-for minutes or hours—or perhaps, I thought at other times, it was the sense that the absence wasn't quite as absent as it now seemed.

I have spoken with people whose eyes gleam at the thought of anaesthesia. 'Oh my god,' said one woman I know, in a tone that was frankly erotic, 'that slide down. That letting go…' Others, probably the majority, don't think about it at all. But a surprising number take on a wary, doubtful look. Early in my research I met a woman who had placed a small newspaper advertisement offering counselling for people facing surgery. This woman dreamed of a fish—more an image than a dream: it was there when she awoke, and there when she went to sleep. A fish being filleted, the knife slicing down the spine. Except it was not a fish: it was her. She had had more than forty operations, she told me, the first in her twenties to fuse her lower spine after a fall ruptured the discs. She shrugged, a small, sweet-faced blonde woman in her early fifties. The fish had come to her during the first operation. The surgery had gone smoothly. She remembered nothing. But in the twenty-four years since, she had not been able to shake the image, and each new operation had reinforced it. 'I don't like to ever touch a fish that's got bones in it. I can't. I can never go to a restaurant and eat a whole fish, because you've got to pull it apart like that, so it's pulling my back apart. It's an awful thing.'

I had heard occasional stories of surgeons stitching up a patient and not realising they had left something inside—a swab or instrument—that could go on to become an irritant or worse. Now I started to wonder, was it possible that other things sometimes got left behind? Words, perhaps. Feelings. Even beliefs?

Then I came across the unrepeatable experiment.

o

Just over fifty years ago, in a small surgery in Johannesburg, South Africa, a little-known psychiatrist named Bernard Levinson staged a strange and disturbing drama. Levinson, then thirty-nine, persuaded a professor of surgery at the city's dental hospital to let him use ten of the professor's surgical patients as unwitting guinea pigs in what would become one of medicine's oddest studies.

The evening before the operations, Levinson selected volunteers from the following day's operating list by taking each aside and asking them to follow a series of instructions. First he counted backwards from three and told them to relax. Then he told them that at his command their right arm would rise effortlessly and touch their nose, and that at this point their eyes would close. Once the patients were in a hypnotic trance, Levinson asked each to go back to a happy childhood memory. Most relived long-forgotten birthdays, he reported, often in surprising detail. Then Levinson instructed them, on the count of three, to wake up, relinquishing as they did any memory of what had just happened. He selected the first ten patients he could easily hypnotise, six women and four men. For the purposes of the experiment Levinson told them simply that during the following day's surgery he would monitor their brainwaves and that later he would again hypnotise them to 'explore their feelings' about the operation. He did not tell them what was going to happen.

The next morning, before each patient was wheeled into theatre, Levinson attached leads to his or her scalp to measure the fluctuations in electrical activity there, and then stood back to allow the anaesthetist, a Dr Viljoen, to administer an ether-based anaesthetic. After the operations had begun, and only when Levinson was confident that each patient was deeply anaesthetised—more deeply than would be usual in such an operation—he instructed the anaesthetist to read out loud the following statement: 'Just a moment! I don't like the patient's colour. Much too blue. His [or her] lips are very blue. I'm going to give a little more oxygen.' After pumping the breathing bag, Viljoen would then say, reassuringly, 'There, that's better now. You can carry on with the operation.'

When the patients awoke a short time later, the theatre staff behaved as if nothing had happened.

One month later, Levinson interviewed the ten separately in his consulting rooms. First he asked what they could remember of the operation. Each said they recalled entering the anaesthetic room and being given an injection. Their next memories were of waking in the ward. Then Levinson hypnotised them. Under hypnosis, he reported later, four of the ten patients could quote some of the anaesthetist's words verbatim. Another four could only remember snatches but became upset and agitated during questioning. One man remembered intense pain. 'One woman said she felt she was spinning,' Levinson wrote later. 'Each time the circle passed the anaesthetist, she could make out a word. Before she could make any real sense out of his words, she spun out again in a circle.' Only two said they remembered nothing.

In the years since, the Levinson experiment has acquired an almost folkloric status, both for what it did and did not do. Critics have dismissed it as breaking basic rules of the scientific method. First, Levinson did not use a control group of patients who were not exposed to a crisis. Second, the experiment was not blinded— Levinson knew exactly what had happened in the operating room before he hypnotised the patients and so, arguably, knew what to expect and may have unwittingly prompted his patients' answers. Yet the great irony of Levinson's experiment was that its apparent success has made it impossible to replicate. Even though his methods were criticised, the fact that under later hypnosis so many of his patients apparently remembered what had been said—or were visibly upset—means it would be unethical to purposely risk subjecting new patients to similar stress.

When I first heard of this experiment, two things struck me forcefully. The first was that I had always assumed, without ever feeling the need to examine that assumption, that having surgery under general anaesthesia meant that I would have no awareness of what was going on within or around me at the time. The second was that in operating theatres around the globe, similar conversations to Levinson's must happen every day.

I came across the first of many references to Levinson's mock crisis not long after I started researching anaesthesia. Often it was discussed in relation to another experiment carried out thirty years later by a famous American anaesthetist who set out to replicate Levinson's study—with intriguing results. Along the way, I also found other studies, some of them very weird—studies in which anaesthetised patients could later identify words read to them during surgery despite having no conscious memory of having heard them. Studies in which unconscious patients who were told to perform particular actions on awakening would later assure researchers they remembered nothing, all the while doing as they had been instructed. Another in which a doctor from northern England used a simple device that allowed him to communicate during surgery with paralysed and seemingly unconscious women—only to find that many of them were awake. Later the women remembered nothing.

o

One of the great puzzles of general anaesthesia is that by definition it is impossible for a patient to report on the experience. Like death, you go there alone; and, like birth, you emerge seemingly empty-handed.

What happens in between might at the time feel like nothing, or it might feel like something. But the you that wakes in the recovery room is in some critical ways not the 'you' that was lying open on the operating table having the experience of being operated upon. The self has been interrupted.

So why might this matter to me or to you or to anyone else? To try to answer this question, I have had to divide myself into two selves, or rather to acknowledge an existing division. The first—the one I recognise as my day-to-day self (the one who goes to work and watches reality TV and thinks about unconsciousness)—would answer thus, possibly in dot points:

- It might matter because there is evidence that what we experience while inert on the operating table—whether or not we remember it—can change the way we feel and behave in the hours, weeks and perhaps years after surgery.

- These changes need not be bad. They might even be good. But they are so little discussed as to be unrecognised by most doctors, let alone the rest of us.

- This carries risks and opportunities.

This is the self I know. A thinking-self. The self I think of as 'me'.

The other self that has been involved in the writing of this book has no need of dot points, or maybe even of language. This self made itself known to me close to twenty years ago when I dimly recognised I had entered an unfamiliar inner realm or state. For many years now I have simply called it 'the feeling' because I have no other words for it, though at times it can seem like grief or fear or anger or even love. Its bodily sense is of a constriction in my chest and throat, a physical unease that, if I can relax or nudge it gently, gives way sometimes to a pervasive, inarticulate sense of loss.

For a long time I treated this feeling-self as something separate from me, an enemy who had arrived uninvited and taken up residence in my chest, an incubus that must be seen off. For a long time I hoped I might be able to do this with magic or by force of will. More recently I have come to see the feeling as a process, a dynamic interplay between intellect and instinct; head and heart. An interior shadow play that continues at times to unnerve and grieve me, but whose outlines and flickering concerns I see expressed in part through my long preoccupation with anaesthesia.

Over that time I have witnessed operations in three continents and interviewed some of the world's best-known anaesthetists. I have seen a heart pulsing in its red pond and watched a womb being snipped from its moorings. I have sat through conferences, scoured professional journals and medical libraries for reports and studies, hounded psychiatrists and psychologists, and cornered dozens of friends and strangers and asked them to talk about their own experiences of surgery.

The world of anaesthesia is a peculiar blend of the mundane and the mysterious: a land of complex, decipherable codes and amorphous, unanswerable questions. As a stranger in this land, I found myself frequently lost in tangles of technology, or pushing uphill through thickets of anaesthetic jargon—a language in which tears become 'lacrimation', a scalpel wound a 'noxious stimulus'. Often I felt like giving up.

Every time this happened, I would find myself somehow in conversation with someone who would tell me about their own (or a friend's or family member's) unexpected anaesthetic experience. And it was these conversations, as random as they were, that in the end persuaded me (the day-to-day me) to continue.

One woman described being able to hear what was going on

during a medical procedure but feeling that she was imprisoned beneath a sheet of glass. Another talked of the vertiginous sensation during surgery of moving in and out of her body. Others described flashbacks, dreams, emotional disturbances. Many had never talked about these experiences before. Several had avoided general anaesthetics ever since.

Most were not the sort of events to make it into the newspapers or professional journals. Often they were not so much anaesthetics that had failed as medical interactions that had failed: confused, anxious patients; absent, unaware doctors. But the repercussions were sometimes profound. Enough to suggest that doctors and nursing staff might markedly improve their patients' surgical experiences, and even outcomes, by changing the way they think about, and relate with, their charges—before, after and even during anaesthesia. And that herein lies an enormous untapped potential—one that some doctors and researchers have already been exploring with surprising results.

But what it also points to is that we as patients might do well to change the way we think, or fail to think, about ourselves under anaesthesia. That we may have the ability to influence our own anaesthetic experience and outcome; that the information and attitudes we take into surgery with us, consciously and otherwise, can affect not only how we wake up from surgery, but how we fare during it: how many drugs we need to keep us unconscious, the length of the operation, even perhaps how much blood we lose while on the operating table.

When I began writing this book I did not know that before I was finished I would have a lengthy opportunity to investigate anaesthesia first hand. Nor did I expect to have the chance to stage an unrepeatable experiment of my own, with myself as its subject. That (entirely unscientific) experiment has helped me draw some of my own conclusions about the extraordinary process that we call anaesthesia, and its significance for anyone facing surgery—in particular the importance of the stories we carry in and out of the darkness. What it took me much longer to understand was that what I was exploring was not just the anaesthetic unconscious, its charted and uncharted realms, but the dumb depths of my own unconscious self.

It began, as things tend to, with a chance meeting.

GOING UNDER

Awake

Many years ago now, in the Blue Mountains outside Sydney, I was invited to a dinner to celebrate the birthday of a friend. There were eight women at the dinner, some of whom I did not know, around a long trestle table covered with a white sheet and many small candles. Between courses one of the women, Rachel, told us the story of the birth of her second child. After she finished, there was silence; it was hard to know what to say.

Not long after that dinner I moved with my family—my partner, our son and me—back to Melbourne. But I kept thinking about Rachel's story. I did not know why, but it was like a bit of grit: I found myself growing ideas around it. I spoke to the friend who had hosted the dinner, who gave me a phone number. For months afterwards I put off calling, afraid she would not want to talk publicly about what had happened. But when I rang her one April evening from my home in Melbourne, she said yes.

Rachel Benmayor's story—of a general anaesthetic that failed; a caesarean birth endured conscious, paralysed and in agony; and a near-death encounter with what she saw as a great, implacable consciousness—became the starting point for this book, although the story had, in the way of all stories, begun long before.

We spoke by phone over two nights: Rachel in the house that she and her husband, Glenn, were renovating in the mountains, me squatting on the floor next to the filing cabinet in our Melbourne home office; she in her soft New Zealand lilt—the flattened vowels and unexpected upward inflections—me in a series of vague half-forays, repetitions and mmmms. It didn't matter. She wanted to talk. She spoke at a rhythmic, even pace, as if describing a familiar dream or film, slowing sometimes, at others clearing her throat or coughing, but rarely stopping except when I interjected. I could not quite remember what she looked like except for an impression, incomplete as it turned out, of softness—brown curls, a shortish figure, an open, appealing face. Something quiet about her, almost arrested. All of which merged over the phone into the steady forward tread of her voice.

'So,' said Rachel, 'I remember going onto the operating table. I remember an injection in my arm, and I remember the gas going over, and Glenn and Sue [*her midwife*] standing beside me. And then I blacked out. And then the first thing I can remember is being conscious, basically, of pain. And being conscious of a sound that was loud and then echoed away. A rhythmical sound, almost like a ticking, I guess, or a tapping that was just like a march and it just went round and round and round and I could hear it.

'And pain. I remember feeling a most incredible pressure on my belly, as though a truck was driving back and forth, back and forth across it.'

Rachel had been admitted to hospital, eight and a half months pregnant, a few days earlier. Her blood pressure had risen rapidly and her doctor had told her to stay in bed and get as much rest as possible before the baby came. But her blood pressure kept rising—the condition, known as pre-eclampsia, is not uncommon but can lead to sometimes-fatal complications—and the doctors decided to induce the birth. When her cervix failed to dilate properly after seventeen hours of labour, they decided instead to deliver the child by caesarean section. Rachel had hoped to have an epidural injection into the base of her spine so that she could be awake for the birth. But she was in a smallish country hospital and that day there was no one available to perform the procedure. Instead she was told she would have to have a general anaesthetic. She remembers her disappointment. She remembers being wheeled into the operating theatre. She remembers the mask, the gas. And then she woke up.

A few months after the operation someone explained to Rachel that when you open up the abdominal cavity, the air rushing onto the unprotected internal organs gives rise to a feeling of great pressure. But in that moment she still had no idea what was happening. She thought she had been in a car accident. 'All I knew was that I could hear things...and that I could feel the most terrible pain. I didn't know where I was. I didn't know I was having an operation. I was just conscious of the pain.'

Gradually she became aware of voices, though not of what was being said. She realised she was not breathing, and started trying to inhale. 'I was just trying desperately to breathe, to breathe in. I realised that if I didn't breathe soon, I was going to die.'

She didn't breathe and she didn't die. She didn't know there was a machine breathing for her. 'In the end I realised that I couldn't breathe and that I should just let happen what was going to happen, so I stopped fighting it.' By now, however, she was in panic. 'I couldn't cope with the pain. It seemed to be going on and on and on and I didn't know what it was.' Then she started hearing the voices again. And this time she could understand them. 'I could hear them talking about things, like about people, what they did on the weekend, and then I could hear them saying, *Oh look, here she is, here the baby is*, and things like that, and I realised then that I was conscious during the operation. I tried to start letting them know at that point. I tried moving, and I realised that I was totally and completely paralysed.'

It occurred to Rachel that she was close to death. 'I was just beginning to go mad with the pain, and I knew that it was going to kill me. It was a funny feeling, I just knew that I couldn't cope. And I knew that they weren't going to hear me, or realise what was happening.'

Then she remembered something someone had said to her many years before. Faced with great pain, the only thing to do was to go into it, not to try to get away from it. It is not the sort of advice most of us want to follow—until, perhaps, there is no choice. 'So I consciously turned myself around, and started feeling the pain and going into the pain, and just letting the pain sort of enclose me. There was a feeling of going down, a feeling of descending, and I just went further and further down, deeper and deeper into the pain.'

I asked her if the pain lessened as she went into it. Rachel laughed, but not humorously. No, she told me, if anything the pain got stronger. 'But I just kept on going down, down, down. And then I started feeling like I was going through something, like through the pain, and then I got to a point where the pain was there, and nothing had changed, except I no longer really cared about it.

'It was like I could be conscious to other things, because my consciousness had turned itself off from the pain. And then I realised that I was in a really amazing place, and I realised that I was very close to dying. I felt like I only needed to move a little bit deeper and a little bit further and across something, and that I would be dead.'

In that place, said Rachel, she felt the presence of people she had known, and some she had not, all the while still hearing the voices around her in the operating theatre: *Oh look, look, it's a little girl. Just pull her up a little bit higher. Look it's a little girl. Glenn, look, you've got a little girl. Isn't she big? Oh she's urinating on Rachel. Quickly. She's urinating. We'll have to cut the cord.*

But Rachel was gone. 'I was way away from there. I could hear it, but I was just a long way away.' She felt safe. 'I was so relieved to not...to have found this place where the pain was happening in my body but I knew that I couldn't tune into it—that I had to stay where I was, otherwise I wouldn't survive, so I stayed in that space.'

Some years after this conversation I visited the Melbourne office of an anaesthetist called Kate Leslie. She was crouched in a tiny cubicle furnished with twin filing cabinets in pink and taupe. Her windows looked out along a diminishing cream brick wall punctuated by other similar windows. It was a room distinguished mainly by its drabness, though brightened on this particular day by the strains of classical music drifting from further down the hall.

'Elgar,' said Leslie, dipping her head in the direction of the sound. She was not actually crouched. It was more that there was something about her that made the room seem small around her. Not only was she quite tall, but she had a vitality that made her seem bigger still, so when I think of her now I have the impression of her scrunched like an oversized Alice into a space she had already outgrown. There was something rakish about her, too, with her denim jacket, hippy skirt and tall black boots: you might have picked her as a rock chick. In fact, she had recently been involved in a study that would help make her quite famous in anaesthetic circles, at least in the circle interested in experiences such as Rachel Benmayor's. None of which you would have known from her office, or her demeanour, which was appealingly direct and forthright. If I was going to have an anaesthetic, I decided, Kate Leslie would be an excellent person to do it.

So, imagine for a moment that I'm the patient and that Kate Leslie is indeed my anaesthetist. Once I have been wheeled into the operating theatre (I may already have had a sedative pre-med to relax me), Leslie will attach a cuff to my arm to measure blood pressure, a small clip to my thumb to measure the amount of oxygen in my blood, and leads to my chest to monitor my heart rate. Then she will hook me up to a drip that will deliver an infusion of drugs designed to put me to sleep, make sure I don't feel pain and relax my muscles.

'So [*this is Leslie*] as depth of anaesthesia gets deeper, the first thing is that you start giggling a bit or your voice is a bit slurred; you know it's like you've had a couple of drinks—or a few drinks actually—and if I say to you "Hey Kate," and you go, "Huh?" you're awake. Your eyes aren't closed, there's nothing I have to do to bring you into consciousness. But you won't remember anything. You won't remember a conversation. But if I stick a knife in, you'll remember.

'And then the next thing is that your eyes close, but if I go, "Kate", you'll wake up.

'And the next thing is, your eyes are closed, but if I went [*poking motion*] "Ka-ate" you'll wake up (we poke them, you know, and they wake up). All of those things are conscious. You're unconscious when you don't respond to command or mild prodding.'

'So you *poke* them?'

'All the time,' said Leslie. 'When they're going to sleep, we say, "You're going off to sleep now," we stick the anaesthetic in and then we go, "Ka-ate"; we test your eyelash reflex'—she brushed the tip of her finger across her eyelashes—'and it's gone.'

From the patient's perspective—mine—in about thirty seconds I, or at least the 'I' that I know, should cease to exist. Once I am unconscious Leslie may switch me to an 'inhalation' anaesthetic (a gaseous mixture of, say, nitrous oxide, oxygen and another drug called sevoflurane) that I will breathe in through a mask. A tube will probably be put down my windpipe: this is known as intubation. I may also be attached to a ventilator that will breathe for me during the operation. When I am unconscious and can feel nothing, the surgeon will begin. This, at least, is how it is meant to be.

o

Later, after she had re-entered her body, and after her daughter, Allegra, had been lifted from her womb; after she had been stitched up again ('I could feel them stitching, and then they'd push down. Push, like tapping and pushing down on my uterus.'); after the nurse had bellowed at her, and her husband had finally come, and she had told him to write down the 'messages' she had received; after she had told her family doctor ('the conversations they'd had, and the fact that they'd found a fibroid in me') and her doctor had started to cry; Rachel Benmayor began to shake.

'I started feeling my body just going into spasm from shock, and I started shaking. And they got really scared and they took me over to—I asked to see Allegra, all I wanted was to see Allegra—so they took me over and they gave me Allegra and I just remember holding her. And you know that newborns have such a black stillness in their eyes, and I just sort of held her in my arms and I felt like she'd just come from where I had been.'

The chances of this happening to you or me are remote— and, with advances in monitoring equipment, considerably more remote than twenty-five years ago. Figures vary (sometimes wildly, depending in part on how they are gathered) but big American and European studies using structured post-operative interviews have shown one to two patients in a thousand report waking under anaesthesia. More, it seems, in China. More again in Spain. Numbers are impossible to come by, but twenty thousand to forty thousand people are estimated to remember waking each year in the US alone. Of these only a small proportion are likely to feel pain, let alone the sort of agonies described above. But that tiny figure far exceeds the number of people having operations at all prior to 1846. And the impact can be devastating.

For Rachel, sleepless and terrified in her small room in the small hospital in the Blue Mountains, it was the beginning of years of nightmares, panic attacks and psychiatric therapy. Soon after she gave birth, her blood pressure soared. 'I was in a hell of a state.' At times, she said, she felt the only thing keeping her on the planet was Allegra, who she clung to as if for her life. 'I'd just hold her and look at her and feel calm.'

Then the fear would start again, and with it her blood pressure would soar or plummet, making her even more afraid. 'At one o'clock one morning I remember them calling Elizabeth, my GP, and her holding me all through the night because I was so scared. And then finally I got up and I rang my mother in New Zealand and I just started crying. I howled and howled.' For weeks after she returned home she would have panic attacks in which she felt she couldn't breathe. Although she says the hospital acknowledged the mistake and the superintendent apologised to her, beyond that she does not recall getting any help from the institution. No explanation or counselling or offer of compensation. It did not occur to her to ask.

I have wondered a lot over the years in which I have been exploring anaesthesia what it was in Rachel's story that not only drew me but has kept me pinioned to a topic about which, eighteen years ago, I knew and cared next to nothing. I wonder too, though not as deeply or as often, about what happens when a person like Rachel hands her story over in good faith to a person like me. It is a transaction in which we have both invested a degree of trust. But in the end her investment has been greater, as has her risk. Her story is hers—but in my retelling of it I have also made it mine. I will endeavour to represent it fairly, but I have chosen it and framed it through my own lens. I have made it fit my own purposes, or at least the purposes of the story I want to tell—that wants to be told. Rachel's story in turn has its own percussive force, a vibration that has minutely and conclusively reordered the particles from which I assemble, moment by moment, my own sense of self. It is a story that has grown on the back of other stories—hers, her daughter's, those of the anaesthetists and scientists and patients I have since spoken with, my own—and that has changed each of us in the telling.

The psychologist who I saw regularly in the lead-up to my spinal surgery once said she felt that the process of writing this book functioned in my life both as an anaesthetic and as the means to wake myself up. The form massaging the content, she said, or the other way around. That content (this content) has announced itself insistently and in ways and forms that I—or the part of myself that likes to think I am in charge—would not have chosen. But part of the process of both the counselling and the writing has also been the realisation that it is not always 'I' who makes the choices—and along with that realisation, the slow erosion of my faith in the ascendancy of my conscious mind.

o

A counselling room in Darwin. I am in my early thirties. I have come to talk about—*what*? I don't remember now. It doesn't matter, because it is not what I talk about anyway. The counsellor is a young woman (it is a women's health service), and instead of the thing I thought I was coming to discuss I start to tell her about something that happened when I was a child. I tell her that in the week of my second birthday my parents—he twenty-six, she twenty-five and four months pregnant with my younger sister—went on a holiday to Europe and left me for ten days with another family. Like my parents, they were Australians living in London, and he, like my father, was a journalist, and they, like my parents, had one or two small girls, and were kind, so there was a connection. I remember none of it. This is a story told to me by my parents.

Yet as I surprise myself by telling this small story to the rather startled young woman at the Darwin women's heath centre, a wail rises out of me and keeps on rising, a serpentine eruption that once it has begun takes over entirely, an umbilicus of grief that coils into the room, silencing the counsellor and leaving me slippery and panting with fright and mucus and tears. When it is done, the young counsellor looks scared. She does not know what to say and nor do I. She suggests that I find someone with more experience.

I tell this story because throughout the process of writing this book I have felt, obscurely, persistently, the tug of other stories/part stories/fragments, that have lain submerged in my own memory or perhaps in my body. Eroded landmarks (or watermarks) around which I have navigated; through which I have organised my story of self; whose presence remains all the more potent for their near-invisibility.

Embedded in this remnant topography, sometimes in the foreground, often far off, are recognisable features: that counselling room in Darwin, a love affair, an illness, a birth, a death. Stories that go back further, too; that concern my mother and my father and their parents before them. And eddying around them the ghosts of feelings: guilt/grief/loss.

I did not invite them. But I name them here because these are the ghosts I bring to the writing of this book, and without them this book could not, does not, exist. And because, in the end, while I go on about 'anaesthetists' and 'patients' and 'scientists' and 'subjects' and all of the rest, these neat segmentations are simply people who carry with and within them their own remnant topographies, their own memories and fears and propensities that influence the decisions they make every moment of every day, including the ways in which they might offer or administer, or analyse or conceptualise, or research or study, or submit to or embrace the process we know as general anaesthesia.

o

When I first did an internet search of the term 'anaesthesia awareness' more than a decade ago, I found this quote in an introductory anaesthesia paper on a University of Sydney website: 'There is no way that we can be sure that a given patient is asleep, particularly once they are paralysed and cannot move.'

Last time I searched, the paper had been adjusted slightly to acknowledge recent advances in brain monitoring but the message remained the same. Just because a person appears to be unconscious does not mean they are.

Equipment can fail—a faulty monitor, a leaking tube. Then there are certain operations—caesareans, heart and trauma surgery—that require relatively light anaesthetics: there the risk is increased as much as tenfold. One study in the 1980s found that close to half of those interviewed after trauma surgery remembered parts of the operation, although these days, with better drugs and monitoring, the figure for high-risk surgery is generally estimated at closer to one in a hundred. Certain types of anaesthetics (those delivered into your bloodstream rather than those you inhale) raise the risk if used alone. Certain types of people, too, are more likely to wake during surgery: women, fat people, redheads; drug abusers, particularly if they don't mention their history. Children wake far more often than adults, but don't seem to be as concerned about it (or perhaps are less likely to discuss it). Some people might simply have a genetic predisposition to awareness. Human error plays a part.

But even without all this, anaesthesia remains an inexact science. An amount that will put one robust young man out cold will leave another still chatting to surgeons. 'In a way,' continued the original version of the introductory paper, 'the art of anaesthesia is a sophisticated form of guesswork. It really is art more than science...We try to give the right doses of the right drugs and hope the patient is unconscious.'

I tracked down the paper's author, anaesthetist Chris Thompson, at the Royal Prince Alfred Hospital in Sydney. It was a quick encounter, as he was in surgery that day. We met in a small waiting room outside the operating theatre. He was still in his scrubs and surgical mask, and my first impression was of a pair of eyes so startlingly intense that for a moment I could not speak. Without the mask, Thompson turned out to have a handsome regular face in which the eyes—I think they were blue—assumed more manageable proportions. He was quick to reassure me that anaesthetists are very good at giving the right doses of the right drugs. Today's specialist anaesthetists train for twelve to thirteen years. They can put you to sleep in seconds, keep you that way for hours and wake you up again in minutes. They administer increasingly specific drugs in increasingly refined combinations; they have equipment to monitor your physical responses and are trained to look out for signs—such as tears or sweating or increased heart rate or blood pressure—that you might be more awake than you look. Applied anaesthesia, he said, was a blend of technical skill, compassion and science. 'Experience is far more important than knowledge alone.'

Chris Thompson was in every way reassuring. He was knowledgeable and articulate and engaged. But a strange thing happened on both of the occasions that I spoke with him. I went into a kind of trance. I don't think it was just his eyes; perhaps it was the cadence of his voice, or the rhythms of his speech, or the things he was saying, some of which were quite technical. He would talk and I would try to focus, to lean in, to concentrate, and instead I would find myself drifting. When I tried to form words or sentences they sounded as if they came from somewhere else, or as if someone else were saying them. It was bizarre. When I think of Chris Thompson I think of him as Mr Anaesthesia.

Anyway, all of this training helps explain why the death rate from general anaesthesia has dropped in the past thirty years from about one in twenty thousand to one, maybe two, in two hundred thousand; and the incidence of awareness from one or two cases per hundred to one or two per thousand. But it doesn't change the fact that anaesthesia is still, in some senses, as close to alchemy as to arithmetic. 'Obviously we give anaesthetics and we've got very good control over it,' another senior anaesthetist told me early in my research, 'but in real philosophical and physiological terms we don't know how anaesthesia works.'

Things have moved on since then (in physiological if not philosophical terms), but while 'anaesthetic cocktail' seems a whimsical euphemism for a potentially lethal sleeping draught, it is closer to the truth than we might like to imagine. Anaesthetists have at their disposal a regularly changing array of mind-altering drugs—some inhalable, some injectable, some short-acting, some long, some narcotic, some hallucinogenic—which act in different and often uncertain ways on different parts of the brain. Some, like ether (a volatile liquid that vaporises into a gas), nitrous oxide (better known as laughing gas) and, more recently, ketamine, moonlight as party drugs. ('If you have an inclination to travel take the ether—you go beyond the furthest star,' wrote American philosopher–poet Henry David Thoreau after inhaling the drug for the fitting of his false teeth.) Different anaesthetists mix up different cocktails. Each has a favourite recipe. An olive or a twist. There is no standard dose.

That said, today's anaesthetic cocktails have three main elements: 'hypnotics' designed to render you unconscious and keep you that way; analgesics to control pain; and, in many cases, a muscle relaxant ('neuromuscular blockade') that prevents you from moving on the operating table. Hypnotics such as ether, nitrous oxide and their modern pharmaceutical equivalents are powerful drugs—and not very discriminating. In blotting out consciousness, they can suppress not only the senses, but also the cardio-vascular system—heart rate, blood pressure: the body's engine. When you take your old dog on its last journey your vet will use an overdose of hypnotics to put him down. Every time you have a general anaesthetic, you take a trip towards death and back. The more hypnotic your doctor puts in, the longer you take to recover and the more likely it is that something will go wrong. The less your doctor puts in, the more likely that you will wake. It is a balancing act, and anaesthetists are very good at it. But it doesn't alter the fact that people have been waking during surgery for as long as other people have been putting them to sleep.

○

Some years after meeting Chris Thompson I would find myself following an archivist in a red cap to the top of a white building on the grounds of the Massachusetts General Hospital. Jeffrey Mifflin, a courtly man with a meandering sentence structure and slow, sweet smile, had agreed to show me the domed amphitheatre that from 1821 until 1867 functioned as the hospital's sole operating theatre. 'They liked to have operating rooms on the top floor,' he explained, 'because patients, before anaesthesia, tended to scream and the other patients found that unsettling.'

It was here, on Friday October 16, 1846, that a packed, sceptical audience witnessed the first successful public demonstration of ether anaesthesia. It was also, as it turned out, the occasion of the first recorded incidence of what is known today as accidental intraoperative awareness—not that the audience would know it.

Dentist William Thomas Green Morton, who had rushed in late after putting the final touches to his newly built gas inhaler, hurriedly administered ether to twenty-year-old Edward Gilbert Abbott. The boy duly passed out, after which surgeon Dr Warren made an incision several inches long in the left side of his neck and inserted a ligature to stop the blood flow to a benign tumour, before stitching him up. 'Gentlemen,' he announced triumphantly, 'this is no humbug.'

That comment was aimed at the previous person who attempted to demonstrate the possibility of pain-free surgery, Morton's former business partner Horace Wells. Recognition for the discovery of surgical anaesthesia entailed a bitter struggle among claimants—variously naïve, venal, pompous and idealistic—from around the globe. For most of them it ended very badly, and you won't meet them in this book. The matter is still not settled. But if life were a little kinder it would be Wells credited as the founder of modern anaesthesia, not Morton—who, confided Jeffrey Mifflin, 'if the truth be told, was not very knowledgeable about anything'.

Mifflin himself was knowledgeable about many things. The next day I followed him on a tour through the nearby Mount Auburn Cemetery, past the grave of the poet Henry Longfellow, whose wife Fanny was the first woman to use ether during childbirth, and who the following day would take himself back to the same practitioner, a dentist named Nathan Keep, to have a tooth pulled ('My brain whirled round and I seemed to soar like a lark spirally into the air'); past the grave of Charles Jackson, Morton's mentor and another claimant for the title ('An unpleasant and irascible man,' said Mifflin, 'though I shouldn't say so'); past graves marked by lambs for children, and broken staffs for young men; (his own grave, said Mifflin, would have a dog and a book, 'because I love dogs and books'); and finally to the grave of William Thomas Green Morton, a suitably overbearing column with the inscription: *Before whom in all time surgery was agony*. Horace Wells' body is interred beneath a different monument in a different cemetery some distance away, where his son placed him as if to keep the pair apart.

It was Wells who, nearly two years before Morton's great day, sat fascinated in a hall in Hartford Connecticut where a Dr Gardner Q. Colton was demonstrating the 'amusing' effects of laughing gas to an appreciative audience. After a brief lecture on the properties and effects of nitrous oxide, Colton invited some of the men onto the stage to try for themselves, among them Wells and a Samuel Cooley. Fifty years later Colton would recall that, 'When Mr Cooley got under the influence he began to dance and dash around and ran against some wooden settees and thereby jammed his legs.' Wells asked after him. Cooley said that he had felt nothing. At the end of the performance, Colton recalled Wells approaching him. 'Dr Wells came to me and said, "Why cannot a man have a tooth extracted and not feel it under the effects of the gas?" I said I did not know. "Well," said he, "I believe it can be done."'

Wells, reputedly an excellent dentist, proposed that they test the theory on one of his own decayed teeth, and the next day Colton took a bag of gas to Wells' office, where he was also met by another dentist, John Riggs. 'I gave Dr Wells some of the gas,' recalled Colton, 'and Dr Riggs took out his tooth. Wells clapped his hands and exclaimed, "It is the greatest discovery ever made. I did not feel it so much as the prick of a pin." That was the first tooth ever drawn without pain.'

Today, nervous patients can still find dentists who will administer nitrous oxide—laughing gas—to ease the stress and pain of dental procedures. But for Wells, the pain was to come. Soon after the tooth-pulling experiment, and having practised on several other patients, he arranged a public demonstration of his new technique before a group of students at a rented hall in Boston. The demonstration was a disaster. A nervous Wells set out to extract a tooth from the mouth of a student volunteer but seems to have given too little of the gas. The student moaned or cried out as the tooth was pulled and the audience, dubious from the start, now heckled and jeered. 'Humbug!'

Morton, a former student and one-time partner of Wells, was in the audience that day; he had even lent Wells some tools for the occasion. Entrepreneurial, persuasive, with the mercenary acumen of a modern pharmaceutical company, Morton already had behind him a series of questionable business transactions and angry creditors. 'He was kind of an opportunist,' said Mifflin, 'and not very well educated, always seemed to be looking for some angle [whereby] he could make money.' Wells' supporters would later argue that Morton had not only learned from Wells' mistake, but had appropriated the idea itself, only modifying it to be used with ether. Morton insisted he had come to his realisations independently; his mentor Charles Jackson later claimed to have given him the idea. Either way, on Friday, October 16, 1846, beneath the glass-domed roof of the circular operating theatre now known as the Ether Dome, Morton succeeded where Wells had failed. By December that year, ether anaesthetics had been administered in Paris and London. By January, even the sceptical French surgeon Velpeau had acknowledged it 'a glorious conquest for humanity'.

o

It is a beautiful room, the Ether Dome, light settling in a sphere upon the tiers of curved benches and the empty space at the centre. The event is depicted in a large gilt-framed painting that hangs there today. A group of dark-coated men is gathered around an unconscious Gilbert Abbott—his mind having been chemically detached from his body in the service of medicine—while others in frock coats and flouncy ties look on from the benches above. The painting was finished in 2001, commissioned by the hospital from an artist named Warren Prosperi. This was not, Mifflin explained, the famous 1882 work by Robert Hinckley that depicts the same event and now hangs several kilometres away in the portly opulence of the Harvard Medical Library. That painting, while dramatic, was not entirely accurate. Hinckley, perhaps carried away with the sense of occasion, had added a few extra observers.

Mifflin had helped with the research for the new painting, going through various archives including the one at Massachusetts General over which he presided, digging out old drawings and portraits of the men known to have been there on the day. He was also among the modern-day hospital staff who in 2000 dressed up smartly and posed as surgical staff and onlookers to help the artist recreate the moment. 'I'm in the top row there, on the far right in the last row,' he told me, pointing. Then, almost as an afterthought: 'My head is cut off.'

If you look you will see a torso that may well be Mifflin's, though it is hard to tell. The distinctive Mifflin head with its tufts of grey and its opinions and musings ('Under a spreading chestnut tree,' he murmured absently at Longfellow's grave) had been detached, this time in the service of art.

In the excitement following Morton's coup, the newspapers were full of it. What they didn't mention, which surgeon Henry Bigelow would later record in an article in the *Boston Medical and Surgical Journal* was this: 'During the operation the patient muttered, as in a semi-conscious state, and afterwards stated that the pain was considerable, though mitigated; in his own words, as though the skin had been scratched with a hoe.' While there was no doubting that it was a great improvement on the alternative, Gilbert Abbott's mind had not, as it turned out, been detached from his body; not fully.

o

Paradoxically, anaesthetic awareness—at least the sort of awareness experienced by Rachel Benmayor—is a side effect of progress. Until the 1940s it was very easy to know if a patient was conscious or in unendurable pain. If you cut into a person who was not fully anaesthetised, they would let you know. In fact, the likelihood of awareness was pretty low, because doctors had to give a lot of anaesthetic to quell the body's unconscious reflexive movements. 'It's much easier to make someone unconscious than to make them stop moving,' the Royal Prince Alfred's Chris Thompson told me. Long after a person loses awareness, their body may still flinch from the knife. The problem for early anaesthetists was how to keep the patient still enough to operate safely, without giving so much anaesthetic they killed them.

It took until 1942 for Canadian anaesthetists to act on what Sir Walter Raleigh had known in 1596—and the indigenous people of South America for much longer—that the poison curare, derived from a native plant, caused paralysis. The neuromuscular blocking drugs developed since then have revolutionised surgery, particularly abdominal and chest operations where muscle contraction had made cutting and stitching almost impossible. The brain/body still broadcasts its storm warnings along the wiring of the central nervous system, but the blocking agents prevent the muscle from getting the message. By deactivating the muscles, anaesthetists can use lighter, safer anaesthetic doses, while still keeping the patient unconscious.

Muscle blocks are now common: they are used in nearly half of all general anaesthetics in Britain alone. But there are trade-offs. The drugs disable the muscles between the ribs so that patients are no longer able to breathe for themselves and must be 'ventilated' with a machine (basically a hi-tech bellows), meaning the anaesthetist needs to insert a breathing tube into the patient's windpipe. And, in quelling the body's unconscious reflexive movements, the blocks also make conscious movement impossible.

This doesn't have to be a problem, particularly if you are not in pain. About half the people who wake unexpectedly during surgery are apparently OK with it. Some are intrigued. One Italian woman who woke peacefully during the caesarean birth of her first child told researchers she had been happy simply to have been present for the arrival of her baby. But the muscle blocks also take away the ability of people like Rachel Benmayor to defend themselves. To compensate, anaesthetists still routinely overestimate the amount of anaesthetic that should be given by an estimated thirty per cent. This has costs, both financial and physiological. And even then it does not guarantee that no one will be aware.

o

In my study I have a row of old glass photographic negatives that lean against the window, a series of blurred and receding landscapes I picked up at junk shop. Individually they are hard to read, but grouped together they make patterns I find pleasing and restful. If I now take the glass plates and lay them on top of each other, something else begins to happen. Plate by plate the patterns deepen and darken, an accumulation of negatives that might in time reveal itself in a three-dimensional outline—a boulder, a heart, a horse's head— or alternatively and eventually darkness.

When I think about anaesthesia I think sometimes about darkness, but I think also about that dark reveal. I think about layers of silvered glass that in time will blur or liquefy (and eventually fragment and float apart); a lipid emulsion that both sinks and separates, and that must in the end rise and be reconstituted. A fluid mosaic.

This is not what I think about when I think about Rachel Benmayor. When I think about Rachel I imagine a single clear pane pressing down on her, through which she can see and hear and feel but through which she can neither be seen nor heard nor felt. It looks like anaesthesia but it is not.

Denial

My favourite story about anaesthetists, told to me by Peter Bishop of the Varuna writers centre in New South Wales, is about being at a dinner party with a group of doctors. Somewhere between the kitchen and the dining room, the pasta dinner slid off its platter and hit the floor. By the time Bishop arrived on the scene, two guests were hastily scraping up the mess and reassembling the food on the platter. 'It's OK,' said one, glancing up at him. 'We've all been anaesthetists.'

I love this anecdote. Its ambiguity, its understatement, its suggestion of disasters made quickly and discreetly good. It is a funny story, but not entirely.

In the early 1990s, *New Idea* invited readers to write in with their experiences of accidental awareness under general anaesthesia. Of 187 writers, about half reported that their claims were disbelieved, ignored or badly handled. 'I told the doctors and nurses. They did not believe me until I told them they were talking about horse racing...I refused to pay the account,' wrote one, who'd had a fractured foot pinned in 1989.

'I was told I must have been dreaming it all,' wrote another woman of her caesarean. 'I have always had the feeling that they thought I imagined it all.'

She was probably right. Anaesthetists have a history of recasting unwanted events. Surveys have shown that they greatly under-estimate the chances of patients—particularly *their* patients—waking up under the knife. The authors of a 2014 British study wondered if the fact that only twelve of around 360 hospitals in the UK had any specific guidelines to manage accidental awareness constituted a 'form of collective denial'. And despite a growing emphasis in today's medical schools on the importance of talking, the lack of empathy is sometimes stark. A recent report from a North American registry of awareness patients found three-quarters of respondents less than happy with the way their concerns had been handled. While the authors acknowledged the sample may not have been representative, half the patients said that neither their anaesthetist nor their surgeon had expressed concern. Only ten per cent got an apology. Two-thirds of these cases had happened since the year 2000.

I had been struck by a 2005 interview in which Frank Guerra, a clinical professor at the University of Colorado School of Medicine, noted that anaesthetists tended not to think in psychological terms, nor to spend much time with their patients. 'I have tried to teach [anesthesiologists] that when awareness happens they need to lean into the problem and make themselves very available to the patient,' he said. 'In the real world, the [anesthesiologist] gets freaked out and runs away from it.' More than a decade later, speaking from his home in Denver, he conceded that the bit about freaking out and running away was perhaps overstated. 'But not a whole lot.'

Guerra is in the unusual position of being both an anaesthetist and a psychiatrist. These days he works mainly with patients under-going electroconvulsive therapy. He makes it his business to talk to them. Before each anaesthetic he tells them in detail what to expect. And, he says, when it happens pretty much the way he says it will, his patients come to trust him. 'It's kind of like abracadabra, you know. There's a certain magic in that.' The word abracadabra, he added, could be sourced back to the Aramaic: as it is said, so it will be.

Unfortunately, many of his colleagues didn't, or couldn't, see things the same way. 'Physicians, as a rule, are perfectionists, and physicians, as a rule, don't like to make mistakes. And when physicians make mistakes it is very difficult to admit that a mistake has been made.' This was partly because of their personalities and partly because they were afraid of being sued (an issue that was improving with new laws). When it came to anaesthetists, he said, yes, there were plenty of capable and communicative practitioners out there, but for many the first inclination when things went pear-shaped was still to look out for number one.

Even when the patient is an anaesthetist.

One of the saddest stories I was to hear while researching this book was at a conference in Hull in northern England in 2004, where an American anaesthetist spoke about his own childhood experience of anaesthetic awareness—and about the treatment he had later received at the hands of his profession when he tried to discuss what had happened. When I saw him speak, more than a decade ago now, Anthony Messina looked like a slightly stouter version of Al Pacino. He talked a little like him too. Brisk and contained. A deep pleasant voice. Nothing superfluous. Just a small, dry cough that punctuated his presentation. Messina had had a series of operations as a child, and it was the last of these, for a hernia, that he still remembered. He had found himself paralysed but conscious in the early part of the operation. He recalled the room going black, a choking sensation, his attempts to scream, and the sense of having been buried alive.

'That was the first phase of my becoming uncomfortable. But I had inadequate anaesthesia for the skin incision and was in a lot of pain before I ultimately fell asleep. And I had nightmares about this event for years.'

Messina said no more about what had happened to him in the operating theatre, but he went on to speak about the effect his experience had on his young self—some of which he remembered, and some of which he had reassembled as an adult with the help of his family. At the time, perhaps with the curious fatalism of childhood, he had not told his parents, or anyone else, what he remembered. But, he said,

> Basically my behaviour changed after my last experience. I remember specifically having this obsession that for some reason my parents were going to die. I had just a total change in terms of an acute sense of fear and anxiety, a severe sleep disturbance, nightmares. I was unable to stay in school by myself. My mother would have to be called from home, take me out of the class and sit me down, [*as he spoke he cleared his throat two or three times*] and this went on for months.
>
> And this was a shock departure from my previous behaviour. It was also [*he coughed*] not consistent with the behaviour of my other seven brothers and sisters. I never told anyone of this experience until I was an adult. I still have flashbacks—very infrequently but they still occur. And I refused all elective surgery as an adult.

Messina did not on this occasion reflect on whether his childhood trauma had gone on to influence his choice of career or specialty (he came from a family of doctors), but even if it had, it seemed that the attitudes of his colleagues might have aggravated rather than alleviated his difficulties.

'In general,' he told a sympathetic audience, 'I don't talk about my experiences with anesthesiologists because scepticism about this topic causes various forms of re-experiencing the experiences myself.'

In the mid-nineties, he said, 'I made the misjudgment…of agreeing, after great reluctance, to doing a TV interview on this topic by some supportive people who knew me, who felt that it may help with the issue [*again the cough*]—and it was a mistake.'

Although the interview had been very pro-anaesthesia ('very supportive of the whole topic'), the response from some colleagues was swift and apparently brutal. 'I was told by the chairman of a major teaching institution that if I continued to give interviews on TV I would be blacklisted in my career.' He said that offers of at least three jobs at major teaching institutions had been withdrawn following the airing of the show, after complaints from other faculty members. 'I was specifically told on a number of occasions that it was felt that my positions on awareness would be divisive in the faculty and other departments. That is my experience as an adult.'

o

Denial is one of those wonderfully pliable terms that has come to mean all sorts of things to all sorts of people. I might deny having knowingly exceeded the speed limit coming along Bell Street the other day. My son might deny having promised to walk the dogs. Either of these claims might be true. But when I talk about it here, I am talking not about a denial of action, but of experience: other people's and our own. In psychoanalytic theory it is known as a defence mechanism. It protects the day-to-day part of ourselves from remembering or even knowing things that we don't want to know. It is a way of forgetting or deflecting things that might make us unpleasantly anxious. The most obvious real-world example right now is the curious inertia with which we regard the growing evidence and implications of climate change. Sometimes denial enables us to blame someone else for our own actions, or lack thereof. But in the end it is a denial that, while it may be applied to other people, begins with ourselves. It is a fluid and elegant compartmentalisation of the self. We do it a lot.

My father was evacuated from the place of his birth, Borneo (then British North Borneo) during the Second World War. He got on a boat with his younger sister and pregnant mother and her mother-in-law. They left behind—to raise the white flag and then die in a camp as the Allied planes flew over to liberate him—his father. The day my father learnt of his own father's death he was eight and had already been at boarding school for two years. He remembers the moment in painful detail and has written about it movingly himself. What he remembers most is not grief but an awful improbable shame, the shame of the son who can no longer remember his own father— and who, or even what, it is that he must now commence grieving. I suspect that my father has spent his life trying to make up for, or punish himself for, that one terrible betrayal: forgetting the face of the father he had not seen for four years. I also suspect that this shame has prevented him from ever fully acknowledging or inhabiting his own grief, which still seeps out of him at unexpected moments. It happens at the table, in the lounge room, on the street: a poem, a piece of music, the witnessing or recounting of some small kindness, some small success, something that has been generated by or befallen someone else; perhaps something that might have befallen him in another world in which he had a father who had not died (necessitating the mutual betrayal) and a mother who had not soon remarried and left him and his siblings in boarding school in Australia.

I say this, but he would not. Ask my father about his childhood, which to a generation such as mine, relatively unscarred by war and its curtailments, seems very sad, and he will say he had a perfectly happy time; that he enjoyed school and that he understood that his parents, his mother and stepfather, loved him and that these were simply the circumstances in which they found themselves. I understand that this is on one level true. But it would be easier to believe him were it not for the leaching sorrow, the imminence of tears (never quite shed). In my family we rarely comment on my father's ghostly grief. (Our denial sitting softly on the shoulders of what has already been denied.) It leaks out day by day only to be refilled overnight.

I too have my forms of denial.

Thinking about those glass negatives against the window in my study, I have wondered recently about a different set of negatives I have stashed in a cupboard or a box or a filing cabinet, or somewhere— *Why am I never quite sure where?*—around the house. These are the X-rays that over a thirty-five-year period plotted the gradual collapse of my spine.

My form of scoliosis—adult onset or idiopathic scoliosis—is, like anaesthesia, something of a mystery. Idiopathic basically means 'cause unknown'. It manifests at the onset of puberty in up to four per cent of people, in a gradual but insistent sideways bowing and twisting of the spine that will in turn distort the ribcage, often displacing the hips. Fortunately, this process will usually resolve itself by the time the adolescent stops growing and the spine stabilises in its new shape. In milder cases, massage and exercise can even reverse the process. Doctors have traditionally tried to treat the more serious cases first with external bracing then, if that failed, with the internal option: open them up and pull them straighter; fix them that way with metal rods and screws. By fifteen, when my parents first noticed my meandering spine, I was deemed already beyond the brace, and in the end my doctors judged that while surgery was an option, my back appeared to have stabilised, albeit with a curve bulging into my right ribcage like a bony question mark. I didn't care. I didn't want surgery and my condition, while sometimes painful, was easy enough to ignore, so I did.

Somehow over the next two decades I managed to overlook the fact that my back just kept on bending. In my mind my spine had, as decreed in my mid-twenties, 'stabilised'. By definition, I decided, it could no longer continue its slow spiral. Looking at it now, and at myself in this process, I am still unsure how that happened. How—despite regular, then intermittent, X-rays that show (if I can find them) a clear and consistent trajectory—I failed to notice or understand or perhaps simply accept each incremental progression. Of course each change in itself was fairly small, a matter of one or two degrees. What I, and perhaps my specialists, failed to do was connect those degrees and see that my spine was looking increasingly like the Sydney Harbour Bridge.

Or perhaps they did. Perhaps they even told me, or tried to. I don't remember, although I do suspect that the process accelerated after my son's birth in my mid-thirties. The situation may also have been muddied by a false reading some years later when one doctor incorrectly measured the angle of the curve and concluded things were better than they were—information I chose to believe despite the growing evidence of my own body. I think that too counts as denial.

It is a remarkably effective system.

It is also at times a necessary system. Among anaesthetists and surgeons it can be what allows them to do their jobs. The day I watched my first operation close up, the anaesthetist observed beforehand that if I were to faint it would probably be at the moment of incision—that first cut. I have witnessed this moment several times now without fainting, and each time have been aware of a building sense of anxiety, replaced, almost immediately, by a feeling that is almost buoyant: relief, yes, but also a sense of something like excitement. It is the same sort of feeling I get each time a plane takes off with me inside it. The thing that has just happened is so improbable it is almost laughable. I have been thrust into a new world with new rules that would be nonsensical to my old self.

This is the moment, an American anaesthetist once told me, in which surgeons transform their patients, you or me, from subject into object. It is a form of denial that enables them to act upon us in ways that would otherwise be unthinkable. To ignore the ghostly griefs and joys and hopes that trail each of us into the operating rooms, and to get on with the vital business of slicing, splicing and excision. 'When you have somebody who has been anaesthetised, the person is no longer regarded as a subject,' the anaesthetist said. 'I mean it is that simple. How could you really regard somebody as a subject and start surgery on them?' Denial is what allows doctors to reduce to manageable proportions the magnitude of what they do each day, the risks they must take, and the stakes.

It is a denial embedded in the very structures and assumptions of the Western medical system. Let's blame Descartes: the Western hospital as a physical representation of Cartesian dualism. Mind and body neatly divided into departments and specialisations, exiled one from the other. It is a segmentation signified in the way hospitals are laid out and the way most doctors are taught to think, and that has its most perfect expression in the process known as general anaesthesia, the chemical separation, albeit temporary, of body from mind. *I don't think therefore I am not.*

I am not.

Although right now, of course, I, the person who calls herself Kate, *am.* I am thinking. And I am being. And I want to keep doing both. The idea of not being disturbs me. I understand that this is not rational. If I don't exist there will be no 'me' to fear anything. (All these thoughts chug dutifully through my head.) But it is not the me who no longer exists who is feeling disturbed. It is me, now, sitting at my desk, contemplating non-existence. It's a circular, point-less conversation. Entirely manufactured by the part of me that can manufacture such conversations. A didactic, pedantic, possessive me, the me who basically runs the show. Or thinks she does.

In the room with me as I think these thoughts are two dogs. One blonde, one black. The blonde is trying to lie as close as she can without my noticing and pushing her away (the blonde exhausts me, I swear *she* thinks too much; everything with her is strategy, advancement, entitlement); the black is stretched out on the floor-boards a little way off, biding his time. When the blonde finally gives up and wanders off, he will materialise silently at my side, place his head gravely, weightily on my knee, and I will let him. I may even run my fingers over his skull, pressing gently into the tiny muscles above his ears. I don't know why but I find him easier to love. I say this in the knowledge that I am hers. (She too is possessive.) I doubt, however, that she spends her time fretting over non-existence. That seems to be my job. I even do it on their behalf; I fret about the dogs' non-existence, if not for them then for the children—who are not even children anymore but who will grieve for them. Technically, they are not even my dogs. They belong to the kids. In the day to day, I consider the dogs to be fairly low in my hierarchy of needs. I make it clear that there are unlikely to be further dogs once these are gone. And yet, in my dreams…

It is the blonde I dream about. She has fallen in a river. She has disappeared. This yawning grief.

o

In 2004, and against a backdrop of growing public and media concern, America's Joint Commission on Accreditation of Healthcare Organizations finally issued an alert to more than fifteen thousand of the nation's hospitals and healthcare providers. The commission, which evaluates and accredits healthcare providers, acknowledged that the experience of awareness in anaesthesia was under-recognised and under-treated, and called on all healthcare providers to start educating staff about the problem.

The American Society of Anesthesiologists subsequently acknowledged that accidental intraoperative awareness, while rare, might be followed by 'significant psychological sequelae...and affected patients may remain severely disabled for extended periods of time'.

Before that, however, then ASA president Roger Litwiller made a small but telling observation. Despite his organisation's concern about anaesthetic awareness, he did not want the issue to be blown out of proportion. 'I would also like to say that there is a potential for this subject of awareness to be sensationalised. We are concerned that patients become unduly frightened during what is already a very emotional time for them.'

This is the anaesthetist's dilemma. The prospect of even the most routine procedure makes even the most relaxed patient anxious—often more anxious than they think. Under stress—which just about everybody facing a general anaesthetic is—we lose our ability and often desire to process complex information. More than half of all patients worry about pain, paralysis and distress. High anxiety or resistance to the idea of anaesthesia may even contribute to anaesthetics failing, or at least increase the chances that we will remember parts of the operation. The more anxious we are, the more anaesthetic it may take to put us to sleep.

This creates a quandary for doctors—how much to tell? When we are anxious our bodies increase production of adrenaline-type substances called catecholamines. These can react badly with some anaesthetic agents. So what does an anaesthetist tell a patient who, because of the type of operation, or their state of health, is at higher than average risk? 'I mean we're trying to make people not worry about it,' said one Australian anaesthetist I spoke with, 'but in the process I think we blur it so much that people hardly ever think about it and that's probably not right either...Should I be telling you that you've got a high risk of death? Is that going to frighten you to death?'

Death, of course, is the mother of all denial. We build civilisations around it. Sporting codes, haciendas, family trees: all constructed around the refusal to countenance impermanence, obsolescence, extinction. And we devote an extraordinary amount of energy to maintaining the pretence. The psychologist who counselled me in the lead-up to my spinal surgery was very clear on this. She set me homework: a book by existential psychiatrist Irvin Yalom that takes as a starting point a quote from seventeenth-century French writer François de la Rochefoucauld. 'You cannot stare straight into the face of the sun or death.'

Yalom writes about the impossibility of living a life 'frozen in fear', and the strategies we employ to distract ourselves: 'We project ourselves into the future through our children; we grow rich, famous, ever larger; we develop compulsive protective rituals; or we embrace an impregnable belief in an ultimate rescuer.'

As I write, I have just received a text message from one of my sisters to tell me my mother is being taken through into surgery to remove a small tumour on her remaining kidney. The other kidney was removed a month ago, having been occupied by a larger, aggressive tumour. My mother of course is impregnable. Just as my own death is unthinkable from this side of that divide (the only side, presumably, from which one can actually think), my mother is, in my mind, immortal. I understand in theory that she is not permanent, that at fifty-plus I have already had her for longer than many people have their mothers. Far longer than she had her own. But contemplating her death is like contemplating my own. I simply cannot stare at that sun.

Perhaps this is why so many of us fear anaesthesia. Because it feels like death, or at least what we imagine death might feel like, and reminds us that non-existence is always there, waiting.

Outside the operating theatre with my parents, before my mother was taken into her first surgery, I tried to remember everything I had learnt about anaesthesia and preparing for surgery, to find something useful to tell her. I could think of nothing. My mother seemed too small on the metal bed. Too forbearing. My mind felt flat and rect-angular and stretched, like a canvas waiting to be drawn upon by someone else. The anaesthetist when he arrived was a middle-aged man who spoke quickly and softly, with a strong Chinese accent that I found hard to understand. At first I was apprehensive, but as he chatted I began to focus not on what he was saying, but on how he was saying it, and what I felt then was a sinewy sense of compe-tence and care, and a bright, agile intelligence. Perhaps I was wrong about these qualities; perhaps I just wanted it to be the case. But I am learning to trust my instincts on these things, and I believe it was so.

o

Today the profession makes much of the emergence of a new genera-tion of anaesthetists more attuned to the experiences of their patients. But the reality is that anaesthetists remain for the large part the invisible men and women of surgery. Many of us still don't meet them until just before or sometimes after our operation, and many, muffled in a fug of drugs, may not even remember these meetings. Nor do anaesthetists generally leave anything to show for their work: no slick scars or bold prognoses; just a bill. When they do leave evidence, it is invariably unwelcome—nausea, a raw throat, sometimes a tooth chipped as the breathing tube is inserted, sometimes a memory of the surgery. Unsurprising, then, that by the time an anaesthetist makes it into the popular media he or she is generally accompanied by a lawyer.

At this point I have to say that, having now had considerably more personal experience of anaesthesia than when I began this book, my recent impressions of anaesthetists have been uniformly positive. I have found each to be accessible, intelligent and more than happy to talk about what it is that they do, and are proposing to do to me. Perhaps this is because they know I am already interested in the subject, but I suspect that a lot of people simply don't ask.

For the doctors who each day make possible the miraculous vanishing act at the heart of modern surgery, this invisibility can be galling. It is not surgeons who have enabled the proliferation of surgical operations—numbering in the hundreds 170-odd years ago and the hundreds of millions today. It is anaesthetists. In hospital emergency rooms in Australia and other countries, it is not surgeons who decide which patient is most in need of and mostly likely to survive emergency surgery: anaesthetists increasingly oversee the pragmatic hierarchy of triage. And if you have an operation, although it is your surgeon who manages the moist, intricate mechanics of the matter, it is your anaesthetist who keeps you alive.

In 2006 I met Greg Deacon, then head of the Australian Society of Anaesthetists. It can be a tricky job, balancing the interests (pecuniary and otherwise) of Australia's anaesthetists with the need to maintain their public professional standing. On the day I met him, in the library of the ASA's Sydney headquarters, he looked the part. Black suit, grey-and-white striped tie, slightly greying hair and a neatly trimmed beard. He did not look at all the sort of person who would knowingly allow a man to have his chest cut open without anaesthetic.

Throughout the interview he was polite and helpful, although at times barely concealing frustration at the media attention surrounding the question of anaesthetic awareness, which he said was extraordinarily rare. The point he wanted to make, and to which he kept returning during the interview, was that on a scale of the things that could go wrong in anaesthesia, awareness was by no means the worst. Sometimes, said Deacon, when patients asked him if there was a chance they might wake up during their operation, he wanted to say to them: 'If you purely want to worry, worry about *not* waking up: don't worry about waking up!'

One of the problems, he said, was that modern anaesthesia had become so safe we now took it for granted. Fifty years ago, if Grandma didn't wake up after her anaesthetic, well...sad, but not so surprising. Or if she woke up, but was never quite herself afterwards. 'Again, that wasn't considered unusual.' Those were the risks you took. These days, he said, 'they expect perfection'. Sure, awareness was an issue. 'But it's not the main thing that I would be worrying about when I have an anaesthetic.' He paused, then added: 'I've had an episode myself.'

At first I thought he himself had woken during an operation. But he meant that one of his patients had, a man waiting to have open heart surgery. Deacon had been preparing to anaesthetise him, he said, when the man went into cardiac arrest. The team managed to restart the recalcitrant heart then raced the patient into surgery where they operated immediately. It was only once the operation had begun, the man's heart now beating steadily, that they could safely administer an anaesthetic. It all went well, said Deacon, and the man made an excellent recovery. Some days later, the patient told doctors he remembered the early parts of the procedure before he was given the drugs.

'That is a sort of incidence of awareness which was thoroughly understandable and acceptable,' Deacon told me: he had not even known if the man's brain was still working, let alone whether he would survive an anaesthetic. 'We were trying to keep him alive.'

This is not denial. This is the tightrope that anaesthetists walk every day. They just tend not to talk about it.

In any event, denial works both ways.

Before I became fascinated by anaesthesia, I didn't think about it at all. The process existed in my imagination largely as an absence, a blind spot. When I thought about hospitals and operations, I thought about surgeons and nurses and *House* and *Scrubs*. I didn't think about the fact that for any of this to take place, I would have to put myself— not just my body, but the very essence of what made me myself, my consciousness—in the hands of a stranger who would...*what?*

'Without a doubt, most people don't appreciate the risks,' one senior anaesthetist told me. 'And even when the risk is explained, most people still don't appreciate it. We've still got the inheritance of a generation of very paternalistic medicine...I regularly come across patients who I tell there's a very small risk associated, and they say, "I don't want to know. Don't tell me."'

And it is not just doctors who sometimes find it hard to admit it when a patient wakes during anaesthesia. In the early nineties a Dutch team tracked down and interviewed twenty-six people who had reported waking during surgery. Most of them had mentioned the experience in preoperative interviews before subsequent operations. The records of the initial operations were unremarkable: experienced anaesthetists who later examined them—side by side with records of other, uneventful surgical procedures—were unable to reliably pick which patients had been aware. But what startled the researchers was that only nine, or just over a third, of these patients had ever told their original anaesthetists what had happened. 'Anesthesiologists may well ask themselves,' they wrote, 'whether they really know what happens to their patients...'

As it turned out, all the patients they approached were grateful, even eager, for the chance to talk. But other patients don't want to talk at all. Some are afraid of being disbelieved. Some don't want to make trouble. Some feel guilty, as though they have been a bad patient. Some can't see the point. Others may be too traumatised to revisit the experience.

Michael Wang is a British psychologist who has built a career investigating the impact on patients' lives of being awake when they are supposed to be under anaesthesia. He was one of the first writers I came across when I started investigating stories about people waking under the knife. As a psychologist, he is already an outlier in a conversation dominated by technicians and theoreticians. Some people think he—or at least his area of interest—is a bit wacky. That he is slightly obsessive. Certainly he has been a persistent and outspoken advocate for anaesthetised patients. 'It is difficult to imagine a more exquisite form of torture than major surgery with consciousness, pain perception and complete paralysis,' he wrote in a 1998 paper. 'Clinical psychologists and the patient's family are then left to pick up the pieces.'

In a 2005 interview, Wang, who was by then working at Hull University, recounted an incident in which he had been called to the Hull Royal Infirmary after staff realised that a ventilator supposedly delivering anaesthetic gas to surgical patients had been dispensing only oxygen. Two patients had already undergone operations with the faulty equipment, one a woman having her stomach stapled, the other a man having a hernia operation. Both had been paralysed. Wang spoke first to the woman. 'I went to the ward to meet her and she was extremely distressed,' he said. 'She was completely awake during the operation, but couldn't move. She felt every one of those staples going in.'

He never got to speak to the man. 'I got to the ward about twenty-four hours after his operation had finished, but he'd already discharged himself against medical advice and all attempts to contact him failed,' said Wang. 'It might be that men assume they're going to experience some degree of pain and distress if they're having an operation, but my suspicion is, they think it's somehow not very macho to complain.'

Even in those patients willing or able to talk about their experiences, the events can be strangely elusive. In a study published in *The Lancet* in 2000, a team led by Swedish anaesthetist Rolf Sandin interviewed nearly 12,000 people who had just undergone general anaesthesia, and asked them if they remembered anything of their surgery. Three times they asked. First, shortly after the operation; then again one to three days later; and again seven to fourteen days after the event.

They found eighteen patients they were confident had been aware—and who themselves reported having been awake—for at least part of the surgery. ('Saw people dressed in green, saw tombstones, thought she was attending her own funeral.') What seemed odd was that only six had mentioned—and, it seemed, even remembered—this when they were first asked soon after waking. In fact, the patients' responses were all over the place. Five reported no memories until the third time researchers inquired. One patient who remembered nothing at the first interview, at the second recalled hearing voices and noises from surgical equipment, trying to get the attention of surgical staff but being unable to speak or move. By twelve days after the surgery she had forgotten again but, at a follow-up interview twenty-four days after the operation, could remember it all in detail. Less than a third reported memories at all three interviews.

It seemed very strange, I thought, that you might be able simply to forget an event as compelling as finding yourself a surprise guest at your own surgery. It suggested for a start that people's experiences of awareness might be significantly underreported, depending on how long or how often after their operations they were questioned. Then there was the matter of what happened to these erratic memories when they weren't in the process of being remembered. Where did they go? How long did they stay there? And what, in any case, were they?

o

February 2010. My psychologist, the one who has been helping to prepare me for my surgery, has asked me a question. I no longer remember what it is, but I have answered in the negative. My psychologist is talking quietly. She is talking perhaps about my habit of using my intellect to avoid my emotions. 'You look upset,' she says. I say that no, I am not upset. If I am not upset, she asks, then why am I crying? I put my hand to my cheek and feel that it is wet. 'No!' I say, annoyed. 'I am not crying. I'm not even upset. My eyes are just leaking.'

Paralysis

It was in the early sixteenth century, as explorers and adventurers set out to seek riches in the New World so recently stumbled upon by Christopher Columbus, that reports started trickling back to Europe of the terrible and deadly poison with which the indigenous people of South America anointed their arrows. Among the vivid tales that filtered home, few were more lurid than those of the 'flying death' that helped natives dispatch their prey—and the occasional pale-faced intruder. In his book *Poison Arrows*, retired anaesthetist and historian Stanley Feldman lists early reports of staring eyes, convulsions and exploding bowels. British poet-explorer Sir Walter Raleigh, on his return in 1595 from what is now known as Guyana, wrote that 'the person shot endureth the most insufferable torment in the world, and abideth the most insufferable death...'

What early observers did not realise was that they were watching a form of suffocation. It took experiments on animals back in Europe to prove that the poison, extracted from native plants, killed neither through its fumes nor through ingestion; nor did it directly affect the brain or heart. In 1812, British surgeon Sir Benjamin Brodie demonstrated the effects of the substance he called 'woorari' before the Royal Society in London by injecting it into a donkey. He waited until the animal collapsed and stopped breathing then made a small incision in its throat to open up the windpipe. For the next two hours he kept the creature alive by pumping air into it with a bellows. Eventually the woorari wore off and the donkey recovered with no ill effects. Brodie had proved that the toxin worked by disabling the muscles that expanded and contracted the lungs.

Scientists now know that curare causes paralysis by blocking the chemical transmission through which motor nerves cause muscles to contract. By keeping patients still it lets doctors reduce dramatically the amount of anaesthetic needed to operate. Its introduction in 1942 and the advances that followed have changed anaesthesia forever. Within ten years, anaesthetic deaths had dropped by a third. In deactivating the powerful muscles of the torso, curare gave surgeons safe access to the fortified cities of the chest and the belly. It allowed doctors to operate on old, frail and ill patients who would not otherwise be eligible for surgery due to the risk of death from the anaesthetic.

But the advance has come at a cost.

It was the French physiologist Claude Bernard who in the mid-1800s first worked out how curare actually paralysed its victims. Through a series of quite horrible experiments involving frogs, he established that the toxin did not affect the sensory nerves, meaning that while his frogs could not move, or breathe unaided, they could certainly feel. Animal activists, including writer Mark Twain, were horrified at Bernard's description of the resultant suffering: 'The apparent corpse before us hears and distinguishes all that is done. In this motionless body, behind that glazing eye, sensitiveness and intelligence persist in their entirety. The apparent insensibility it produces is accompanied by the most atrocious suffering the mind of man can conceive.' Even so, there are harrowing early references to doctors operating on paralysed patients who were awake, in the belief that they were unconscious. It took until late 1946 for American anaesthetist Scott Smith to settle the matter by submitting to four hours of complete paralysis under a high dose of a curare derivative, eventually emerging to report on what had happened. Apart from having been fully aware of everything around him, he detailed his feelings of suffocation and choking. 'Pain,' he said, 'touch, and other modalities of cutaneous sensation remained normal throughout.'

All this, of course, is known to Rachel Benmayor.

There is a hand-written entry on quarto paper in the patient files of the Blue Mountains Hospital that reads: 'She has convinced me that awareness occurred and that it occurred for much of the operation...I have never heard of such a complete description.' It is signed by a hospital anaesthetist, though not the one who worked on Rachel that day. 'I have apologised on behalf of the hospital and anaesthetists. I have told the patient that all [*notes?*] are available to her. Mrs Benmayor feels that this discussion has been helpful.'

o

But the pain may not be the worst of it.

Take that Swedish study in which people who had reported remembering nothing when they first woke from surgery could then go on to recall details if the interviewers put the same questions to them days, or even weeks, later. When Rolf Sandin and his team analysed the data from the eighteen patients they were confident had been conscious for at least part of their surgery, they found some other surprises. The people who were the most distressed by their experience were not, as you might expect, the ones who had been in pain, but the ones who had been paralysed. None of the four patients who had *not* been paralysed during their operations—even the ones who had felt parts of their operation—said they had been worried at finding themselves awake. Nor did they go on to have nightmares or anxiety in the weeks after the surgery. But ten of the fourteen who had been chemically restrained reported that they had felt anxious at awakening during the surgery—and four went on to show what the researchers called 'delayed symptoms'.

One of the first articles I came across when I started researching this book was a 1998 paper by Michael Wang (the British psychologist) entitled 'Inadequate Anaesthesia as a Cause of Psychopathology'. Wang pointed out that pain—'even unexpectedly severe pain'—did not necessarily lead to trauma. Post-traumatic stress seldom followed childbirth, for example. What could be devastating, he said, was the totally unexpected experience of complete paralysis.

Even today, most patients undergoing major surgery have no idea that part of the anaesthetic mix will be a modern pharmaceutical version of curare. Few will be aware either that during surgery their eyes will be taped shut, that they may be tied down, and that they will have a plastic tube manoeuvred into their reluctant airway, past the soft palate and the vocal cords, overriding the gag reflex, and into the windpipe.

For the patient paralysed upon the table, said Wang, '[t]he realisation of consciousness of which theatre staff are evidently oblivious, along with increasingly frenetic yet futile attempts to signal with various body parts, leads rapidly to the conclusion that something has gone seriously wrong. The patient may believe that the surgeon has accidentally severed the spinal cord, or that some unusual drug reaction has occurred, rendering her totally paralysed, not just during the surgery, but for the rest of her life.'

Two years after their original study, the Swedish team decided to follow up the same group of eighteen awareness patients. In the end they could only speak to half of them. Six refused, and another two simply failed to respond. Of the nine who agreed, four were still badly affected by their experiences, fulfilling the criteria of post-traumatic stress disorder (PTSD). They recalled the events in detail and variously found themselves prey to flashbacks, panic, sleep disturbance, nightmares, difficulty concentrating and irritation. Three others had less severe symptoms, with which they could cope 'in daily life'. Again, what was clear was that by and large it was not those who had been in pain during their operations who were still suffering two years later. It was those who had been terrified. Of the five who had woken during surgery and lain there paralysed and afraid, only one did *not* have PTSD. The fact that six others had refused to take part in the follow-up was in itself disturbing, said the researchers, as the very act of avoiding situations that might trigger distressing memories is considered a symptom of PTSD.

o

At the newspaper where I work, I sat for several years at a desk next to the third-floor exit that led downstairs to the second-floor canteen. This meant that a lot of people passed my way, and sometimes they stopped. A while back, a colleague called Clay Lucas paused to chat. He asked how I was, and I had just launched into a summary of my fascinations and frustrations with what I was by then referring to as 'the anaesthesia thing', when Clay interrupted. 'That happened to my mother.'

Clay's mother, Jan, had moved to London in the late 1950s. Shortly after her arrival, doubled up with severe abdominal pain, she got herself to the nearest hospital where she very soon found herself lying on an operating table about to undergo emergency surgery for appendicitis. In went the anaesthetic. On went the preparations. Jan lay there waiting for oblivion. Nothing. She tried to move. A different sort of nothing. 'She seemed to think she was probably lying there for a few minutes,' said Clay. 'Enough time for her realise what was going on. Enough time for her to get really really scared.' Seconds before the surgeon started cutting, someone realised she was awake.

In went the anaesthetic. This time, it worked.

Clay said his mother had only recently told her children what happened that day, but, growing up, he remembers her distress whenever anyone in the family faced surgery. For forty-five years after her London experience she refused to have an operation under general anaesthesia. It wasn't until 2008 when, faced with a life-threatening illness, she finally told doctors about her fears and reluctantly submitted to another general anaesthetic, this time with no drama.

After Clay wandered off, I sat silent, thinking about similar stories I had heard, one from a dear schoolfriend, Harriet, which she shared with me for the first time only after I mentioned this book. Then from the seat immediately behind mine came a voice. 'That happened to me too.'

Rachel Gibson was a friend with whom I had shared a cubicle for at least a year. We talked a lot. Now she told me about the time in the early nineties when she'd had her wisdom teeth removed. This time the paralysis came not at the beginning but as she woke after her surgery. She was cold. There was a tube up her nose. She couldn't speak. Again, it was only minutes. She felt the trolley being shunted into the recovery room. When she could, she began to whimper, until a nurse told her to stop disturbing the other patients. It turns out that about two-thirds of awareness cases happen like this—either as people are put under or emerging from general anaesthesia. For Rachel, the experience was so frightening she too simply determined never to have general anaesthesia again. 'It was awful, it was absolutely terrifying.' She too stuck with her decision for many years until finally, following complications after the birth of her twin boys, she had no choice. Even then, she said, 'right up until they were wheeling me in to the surgery I was insisting I'd have a local'.

The worst of it, she said, was not being able to tell anyone what was happening to her, first in the operating theatre and then again in the recovery room. 'It's a bit like being in a dream and wanting to scream and being unable to, and wanting to run away and you can't.'

American psychologist Peter Levine has written a lot about paralysis. In the face of what appears to be life-threatening danger, he says, humans and other mammals and reptiles are hardwired to react with any of three instinctual responses: they fight, they flee or they freeze. We're all familiar with the fight or flight mechanism—the rapid and purposeful movement either into or away from the problem. But the third, the immobility response, gets far less, and less favourable, attention. It is here, argues Levine—in a state of total and involuntary paralysis in the face of overwhelming threat—that a virulent and particularly human form of suffering is born.

To explain the freeze response, and its sometimes toxic effect on humans, Levine looks to animals in the wild. He notes that an impala that sees a cheetah approaching will use its extraordinary speed and agility to try to run away; but if it cannot escape and death seems imminent, it may collapse motionless to the ground. It looks dead, but what is really happening, argues Levine, is a last-ditch strategy hardwired into the animal's nervous system—the body shuts down. This response can be seen in all animals including humans, says Levine, and is seated in the oldest and most primitive parts of the brain, the bits that perch at the top of your neck and deep in the centre. Paralysis has advantages in the wild—it confuses predators, draws blood from the periphery to the vital inner organs, and may reduce the experience of pain—but in humans, Levine argues, there can be debilitating side effects. He likens the freeze response to that of flooding an engine with petrol at the same time as slamming your foot on the brake: all the energy that has been summoned to fight or flee is suddenly frozen in the body. For the organism to recover, it must discharge it—which explains, he says, why in the wild, when the threat has passed, animals twitch and shake for a while before continuing peaceably with the business of living.

In humans, however, the clever front parts of the brain, tucked behind the forehead, can get us into trouble by trying to override this response. Among the complex mores that govern most human societies are sanctions against showing fear and its physical manifestations such as shaking and crying. We are embarrassed by our animal responses and work hard to hide them and their connotations of weakness by suppressing our natural recovery mechanisms. Levine speculates that one of the reasons we habitually quash the freeze response is because it reminds us of death. In any case, he argues, it is the failure to discharge the build-up of energy that causes post traumatic stress, and with it chronic fear, rage and helplessness.

I do not know whether Peter Levine's theory has been or can be proved, but I do know the particular creeping awfulness of the freeze response he talks about. Once in my late twenties I was staying with a group of friends at a house in a country town. The house had a wide covered terrace at the front and a small rickety balcony off the kitchen with a door that we rarely used. It was daytime, and several of us were standing in the kitchen. I felt the shift in the atmosphere before I realised what was happening, and when I looked up a strange woman had appeared in the room, seemingly from nowhere. She was moving purposefully towards me—not a big woman, but she brought with her a roiling, chaotic energy and she was talking loudly, unconstrained by the usual delineations of personal or social space. It was as if a small, mad tornado had risen suddenly through the floor and was now churning towards me with the slow inevitability of nightmare. I have no idea what anyone else was doing. I stopped hearing. Time and colour distorted, the room was whirling slowly around me and I was utterly still. I was aware that I was unable to move or make sound, but the awareness seemed to come from a long way away and the woman kept talking at me, very close, into my face. It probably took seconds. Then the others took control, escorted the woman firmly back to the door and pointed her towards the driveway. I'm not sure if anyone even noticed my absence. I came back to myself slowly, my heart still thumping, body cold and slightly nauseated in the tidal pull of adrenaline; suffused with a sort of shame, which I hid as well as I could. At no point that day was I in immediate physical danger yet I still recall vividly the particular dull terror: the helplessness.

It was not the first or last time I would have such a reaction, and it left me with lingering concern that in the face of real danger I would neither fight nor flee but stay rooted to the spot. So when, some years later and living in Darwin, I came across an advertisement for a women's self-defence course, I signed up. At our first session one of our instructors, a lean and striking young woman, told us that she had taken up martial arts after being attacked in her early twenties. In the coming weeks, as we learned how to free our voices, to make loud *huh* sounds as we kicked and chopped at large stuffed bolsters, she let slip more about her ordeal. In fact, as the course progressed I got the feeling that the whole program was organised around this ordeal and her determination that other young women be better prepared than she had been. She was insistent that the best strategy was constant vigilance. Don't walk by yourself after dark: if you have to, always make sure you have a key gripped between your knuckles; if you find yourself under attack, aim a quick strong kick at his shin or thigh or balls and then run.

'So this is what he'll do,' she would say, eyes glinting, 'when he gets you. He'll push you back like *this* [*bam!*], and you won't have time to think. Your head will slam into the wall [*thud*] and you'll be dizzy, and then he'll come at you—like *this,* and what you have to do, if you're still conscious, is *this.*' It was vivid and visceral. The only problem was that the more she talked about all the terrible things that might happen to me, and the more I thought about them, the more anxious I became about my ability to prevent them from happening (like *this* and like *this...*).

And then there was graduation night to look forward to, a mock attack by an obliging group of local bikers whom we, for our part, would fight off. This is a true story. In class we heard a lot about how previous women had fared, the one who had driven off her attacker by spitting in his face and others who had landed blows. But the story I could not forget was the one about the star pupil, a tough, energetic young woman who had mastered every technique demonstrated in class and squared up for each challenge. On the evening of the graduation, as the group was assembling in the park, she ran off to use the public toilet. There, as she sat in her cubicle, an over-enthusiastic biker came in over the top of the door and dropped down beside her. Shortly afterwards, when the instructors arrived at the man's bidding, they found the girl still frozen in foetal position in the corner.

I have various attributes I think I can be proud of, but physical bravery is not among them. It is not the being struck or even hurt that frightens me, however, so much as the prospect of that terrible state of suspended animation. Paralysed and abandoned and alone.

As graduation day drew closer, I started to feel more and more sick at what was to come. I started seeing threat everywhere. I stopped wanting to go to classes. And when, about halfway through the course, I discovered that I was pregnant, it was with intense relief that I dropped out.

Two hearts

One summer's day late in 2000, I made my way with a photographer from the *Age* newspaper through the lobby of Melbourne's Alfred Hospital. The foyer had recently been renovated and visitors entered through sliding glass doors into a cavernous entrance hall with faux-marble floors and a faux-Parisian sidewalk cafe (wrought-iron tables beneath a white neon sky) through which doctors with beepers and mobile phones moved purposefully and without effort. On the concrete outside, smokers with dressing gowns and drips gathered like injured birds to warm themselves in the sun.

The real hospital was upstairs. We took the lift and then made our way as directed along corridors of mottled linoleum the colour of old bones to a cubicle window where a woman greeted us, opened a side door and pointed us to the change rooms. Inside, we undressed to our underwear and pulled on loose blue surgical pants and shirts, as well as disposable caps and face masks.

The operating theatre was a rectangular room with more lino, and brown stains on the walls. It was clean but threadbare, as if the varnish had lifted after years of scrubbing. Only the equipment in the centre of the room gleamed. It was like walking onto a film set: most of the space was irrelevant, a receptacle for the action taking place at its centre. Here, the costumed medicos, the gleaming instruments, the white lights seemed as familiar and calculated as the ones on television. And everything, even the draped green shape on the stainless steel trolley, seemed crystalline, unreal.

The operation was already underway. Up close, where the surgeons were working, the green drapes had been positioned to reveal a rectangle. It did not look like a person. The skin, painted in brown antiseptic and covered in plastic wrap for warmth, did not look like skin. It looked like something you would find in the fridge. Then the wound—a meaty gash in the middle of the chest that appeared as if someone had put a cleaver through it.

When we arrived, this first operation was almost over. The surgeons had removed a chunk of the man's lung to try to slow the progress of his emphysema. Now they were sewing up the breastbone with wire, hauling it through with their body weight, lacing up the rib cage like an old footy boot. Suspended above the man's neck was a small green drape. It was there to protect his face, said a nurse. From the top of the trolley, where I moved back to stand with anaesthetist Paul Myles, the drape had sectioned the body in two, and all I could see was the top of the man's head, strands of greyish hair that made me think of my father, and his forehead, on which was a strip that looked a bit like a bandaid. These led along thin wires to a box, too small for shoes, on which was a screen dominated by a constantly changing number located in the top left-hand corner.

In May of that year anaesthetists at Melbourne's Alfred and Royal Melbourne hospitals had launched a 1.5 million-dollar international trial of a new anaesthetic monitor, the Bispectral Index (BIS). Makers of the monitor claimed that it could analyse the brain's electrical activity and translate that into a score from 0 to 100, correlating to the patient's depth of anaesthesia. If proved reliable, the 1.4 kg blue box would let anaesthetists adjust the anaesthetic dose to keep the patient in the ideal range—between 40 and 60—during surgery. While a number of other so-called 'consciousness monitors' (not so-called by manufacturers—they carefully avoid this terminology) were already available, supporters of the BIS claimed it was the most user-friendly and accurate. Myles and co-investigator Kate Leslie (this was shortly before I first met her in her pink and taupe office) had decided to put these claims to the test. Their study, the largest of its kind, would focus on 2,500 patients deemed to be at a higher than usual risk of awareness, many with a history of consciousness during surgery. It would be the first time an independent, large-scale study had ever tested whether a machine could detect and prevent awareness.

Paul Myles was the joint chief investigator on the trial. Back then, when he was not in the operating theatre, he worked from a tiny alcove office on the first floor of the Alfred, hemmed in by top-heavy bookshelves and filing cabinets. Then, as now, Myles was a man blessed with an appearance of chronic, perhaps congenital, satisfaction. The corners of his mouth turned up, his forehead was smooth, he exuded a sense that the world was turning smoothly and unremarkably on an axis both pleasing and appropriate. Despite his greying hair he brought to mind a grown-up Tintin, his disposition at once benign and determined. He was not yet a big name in international anaesthesia circles, but with the BIS monitor's help he was on the way.

Myles was one of those rare people who had known since childhood what he intended to do. From the age of six, he said, he wanted to be a doctor. There was no obvious reason. He had not, like many others in his profession, come from a long line of doctors. Quite the opposite. 'We came from a very working-class, poor, single-mother family.' The family had moved around a lot, he said, in Melbourne and then country Victoria, and Myles, perhaps in reaction to this, had decided he wanted to be a country GP. 'The idea of living in a country community—and an important and valued role in that— that appealed to me.' As a country GP he knew he would need a good working knowledge of obstetrics and anaesthesia, so after finishing his basic training and a residency he went to the UK for a further year of anaesthetics. And it was here, in his first weeks as an anaes- thetic registrar, that he read an article that would change his life.

In August 1979, eleven years before Rachel Benmayor gave birth to her daughter, an editorial appeared in the *British Journal of Anaesthesia*, entitled 'On Being Aware'. 'The following,' read an intro- duction, 'are the unedited recollections of a medically qualified lady who experienced Caesarean section under general anaesthesia which was insufficient to prevent awareness during part of the procedure.'

Like Rachel, the medically qualified lady remembered passing out ('literally as though someone had switched the lights out') and waking in confusion soon afterwards. Unlike Rachel, she was not yet in pain, but as soon as she heard a voice above her mention her bladder, she understood her predicament: 'I was lying there intubated, covered in green towels, my abdomen split open, strange people delving inside me, blood, swabs on the rack, etc.'

Her first reaction, she wrote (with what seems in the circum- stances extraordinary self-censure) was an 'irrational' surge of panic, and 'the absolute desperate necessity to move'.

'I felt,' she added, 'that I had to insert some of my own will on the situation. The closest parallel I can think of is of being in a coffin, having been buried alive. It was only then that I realised I didn't have a body to move.'

Not long after, she heard her baby cry. And soon after that she began to feel pain, first a feeling as though someone was drawing sandpaper across her flesh, and then a stabbing sensation.

In character it was exceedingly unpleasant. The nearest comparison would be the pain of a tooth drilled without local anaesthetic—when the drill hits a nerve. Multiply this pain so that the area involved would equal a thumb-print, then pour a steady stream of molten lead into it. If you imagine the effect of a too-hot pan moved from the cooker on to a plastic surface, then that is what that pain was doing to my non-existent body.

Paul Myles was transfixed. 'I had never heard of the issue in my life,' he said. 'I was fascinated by it, that human experience, how completely terrifying and tragic it was, and I couldn't believe that it was allowed to occur. Not that people wanted it to occur. But the fact that medicine, or anaesthesia hadn't developed to a stage where they could stop it. I was just fascinated by it.'

And here he was, two decades later, still fascinated.

One of the things his patients feared most, he said, was that they might wake during surgery. 'They don't really ask me are they going to have a stroke or a heart attack or a wound infection—which do occur, and can occur more commonly than awareness. They ask me "Will I be awake?"...I smile and reassure them that we will do everything we can to prevent it—but we can't guarantee it. And I want a monitor that can guarantee it.'

He went on: 'I'm an anaesthetist. I monitor at least forty different things during anaesthesia. The patient gets closely watched. The anaesthetist is there from start to finish, looking after their welfare. But the one thing I can't measure is what I do.'

Even back then Myles was talking about the BIS monitor as anaesthesia's possible Holy Grail: a way of finally measuring what it was that he and his colleagues did. Early indications were encouraging. But he acknowledged that the blue box had met with a fair bit of scepticism in the profession. 'If you want to ruin a career in anaesthesia research, you should study depth of anaesthesia,' an esteemed professor had once told him.

Critics pointed out that the trial had been partly funded by the US company, Aspect, that manufactured the BIS. And then there was the number-crunching: if the monitor did prove reliable, the cost of attaching disposable electrodes to every patient, at twenty dollars per operation, would add thirty to sixty million dollars each year to Australia's health budget. Even supporters doubted that it would ever be standard issue. Others were unconvinced by the very notion of trying to allocate numeric values to a concept—anaesthetic depth—that still came as close to philosophy as biology. Like trying to measure happiness with a ruler.

None of this seemed to much concern Myles. He gestured towards the emphysema patient being stitched together on the operating table. 'This is very challenging,' he said cheerfully. 'He could hardly breathe before the operation. It's the perfect sort of operation to test the BIS. We're running at half the level of general anaesthetic, partly with the combination of other drugs but also because the BIS monitor tells us that we don't need that much to keep him asleep, and therefore we know that we can wake him up faster and more reliably.'

Ranged alongside the BIS were the more usual gauges, including one measuring the pressure of air in his lungs and airway. In most operations, said Myles, the patient took five to twenty minutes to wake from the anaesthetic. But patients with severe lung disease needed to be awake faster. They had to start breathing quickly, on their own, or they might end up in intensive care anchored to a breathing machine. Or, or course, dead.

As the surgical team stitched, they chatted. The operation had gone well. There was a buoyant, almost festive atmosphere in the room. No one in the team said anything unkind or inappropriate—although they did say things they probably would not have said if they had thought their patient was awake.

'He told me he played for Melbourne,' said one of the nurses, nodding at the man on the table, whose football days were clearly some time behind him.

'Did he?' said Myles, in a tone that might have been quizzical.

'He'd had a bit of midaz though,' said the nurse, to general laughter. (Midazolam is a potent sedative known to make patients chatty—often chattier than they realise—before they go under.)

'He was just trying to flirt with you I think, there,' said Myles, with good humour.

'He might have played in the under-nineteens or the reserves,' said another man. 'That's the sort of thing people will often tell you.'

'Or in the crowd,' said someone else, drily.

The banter and the stitching continued. 'We've just got one more layer of the skin to go,' reported Myles, as an aside to me. 'We're nearly finishing. And everyone's just sort of gearing up for that I guess. Aside from the anaesthetic and the machine, this case has gone very well. This is as good as it gets really...At the moment we're using a very, very light anaesthetic. Much lighter than I'd normally run because the BIS gives me confidence that he's still asleep.'

In his usual practice, said Myles, he now gave about a third less anaesthetic than he would have previously because he was confident he was still able to keep the patient from waking. This reduced the probability of side effects and increased his patient's chances of a quick recovery. He glanced again at the body.

'This operation,' he said speculatively, 'I'd love it if he's awake in eight minutes.'

As if on cue the body on the stretcher sat up. Like Frankenstein's monster. Or started to: surgical staff pushed him down slowly, firmly, talking to him. 'You're just waking up from your operation. Now lie down. Lie down mate. You're still in the operating theatre.'

'Or maybe two,' said Myles, deadpan, as the man kept trying to sit up and staff kept easing him back.

'It's gone very well, OK? It's gone very well.'

'Breathe through the breathing tube. Now take a big breath for us. It'll be coming out in just a moment.'

'Lie down for us. You're doing really well.'

'Big deep breath for us, in and out.'

The man started moving his leg, which dropped off the side of the trolley. Someone tried to put the leg back, while someone else took the breathing tube out of his throat.

'Well done.'

'Lie down on the stretcher now.'

'Do you have any pain?' asked Myles, going around to the man's side. Myles seemed unperturbed. The BIS had done its job: the patient had been asleep; now he was awake. 'Are you sore at all? Big breath through the mask for some oxygen. That's the way.'

The man kept subsiding then rearing up again, staring around. His eyes, when they opened, were very blue.

o

It is one thing to send a patient to sleep; it is another to know exactly where that is. Early measurements were based on what doctors could see. In 1847 the physician John Snow proposed what he called five observable degrees of narcotism in ether anaesthesia, beginning with exhilaration (the chatty stage) and moving towards (though hopefully never reaching) the fifth stage, where breathing slows then stops, culminating in death. Stage three was generally sufficient for surgery. 'When voluntary movement ceases, with the eyes fixed in an upward gaze during the gas induction of anaesthesia, the patient is protected against the risk of mental suffering.'

These measurements were refined over the years with the advent of new drugs and gases. In time, the development of sophisticated instruments to measure internal states such as heart rate and blood oxygen levels meant doctors could gauge with increasing certainty how their patients were faring. Even today, these sequential stages remain central to many anaesthetists' understanding of their craft and are still used as a practical guide to how deeply anaesthetised a patient is. They are sometimes known as the planes of anaesthesia. When I first heard the term, I thought it was spelt 'plains' and I pictured a vast desert or tundra with a small figure trudging through it. Actually they are assessments based on a series of readily observable physical signs: whether a patient responds when she hears her name, or wakes when pinched; or startles when the doctor touches her eyelashes.

In the early days of anaesthesia the main aim was to ensure doctors did not overdose their patients. By the mid-twentieth century, with improved drugs and methods of delivery, the focus had shifted. Death, still possible, had become far less likely and the challenge facing anaesthetists was to ensure their patients were really unconscious. From time to time in the century after William Morton's triumph in the Ether Dome surgical patients mentioned having been rather more awake than they had expected, but it wasn't until the introduction of muscle relaxants in the early 1940s that this oddity became a problem. The first case of awareness involving muscle relaxants was officially reported in 1950. Ten years later a study put the incidence at an alarming 1.2 per cent. Almost certainly many cases went unreported.

So the search continued for new ways to gauge (un)consciousness. In the mid-sixties a now famous anaesthetist (we'll meet him later) developed a technique to measure the concentration of anaesthetic gas in patients' lungs. It is still regarded by many as the gold standard. The eighties saw the emergence of a score based on the body's autonomic (unconscious and automatic) stress signals: blood pressure, heart rate, sweating and the tears that sometimes slide down a patient's cheeks during surgery and which doctors know as lacrimation. Blood, sweat and tears. But by then the Medical Defence Union of Great Britain was hearing regular complaints from people insisting they had been awake and sometimes in pain during their surgery.

Then, in January 1998, an American musician called Carol Weihrer underwent anaesthesia for eye surgery, and awoke just as doctors prepared to remove her diseased right eyeball. Weihrer's case is famously horrible. Her descriptions of her panicked realisation of what was happening—and her futile attempts to communicate with the doctors before and then during the surgery—are well documented. Weihrer estimates she was awake for between forty minutes and two hours during the operation. During this time she felt her eye being scooped and wrenched from its socket, and then the fibres of the optic nerve being severed. 'Nothing gets much darker than those seconds,' she would tell a conference in 2004.

Weihrer founded the Anaesthesia Awareness Campaign in 1999 to raise the profile of the issue within the medical community, and to have safeguards put in place to protect the tens, maybe hundreds, of thousands of people who wake during surgery each year. By the time of my visit to the Alfred Hospital's Operating Theatre 1 with Paul Myles, and due in part to the media attention arising from Weihrer's website, the question of how to measure anaesthetic depth during surgery had taken on a new urgency. But now, anaesthesia researchers had started looking to the brain itself as a possible guide.

Scientists in the second half of the nineteenth century had already noted the rhythmic electrical activity given off by the brains of rabbits, dogs and monkeys. The following century saw the development of the human electroencephalograph (EEG) which used electrodes placed on the scalp to record the activity within. It's a little like eavesdropping by putting your ear to a glass pressed against a wall: the information is incomplete—picking up the electrical signals closest to the skull—but enough to make out the different bands of activity broadly known as brainwaves. These are translated into squiggly readouts that shift between the shallow spiky waves of the waking mind and the deep slow undulations of sleep or unconsciousness. It was these voltage fluctuations that Paul Myles was measuring with the BIS electrodes.

Today there are various EEG-based monitors in use. Some measure brain activity directly, others gauge the brain's response to a stimulus such as sound. All are based on the fact that while doctors still don't know quite how anaesthetics work, they do know that they cause changes in the brain's electrical activity. But at the time of my visit to the Alfred Hospital, while various commercial monitors were on the market, none had been subjected to the sort of testing through which Myles and his colleagues were now putting the BIS.

o

Back at the hospital, an hour or so after Paul Myles' first patient tried to climb off the table, I watched the start of a second operation in the same room. A middle-aged man was wheeled in on a stainless steel trolley. He had had a sedative 'premed' to relax him, but seemed otherwise alert. Soon, surgeons would open up his arms and his chest to bypass and replace the damaged arteries leading from his heart. But for now he lay on his trolley and watched the medical staff milling around him. Some attached monitors to measure his blood pressure, pulse rate and the amount of oxygen in his blood. Others swabbed him with antiseptic and inserted a catheter into his jugular vein to monitor his heart function during surgery. He had a thick, powerful neck; a boxer's nose.

Paul Myles attached a thin disposable electrode to his forehead. This would provide the readings that the BIS would analyse. The man's eyes closed and opened. Around him blue- and green-suited medical staff were getting on with their jobs. Adjusting monitors, laying out instruments, chatting as he looked on. He followed them with his eyes. Patient. Watchful.

Myles put a mask over his face. 'Big, deep breath.' Within seconds, it seemed, the man was gone. There were more people in the room now. The small talk had stopped. There was quiet except for the opening of plastic packages, the click of instruments and monitors. A woman staffer deftly removed the man's false teeth and his lips wilted inwards. Other medicos adjusted the monitors around his groin. The tip of his penis peeped from the green drapes. A woman reached for it and smoothly inserted a long, white catheter up his urethra. Someone else took some clear adhesive tape and taped his eyes shut; from the sides of the operating table two wooden struts were pulled out at shoulder height. Staff lay the man's arms along the supports and bound his wrists to them, as if to splints or a cross, exposing the soft white skin of his inner arms. This was where the surgeons would get the arteries they would repurpose as bypass grafts for the blocked arteries in his heart. The covers had been pulled back. His body was soft, pink: hairless after shaving. Someone started swabbing him all over with browny-yellow antiseptic liquid. Someone else pulled the green drapes over him, tent-like, leaving only a large rectangle of yellow skin visible.

Myles adjusted the anaesthetic mix to bring the man's blood pressure down. The BIS reading dropped to 19; gradually buoyed itself. 'We're at cruising altitude now,' said Myles. As if in confirmation, someone put on a CD. The Whitlams. Wry, tuneful pop.

I walked around to the top of the table, where Myles and his assistants were adjusting and monitoring the anaesthetic mix and peered over the top of the drape, down at his chest. There were three surgeons working at once. First with scalpels, then with pencil-thin cauterising wands called diathermies, one on each arm, one at his chest. The tiny blowtorches scorched through the layers of skin and yellow fat and flesh, cauterising the capillaries as they went. There was very little blood. Just the smell of cooking. 'Sometimes,' confided one of the nurses later, 'if we're working before lunch, it makes me hungry.' One part Goya, two parts Python. In the background, the Whitlams were still singing: 'There's no aphrodisiac like loneliness.'

Myles checked his monitors. 'This guy's got a good strong heart.' Then, equally conversationally: 'I've only had one case of awareness myself in my whole career—bypass surgery, and they just remembered this bit coming up, they remembered their chest being sawn open and pulled apart.'

'OK,' said a voice from the other side of the screen. 'Lungs are down.' Then there was a sound like a food processor.

'He didn't have pain,' continued Myles. 'He was a really easy-going sort of bloke. He found it interesting. He was amazed by it, not terrified by it.'

On the other side of the drape the surgeon was sawing through the breastbone. Someone clamped the chest cavity open. I peered over and looked down inside, and there was his heart: a small red frog throbbing in the dark. I was transfixed. But even before they began to cut again I could feel part of myself peel away, leaving, to return in increments over the next day or so. Inside the operating theatre, the juxtaposition was so extreme that the mind stopped trying to contain it. A man crucified on a table, chest and arms gaping wide, the victim of some unthinkable transgression, alongside a clatter of voices and work and jokes and music. It was precise, painstaking work. The surgeons separated layers and strands of membrane and meat, burning their way through to the red threads that might help save this man's life.

When I walked out of the hospital an hour later, they were still operating. I felt odd. Fine, I thought, but disconnected. Crossing the road I forgot to look for traffic and had to step back quickly out of the way of a car. I drove carefully. Later I rang and found out the operation had been successful. The patient was well. I felt murky and irritable. In the following days I found myself dwelling upon the operations at the Alfred—the seared flesh of the arm, split like a fruit to the core; the Whitlams in the background marking time. And this was what I came away with most strongly—the sense of opposing realities. The staff, to whom this was familiar, difficult work: their need for teamwork, camaraderie, communication. And the man on the table, to whom something catastrophic had happened, who was silent and completely alone.

THE COLD BOSOM
OF THE OCEAN

Questions without answers

Four years later I encountered Paul Myles again in, of all places, Hull. I had not planned to visit; I had come to England to reconnect with old school friends. But shortly before leaving Australia I had discovered that my visit was to coincide with an obscure but intriguing anaesthesia conference: the Sixth International Symposium on Memory and Awareness in Anaesthesia and Intensive Care.

MAA6, like MAAs 1 to 5 before it, was a curious affair, a triennial thinkfest peopled by a mixed bag of doctors, psychologists and other researchers and practitioners working at anaesthesia's outer reaches—the liminal zone where medicine and its careful demarcations wash up against more open-ended explorations of the nature of memory, consciousness and, inevitably, unconsciousness. This year's conference was to focus on brainwave monitoring.

I arrived on a gloomy Wednesday afternoon with a sore throat and burning chesty cough, having spent most of the past nine hours in cars, planes and trains. I had already missed the start of the conference. After waiting twenty minutes at Hull Station for a taxi I eventually found my way into a lecture theatre at Hull University halfway into the first formal session; and there, sleek and completely grey at forty-five, was Paul Myles. He had had a good year professionally. His team, including co-researcher Kate Leslie, had just published the results of their three-year B-Aware trial in the prestigious medical journal *The Lancet*. The trial had involved 2,463 patients considered at high risk of awareness during general anaesthesia, including those undergoing caesareans and cardiac and trauma surgery. They'd been randomly assigned either to a group being monitored with the BIS or to a control group receiving routine care. Shortly after waking, all the patients were assessed for awareness, then assessed again the next day and a third time a month later.

In the end, the researchers found two cases of awareness in the BIS group compared with eleven in the control group—an 82 per cent reduction in the risk of awareness. The monitoring also reduced recovery time by allowing anaesthetists to give smaller doses of anaesthetic drugs. It was a dramatic result, and one that the assembled anaesthetists and developers and proponents of alternative monitoring machines would spend the next two days (and in some cases years) variously applauding, dissecting or disparaging.

In the years following the Hull conference, the study would propel Myles and Leslie into international prominence among their colleagues, and fast-track their careers at home. The next time I spoke with Myles he would be the head of anaesthesia at the Alfred Hospital; six years after the Hull conference Kate Leslie would become the youngest person to head the Australian and New Zealand College of Anaesthetists. The BIS, meanwhile, would become a star in its own right. The trial would go on to cement the monitor's status as the best known and most widely used depth of anaesthesia monitor in the anaesthetic world—and also promote the use of such devices more generally in procedures with a higher risk of awareness. The small blue box with its secret algorithm would also become the focus for competition, speculation and, in some quarters, derision. Critics would point out that the device could only measure the probability of someone being aware and could not predict the actual moment of waking. Others would also highlight some embarrassing shortcomings, including occasional false readings due to interference from electrical devices such as the diathermy wands used in surgery.

But what was clear as Paul Myles spoke in the auditorium in Hull was that the numbers were in—and they were impressive enough to suggest that using that blue box during surgery, while not infallible, might make things quite a bit clearer when lowering patients into anaesthesia's unfathomable realms.

Right now, however, hunched at the front of the auditorium, trying not to cough, I appeared to be entering an unfathomable realm of my own. Hovering just above me in a throaty, snotty miasma was the question I had been trying to avoid during the long hours of suitcase-lugging: why?

All the previous week, English friends had greeted news of my impending trip to Hull with blank or startled looks and the same question. The answer was that I had no idea—and yet here I was. I had a snazzy blue conference bag and a name tag that said *Kate Cole Adams. Press.* I had met briefly with Michael Wang, who had organised this year's conference and who seemed to regard my attendance as pleasing and unremarkable. I was here; I was a journalist; I was taking notes. But I felt like a figment of my own imagination.

I skipped the evening's talk and the free bus trips afterwards and headed to my hotel. The taxi driver made an odd sound when I told him where I was staying, but would only say that the place was new—which it was. Also ugly, and situated in a bleak corner of the city.

The room, a functional rectangle looking onto a brick wall, did nothing to settle me although, apart from a strange modular bathroom, it was inoffensive. But I knew that I was teetering on the edge of something. I could feel myself starting to collapse inwards; afraid of being lonely, afraid of getting sick, afraid of being afraid—a set of stairs descending to nowhere.

○

I am afraid of dying. I know this is unremarkable but I think about it a lot. How can someone be here and then not? How can that ever make sense? It does my head in. When I was a child I would try to lie awake in wait for the moment—the actual instant—when I would cross from my waking self to that other. I think I believed that if I could only capture the intruder sleep I would be able to prevent it running off with my thoughts and all the things that made me feel like me.

I am six? Maybe seven. A weatherboard house in Melbourne's outer eastern suburbs. It is dark, I am in bed and this terrible knowledge rises and rises around me. I can't remember which realisation comes first: that I will die, or that my parents will. One knowing leads quickly to the next. Either way, there arrives the appalling certainty that I will have to go to this place and I will have to go there alone. No one will look after me. No one can come with me. I will never see my mother or father again. I feel that the bed beneath me and the floorboards beneath it and the ground beneath them have ceased in this instant to exist and that I am plummeting. I simply cannot grasp the immensity of what has happened. I lie here for a long time and the sense of horror does not abate, nor my sense of outrage in the face of it. When I wake in the morning it is still there and nothing is quite the same.

My parents, who both started practising early with the deaths of their own parents, have often seemed to me pragmatic to the point of fatalism about mortality. I grew up assuming they would be dead or close to it by the time I hit my twenties. I worried when they went out that they would not return. I imagined car crashes and roof collapses and absence and loss.

Anaesthesia is not, I understand, the same as death (although sometimes it is; it was for Michael Jackson). But it feels like death. Not so much the experience (although who knows?) but the fact of it. The extinction of self. It worries me. So does the idea of being paralysed. And the idea of being buried alive. Not of course that your doctor is going to bury you alive—but to be paralysed, and unheard…And of course the idea—not just the idea, the certainty—of losing control.

There was a stage in my life, probably a too-long one, when I liked to lose control. I liked drinking, I liked rollercoasters. And I liked getting on airplanes, buckling up and relinquishing myself to the ministrations and constraints, the hot face towel, the regimented, geometric meals, the little screen halfway up the aisle showing obscure or yet-to-be-released films (this was the olden days). The destination set and irrevocable. On a plane I would enter a kind of trance, a perfect passivity born of the almost complete absence of options. So that each little choice seemed delightful. Chicken or beef. Red or white. All the while hurtling through a strangely unreal sky (day night day) perhaps towards some distant, more perfect version of myself. I think that was it. I loved it.

Until one day I didn't.

I was in my late twenties in a plane en route to France when I became aware of an unfamiliar unease that quickly coalesced into dread. Belted into my narrow seat in that inexplicable metal cylinder, what terrified me was not that the plane would plummet or explode or hit another plane, but that any second now, unless I could exercise an unthinkable degree of control, I would start to scream. I could feel my hands and feet twitching with the need to leap up. My throat shrank with the effort of staying silent. It seemed to last hours, though the worst of it was over by the time we stopped to refuel somewhere in the Middle East. There I accosted a Frenchman and begged for one of his cigarettes. He gave me two, which I smoked in succession, drawing the hot grimy air deep into my lungs with gratitude and relief. I have no idea what I would have cried out if I had risen to my feet in the plane and started to yell. But for some years after that, whenever I entered an airport I would begin to feel the same sort of spiralling incapacity as now enveloped me in the anonymous hotel room in Hull.

This is a special way of being afraid / No trick dispels, wrote poet Philip Larkin in his tart, sombre rumination on death, 'Aubade'. Larkin spent most of his working life in the Brynmor Jones Library at the University of Hull, where the MAA6 conference was now being held. I don't know how many of the anaesthetists knew the poem. It wasn't mentioned in the conference material...*no sight, no sound / No touch or taste or smell, nothing to think with / Nothing to love or link with / The anaesthetic from which none come round.*

I took some deep breaths and spoke to myself out loud—sensible soothing words—and after a while I sat at the desk and started to write down the day's events. As I wrote, I began to feel better. Lulled by language, by my version of the day, I started to feel real again. After an hour or so I decided that I needed food, and that it might be depressing eating at the hotel, and that I would go out and find somewhere to have a meal.

The girl at reception directed me to an undistinguished Indian restaurant around the corner. I was the only customer. Two staff, both men, were playing some sort of game—dice or maybe counters—at one of the tables, and in the too-quietness of the dining room my unease again took hold as I ordered. After delivering my food and a glass of wine, the waiter and bartender resumed their game, paying me no particular attention. But a mean, angular fear had closed around me and with each mouthful I became more convinced that something terrible would happen—that, for instance, I would not leave the restaurant alive, that they would hurt me, then kill me and that no one would know where I was. I knew this was improbable, ludicrous, probably racist, but the knowing came from such a long way off that it barely nudged into the bulging membrane of my imaginings. By the time I finally paid and left amid polite farewells, I was almost nauseated with fear—no longer of the staff but of myself, my coiled thoughts.

Back in my room I brushed my teeth and avoided looking at myself in the mirror. I glanced at the abstracts of the following day's events. The keynote address to be delivered by Anthony Angel of the University of Sheffield was about the effects of anaesthetic agents on senses such as sight and sound and touch. In the absence of a single, distinct pharmacological action, said Angel, the best question was not how anaesthetics worked, but where. He pointed to the thalamus—or thalami—which nest like a pair of tiny doves above the brain stem, decoding and relaying messages between the sense organs and the cerebral cortex—that great folded mass that allows us to remember, contemplate and describe our worlds. This pulpy sheath sits directly beneath the skull and wraps around the rest of the brain. With its fissured lobes—temporal to the side, and then, pushing from the rear of the skull towards the forehead, the occipital, parietal and, most spectacularly from an evolutionary standpoint, frontal—it dominates the inner landscape in size and sheer clout. Here are the capacities that gave us Stonehenge, Sudoku and climate change: language, problem solving, analysis, planning, reflecting, as well as high-level sensory processing. Angel, in any event, reminded us that anaesthetics did not shut down sight, sound or touch in the eyes, ears or skin and muscle, but in the brain, and speculated that anaesthetics somehow curtailed the ability of the thalamus to communicate with the cortex. 'And thus,' he concluded, 'for the patients the world goes silent, black and with no sense of touch or taste.'

As it happened, among the fears assailing me that night the most obvious (though to me least apparent) was the prospect—distant, but decreasingly so—that I might one day end up alone in a small white room rather like this one, waiting to be taken downstairs and operated upon. It was the fear I had been holding at bay since my spine began to twist in adolescence. Over the years I had my regular reviews, some of which showed the curve advancing. But it was by now so familiar it was part of me, a distant smudge that seemed somehow to rest always on the horizon. In recent years, however, following my pregnancy and the birth of my son, and presaged by a growing discomfort in my body, the smudge had been gradually becoming less distant, less blurred. I hurt more. I stooped. None of this had I yet allowed myself to know.

In the dining area the next morning a smooth-skulled American pulled out a chair and gestured me to join him and a small group of fellow conference-goers. He had an intense compressed energy, at once hospitable and edgy, and it turned out he was speaking later the same morning. He was a psychologist. I, despite my cough and my general feeling of weirdness, was a journalist. I pulled out my tape recorder and placed it in front of him.

'My name is Hank Bennett. I'm an associate professor at the University of Medicine and Dentistry of New Jersey. I'm not telling you my social security number.' Bennett was what is known in the media as good talent. He was articulate and clearly spoken with a facility for metaphors and thumbnail sketches. He was also the only person at the table for whom English was a first language, and I gravitated to him more or less shamelessly.

The day's program included sessions on the effect of anaesthetics on the brain, and a comparison of the ways in which different brain-wave monitors attempted to measure how deeply any given patient was anaesthetised. But it turned out that Bennett was not at all convinced by the whole premise. The real question, he argued, was not so much *how* to measure anaesthetic depth, but *what* to measure. Rather than anaesthetists simply trying to decipher the jagged fluctuations of the various brainwave monitors, he argued, patients might be better served by a device that also measured the body's responses to pain. Intriguingly, however, he was not just referring to the pain that might be felt by someone such as Rachel Benmayor, undergoing surgery awake but paralysed, but to the experience of patients who remained unconscious during general anaesthesia.

Bennett did not, by the way, use the word 'pain'. Pain by definition involves not only a so-called 'noxious stimulus' (such as a scalpel might inflict) and the body's reflexive response, but the brain's conscious registration of that response. To be in pain, in other words, you have to know that you're in pain.

Bennett instead talked of nociception. Nociceptors are nerves that have evolved to respond to physical damage, or even the possibility of damage, in an organism (such as, for example, a patient). One set of neurons (the 'afferent' ones) shoot these messages along nerve pathways up the spine to the brain; while 'efferent' pathways stream from the brain back to the muscles and glands and other cells, carrying the unambiguous message: *owww*, you are in pain; act now to protect yourself. What anaesthetics—at least inhaled general anaesthetics—do, said Bennett, is disrupt the second part of the process, not the first. The body still broadcasts its storm warnings along the wiring of the central nervous system and into the brain, but here the signal is blocked or scrambled. While the older brain centres sitting above the spinal column register the information, the brain's owner neither perceives pain, nor remembers it afterwards. Instead, as Anthony Angel might argue, the world is silent and black and with no sense of touch or taste.

But how could Angel or anybody else be so sure?

One of the reasons why the discovery of curare, and the paralysing (or 'relaxing') drugs that followed, has been so important is that they make patients lie still. Without paralysing drugs, unconscious patients may still twitch, jerk, wince and grimace as their nerves are dissected by scalpels and diathermy wands. While this doesn't mean that they are experiencing pain in the way that you or I understand it (even a cat whose cortex has been largely removed will arch in response to messages its brain can no longer process or act upon) it shows clearly that at some level the body is still responding to what is happening to it, albeit unconsciously.

So what?

Apply an electric shock to the side of a giant sea slug, and the response of its neurons can be graphed in a single narrow peak. Up, down: *ouch*. Apply the same shock twenty-four hours later on the other side, and you get the same reaction. But repeat the shock at the original site, and the pattern is now quite different. Instead of a single peak, there is a mountain range, a jagged outline of pain stretching to the end of the graph. US anaesthetist Daniel Carr has used this example to support his belief that the memory of pain—the body's memory of pain, that is—can be more damaging than the original experience, conscious or otherwise. I had heard Carr speak in Australia in 2001 when he argued that when it came to the operating theatre it was not enough simply to cloak pain signals with hypnotic drugs. Doctors needed to prevent the messages from getting to the brain in the first place. 'In practice,' said Carr, 'many anaesthetists administer an inhaled anaesthetic gas during the operation with little or no intravenous "painkiller", and then titrate small incremental doses of pain medicine as the patient emerges post-operatively from general anaesthesia.'

When I approached Carr after the conference, he referred me to the work of US anaesthetist and pain researcher Clifford Woolf, who had established that pain, even unconscious pain, could trigger chronic responses in the spinal cord that could later coalesce into pain the patient would be all too aware of months, sometimes years, after the operation was over. Woolf had argued that strong pain relief should be given during surgery and maybe even before (though the evidence for this remains patchy), as well as when the patient was waking up, to avoid 'sensitisation' of the central nervous system. Today most general anaesthetics include painkillers—aiming to dampen the body's stress responses (rising heart rate and blood pressure, grimacing, twitching), if only to reduce the chances that their patients will start to wake up. But Carr, now director of Tuft University's pain research education and policy program, still argues that analgesia during surgery—particularly the ever-more-popular day procedures—is often too little too late, and that this has implications for long-term pain.

Hank Bennett too was convinced that under general anaesthesia, pain—or at least its precursor—was often not so much banished as hiding. Unlike nitrous oxide, which blunts sensation even before people pass out (as Horace Wells noticed at that demonstration), today's potent gases are not generally analgesics. And while most anaesthetic cocktails include a painkiller, there is no way of knowing for sure what an individual patient is feeling in the moment, or might feel later.

o

Spend any amount of time around anaesthetists and you are bound to hear a fair bit about the brain and its constituent parts. Cerebrum, cerebral cortex, corpus callosum, hippocampus, thalamus, brain stem, amygdala, cerebellum—like players in a Greek drama, each contributing its own story, its own viewpoint and version of events.

The best way of visualising the brain that I have come across is a simple exercise that involves lightly clenching both your fists around their thumb and then resting them together, wrist to wrist, forearm to forearm in front of your face. Now you are looking at your brain, or a digital representation (each fist a hemisphere). At the base of this mass, where the wrists connect, pulse to pulse, is the brain stem, the most primitive part of the brain in evolutionary terms, which rises above the spinal cord (running down between the forearms) that carries the multitude of messages, afferent and efferent included, that in any instant tick up and down the nervous system's superhighway.

The brain stem is the survival centre for creatures as diverse as toads, tapirs and tattoo artists. It is the body's autopilot, overseeing the basic functions of life: respiration, perspiration, salivation, heart rate, blood pressure, balance, sleep and waking, for starters. Above, where the thumbs disappear into the fold between the fingers and the palms, is the limbic system—the emotional or so-called 'mammalian' brain, common to humans and other mammals—which modulates functions including emotion and memory, along with the capacities that enable us not only to learn from experience but to live in groups. In humans this buried treasure includes the hippocampus (which lets us remember our car's number plate, dog's name and what happened yesterday, and without which we would have no conscious memories at all), the amygdala (an almond-shaped cluster that helps us store and retrieve emotional memories, particularly fearful ones), the thalamus, and an elegant arc known as the cingulate gyrus that helps in communication and social behaviour, as well as governing sensations such as fear, anxiety and pleasure.

And it is here, in the limbic centre, argued Hank Bennett, that pain signals reaching the anaesthetised mind might be marooned, unable to pass their messages to the outer and most peculiarly human section of the brain, the cerebral cortex (represented by the fingers and backs of your hands) to be translated, acknowledged and acted upon.

○

Back at the university the next day, not a lot of attention was being paid to pain that no one could see or recall. Unsurprisingly, pain that no one knows they are experiencing is trumped by pain that stampedes up and down the afferent and efferent pathways of people who are not only conscious but who can also remember it later. At one point in the conference, during a session on the impact of anaesthetic awareness, I heard from within the auditorium a sharply indrawn breath from the audience and a woman's tight sharp voice. 'No!'

The speaker had just described a paper published in the early 1960s by a doctor who reported operating on paralysed patients without anaesthesia in the misguided belief that once a patient had been sedated and knocked out with a short-acting induction drug, all that was needed to keep him that way was curare—and lots of oxygen. The indrawn breath was, I felt sure, that of Carol Weihrer, the woman whose own eye surgery and subsequent public campaign had helped publicise the prevalence of anaesthetic awareness. Weihrer herself had addressed the audience in the previous session, describing in gruelling detail her experience and its emotional and psychological legacy.

Weihrer's life in the years since her surgery had been consumed by her failed anaesthetic experience and her subsequent activism on behalf of other victims. 'I have not slept in a bed or laid on my back for six years and five months,' she told the silent anaesthetists, 'because I cannot face lying in the same position as the surgery required…I am easily startled, hyper-vigilant, have flashbacks, triggers, temperature flare-ups, mood swings, fatigue…Control becomes an all-consuming necessity…'

After speaking she walked heavily back up the aisle and resumed her seat.

Much later I would come to understand other things about pain. That the *owww* moment is just the beginning. That it is what we do next with the pain that really counts. That, while for any two people each nerve fibre and relay point and electro-chemical jolt may be pretty much the same, each person's experience of pain is unique. That the same stimulus (bee sting, paper cut, scalpel) that translates for one person as a sharp but transient discomfort may, for another, feel closer to torture, and may keep on feeling that way for a long time. And that this does not simply mean that my pain, or yours, is 'in the mind' (although that is part of what it means, but not in a 'get over it' way—although even sometimes partly that). But that each of us brings to our own subjective experience of pain exactly what we bring to the rest of our lives: our culture, our personal history, our previous pain, even our education. And that these in turn not only frame the way we think about pain, but affect the intensity of the pain we experience.

I knew none of this then and most of it, in any case, is beyond the scope of this book. There is a staggering amount that is beyond the scope of this book. (What about memories that don't even happen in the brain? Brainless amoeboid cells have been shown not only to learn but to pass that information onto other cells. What might that mean for the anaesthetised you or me? I don't know. I don't think anyone else does either.) What is worth considering, however, is this possibility, floated by several researchers: if the stimulating effects of surgery are not properly counteracted by adequate painkillers, they may start to push us up towards the waking world. And in that case, what awakens may not be all of us, but a part of us. A part that we don't know about, but that is there all the same, all the time, unconscious. Hidden.

o

By day three, the strange panic of that first night had receded and I felt once more on solid ground. It had all started to feel less like a bizarre hallucination, more like a school camp, and I was rather enjoying both Hull (which, away from my bleak corner, resolved itself surprisingly quickly into wide, pleasant avenues) and the company of my fellow campers. I admit now, in fact, to thoroughly liking almost all the anaesthetists I met in the process of researching this book.

True, it was a very particular cross-section of the profession, as most of those I spoke with had an interest not just in anaesthesia but in some bigger questions. The nature of consciousness. The permutations of the unconscious. What makes people so...*themselves*. They were enthusiasts, quick-thinking, inquiring, often funny and self-deprecating. Not once did I hear anyone discuss the stock market, scuba diving or their golf handicap. I liked them so much that I started regretting my liberal arts background and found myself wishing that I had persevered those extra eight or so years with maths and sciences instead of ditching them as soon as I was able at fifteen (not that I really had a choice), and studied medicine myself. Or failing that, taken the advice of an older mentor who, when asked her advice for young writers, had once suggested, 'Marry a doctor.'

Throughout the conference, however, beyond the talk of monitors and brainwaves and EEGs, of lightness and darkness and shallows and depths, was another, deeper current. Increasingly, the conversations I noticed around me were not just about conscious memories, their impact and how to prevent them, but about a different sort of memory that, like pain, may not be experienced consciously, but which may, nevertheless, linger in the nervous system. Here was British psychologist Jackie Andrade talking about a process called 'priming'. Memory priming happens when, say, you or I are in a lab and a scientist flashes up an image or plays a sound so fast that we don't think we notice it, but later we change our behaviour based on the image or sound we didn't know we had seen or heard. 'It's clearly not going to have any effect as dramatic as being awake during anaesthesia and recalling it afterwards,' Andrade told her audience. 'But I think I might be able to persuade you [...] that it could be a very general phenomenon that affects everybody that you anaesthetise.'

Through it all, largely unspoken but unavoidable, was the tidal pull of Bernard Levinson's 1965 experiment. It was there on the second page of the program in a brief article about the history of the MAA conferences. 'During the early 1960s,' it began,

a South African physician training to be an anaesthetist in London, Bernie Levinson, was concerned by pejorative comments made by surgeons about their patients, ostensibly unconscious, lying on the operating table. He was sure that such remarks were processed by the brain at some level and decided to conduct an experiment to demonstrate this.

It then went on the summarise the experiment: the ten patients; the manufactured anaesthetic 'crisis'; the meetings one month later in Levinson's rooms in which he hypnotised them, and 'took them back to the time of their operation', and in which four of the ten repeated the dentist's words verbatim, and another four became distressed enough to suggest they had been aware of the supposed crisis. Despite methodological limitations, said the article, 'Levinson's findings...

prompted widespread concern and interest in the possibility of cognitive processing during general anaesthesia.'

On our final evening in Hull I ate out with a group including Hank Bennett. Afterwards I sat up in the bar at the hotel with them and tried to flush away my remaining flu symptoms with scotch. Much of the evening has settled in my memory as an amiable blur. But there is one story told by Bennett that stands out. One day back in the 1980s, he had received a phone call from a woman who had read about his work in the *New York Times*. As Bennett recalled, the woman told him about an operation she had previously undergone to remove cancer from her abdomen. She had woken, he said, remembering nothing, but over time had become increasingly uneasy. Something was wrong. She had gone back to her surgeon, who insisted that the surgery had gone very well—he had removed all the cancer, and the remaining tissue had been tested and looked healthy. Instead of feeling reassured, the woman went home convinced she was going to die. She saw a psychiatrist, who gave her drugs. Still she believed she was going to die. She went back to the surgeon a second time. He tried again to reassure her, to no avail. Suddenly she cried out, the words that burst from her surprising her as much as they did her doctor: 'But you didn't get it all! You didn't get it. The black stuff—you didn't get the black stuff!'

There was a pause and then the surgeon turned to her in disbelief. 'Oh my God.'

Of course, Bennett said, all this was a long time ago, and the drugs were different back then. But what the woman told him was that as her surgeon was closing her up that day—the cancer safely excised, the tension over—he made an idle and completely unrelated comment to one of his fellow doctors. 'You know, no matter what I do, I can't get rid of that black stuff in my shower.' He was talking about mould. After her unexpected outburst in the doctor's surgery, said Hank, the woman's anxiety disappeared.

As the evening fragmented, conversation swung wildly through increasingly lurid tales of pharmacological cause and effect—the way the drug angel dust shuts down the brain, section by section; the planes of anaesthesia; the effect of anaesthetics on the nervous system; stories without beginnings or endings—a court case, a child who wouldn't get well after surgery—tales of birth and death and flying saucers. The drinking continued and someone else suggested that unconscious memories of surgery might be linked to antisocial and even psychotic behaviour. There was talk of a murder. A small group of us stayed up late into the night, cocooned in a haze of alcohol, ideas and a sort of reckless bonhomie—wavering circles of meaning that later pulsed through my night and settled finally far beneath the surface, where the world was silent and black.

Things you don't know you know

Johannesburg 1965. It is a month since Bernard Levinson staged his fake crisis on ten unsuspecting patients undergoing dental surgery with the help of anaesthetist Dr Viljoen. Now the psychiatrist has summoned to his rooms a twenty-two-year-old florist, Miss D, whom he is in the process of hypnotising.

'She entered a trance easily and was regressed to the morning of the operation,' Levinson later wrote in his notes.

> She relived the difficulty the anaesthetist had in finding a vein when the anaesthetic began. (This I could corroborate.) Then she signalled with her finger that she was 'asleep'. I gave her the same injunction as the others in the series—'If there is anything that disturbs you, signal to me.' She signalled with her finger.
>
> Miss D: Someone is talking.
> BL: Who is it who's talking?
> Miss D: Dr Viljoen
> BL: What's Dr Viljoen saying?
> Miss D: He's saying that my colour is quite grey—and he doesn't like my breathing—he's going to give my [*sic*] oxygen.

BL: Yes, what's he saying now? What's he actually saying?
  What are his words?
[*Long pause.*]
Miss D: He said that I will be all right now.
BL: Yes?
Miss D: They're going to start again now.
BL: They're going to start again?
Miss D: Yes, he's bending close to me now.

Bernard Levinson has the sort of voice you want to listen to all day, textured and rich, with a slight upward inflection as if he is telling a wonderful story that is unfolding before him even as he speaks. If I was going to be hypnotised by anyone, I would like it to be him. Forty-two years after his famous experiment, I tracked Levinson down with the help of Google and, after a friendly email exchange, rang him one afternoon in his Johannesburg home. In the decades since staging his mock surgical crisis Levinson has worked as a psychiatrist in private practice and public hospitals and has for many years been a prominent sex therapist. He has had numerous books published, including two novels and four volumes of poetry. He is a wonderful storyteller. He is glad he is not an anaesthetist.

As a young doctor in the early 1950s, he spent a year in England working as a resident anaesthetist in a hospital in Chelsea. It convinced him he would never be good at the job. 'I hated it,' he told me in the first of a series of phone conversations. 'I wanted to work with people who were conscious, who could talk to me…I didn't understand it. And it frightened me.'

He had said something similar in Glasgow in 1989 when he was invited to speak to a group of anaesthetists at the first Memory and Awareness in Anaesthesia conference (the same series I would attend fifteen years later in Hull). What stood out most clearly for him about his early experience, he told them, was the distress he felt.

'The year was 1953. It was the year of the Coronation. Hillary has just climbed Mount Everest and I had made the astounding discovery that every time there was a crisis in the operating theatre a current of anxiety flowed between the surgeon and myself via the patient. It did not seem to matter where the crises began or in which direction it flowed, it always involved the three of us. Now this does not sound like a monumental discovery, but it was the bewildering anguish of my entire anaesthetic career!'

By the time I first spoke with Bernard Levinson, it was many years since he had administered an anaesthetic—or stood by as someone else did—but, at eighty-one, he still recounted the 1965 experiment and the events leading up to it with a sort of wonder.

After his year in England, Levinson returned to South Africa, where he practised as a GP and later specialised in psychiatry. It was while working as a psychotherapist in the early sixties that he began to get a sense of what had so upset him during his time in the hospital in Chelsea all those years before. Among Levinson's patients at this time was a young woman, Peggy, who was recovering from a traumatic car accident. Levinson was using hypnosis to help her find the confidence to drive again. Peggy was also seeing a plastic surgeon who was preparing to operate on her damaged face. It occurred to Levinson that if the anaesthetist would agree to play music to her during the operation, he, Levinson, might hypnotise her later to see if she could identify the music. The anaesthetist agreed. On the day of the operation, the anaesthetist applied the ether but before Levinson had even put the music on, he said, the surgeon, who had begun by preparing to remove a cyst from Peggy's mouth, exclaimed, 'Good gracious! This may not be a simple cyst; it may be cancer.'

According to Levinson, Peggy's pulse raced and her blood pressure went up. He waved to the surgeon and wrote on a piece of paper, 'Reassure her please!' The surgeon quickly recanted. 'On second thoughts,' he said, 'it is only a simple cyst.'

A month later Levinson saw Peggy in his rooms. The cyst had been analysed and found to be benign. Peggy knew this. But under hypnosis she seemed not to believe it. She not only repeated the surgeon's exclamation verbatim, said Levinson, but told him she did not believe the surgeon's reassurance. She continued working with Levinson and began driving her car again, but two years later died of uterine cancer. 'I don't know how to understand that,' wrote Levinson later. 'To link this to our experiment would be an appalling thought.'

In the early sixties, at around the same time Levinson was starting to wonder about the effect of anaesthesia on the unconscious mind, Californian gynaecologist and obstetrician David Cheek hypnotised several patients who were making poor recoveries from surgery. None had reported any memories of the surgery, but under hypnosis, he said, several claimed to have remembered hearing negative statements made about them during their operation.

Levinson was fascinated with Cheek's work, and the two struck up an energetic correspondence. 'I remember Louie,' wrote Cheek of one patient.

> He was an asthmatic. I was obsessed in those days trying to understand the body's language. Was his breathing an expression of some deep psychic distress? I was using hypnosis to explore his life and to my astonishment he took me back to an operation he had undergone years earlier. He heard the surgeon say: 'Look at the lung. Have you ever seen anything as black as that?' I knew the surgeon and he actually remembered saying those words.

Cheek claimed to have corroborated this and other reports, although critics argued that his interview methods were dubious.

Cheek, who published a series of papers on the subject, argued that such unconscious learning, if allowed to remain unconscious, could trigger traumatic neuroses in patients. After the memories were brought into consciousness through hypnosis, he reported, the patients' symptoms lessened or disappeared.

As anecdotes go, these were compelling. Then again, this was the sixties—a decade in which American scientists studied inter-species communication with horny dolphins; in which a Yale professor set out to control the mind of a charging bull with an electrical implant; and in which the CIA tried to control the minds of unwitting US citizens through the secret application of LSD and other brain-frying drugs. The mind was a playground. And many of the experiments that took place there were later discredited.

So, anecdotes such as David Cheek's are just that. They prove nothing. But they do invite questions, many of which remain unan-swered, perhaps unanswerable.

Here's one now.

I have a friend who until recently worked as a nurse in a clinic dedicated to the awkward but necessary procedures known as colonoscopies and endoscopies, in which a long probe the width of a finger is inserted up your rectum or down your gullet to examine the lower or upper diges-tive tract. My friend (let us call her Deep Throat) had some engaging stories about the sorts of things that went on in the surgery. There was the surgeon who talked at infuriating length about his overseas holidays, and another who liked to discuss the minutiae of his share portfolio while delving for polyps inside the 'client' on the table. There was the anaesthetist who passed the time making intricate origami figures while the surgeons did their probing. A while ago, my friend came over for dinner and told us this story about a woman who had come in for a colonoscopy.

The woman had been given a light sedative anaesthetic and was lying immobile on the trolley. Staff inserted the probe and the surgeon started looking for any signs of cancerous or pre-cancerous growths in the woman's large intestine. Instead what he found was a live worm. Who knows how it had got there. Perhaps the woman had eaten undercooked meat, or drunk untreated water, or touched the wrong part of the wrong object. But here it was, a small parasitic worm, going about its business in the dark tunnel of the woman's digestive tract. The surgeon duly disposed of it and continued easing the tube, with its tiny light and camera, up and into the coils of the woman's colon. This was when things started getting stupid. On the team that day was a young, inexperienced nurse, whom the surgeon and anaesthetist began to tease. 'Oooh, you've got to look out for those worms. That one was just a baby. Wait till you find the Motherworm. They get pretty territorial.' Everyone was laughing by now, my friend included. But the young nurse was getting nervous. Just as the probe rounded the next curve the surgeon cried out: 'Look out! There it is! The Motherworm!' The young nurse screamed. Everyone else fell about. The patient just lay there looking deadish, which is how we look under anaesthesia. It was funny. But my friend wondered later if it was OK.

So that's one question.

Here's another. What does it even mean to be unconscious? When I last googled 'unconsciousness' I found a link to the classic textbook *Adams and Victor's Principles of Neurology*. While acknowledging the near impossibility of conjuring up a single conclusive definition of either consciousness or its converse, the authors noted that doctors usually adopted a narrow but pragmatic interpretation: 'a state of unawareness of self and environment or a suspension of those mental activities by which people are made aware of themselves and their environment, coupled always with a diminished responsiveness to environmental stimuli'. While this seems a perfectly efficient definition, it tells us little about the range of states and experiences to which we routinely ascribe the label 'unconscious'. And there are so many ways that we can *be* unconscious. We can be fainting, or having a fit, or falling into a coma or being anaesthetised. And within each of these descents are uncertain gradations from deep to light, from very to not-very. And what of the unconscious processes that happen when we are awake? The submerged current of things we know, sense and remember, without knowing that we know, or sensing that we sense or remembering that we remember them, but which help us to juggle or drive a car, or tell if a colleague is upset or a child is falling ill or a stranger is watching us, unseen. And what about Freud's unconsciousness—or the version of the unconscious that he popularised early last century—a psychoanalytic stew brimming with thoughts, memories, emotions and desires, all hidden, perhaps forever, from the conscious self?

Personally, I have never much approved of my unconscious self. By this I mean not the multitude of unconscious, automatic processes that form the substrate of my waking life—reading, writing, riding a bike—but the half-formed, unarticulated thoughts and memories, associations and opinions that together constitute what I think of as my hidden self. I like it in theory, and sometimes in the cinema of dreams, but up close it frightens me. It is unruly and I cannot control it. I feel that it makes me vulnerable. Sometimes it gets in the way of me doing the things I think I want to do. Often it tells me things that I don't want to know. (Once while kissing a man I liked I had the vertiginous sense that his mouth would open and open and that he would swallow me whole.) And too often I push it away. But wherever I go it trails along, insistent and unquiet. Like a small dog yapping behind me. The harder I push, the more insistent the yapping.

Who knows what to make of Freud's psychoanalytic unconscious? What is it? Where does it happen? Is it even a thing? Freud's labyrinthine theories have been pilloried and parodied in part because of their imprecision, as well as their pervasive emphasis on sexuality. Even if we accept the basic idea that there are things about ourselves that we don't want to know (without actually knowing that they are there not to be known)—and that we somehow exile them to an uncertain realm where they settle like silt, if only for a while—the limits of this kingdom remain obscure. As do its laws. As do the means of banishing or retrieving material to or from it.

Yet the evidence of my own life tells me there are parts of myself that I do not recognise or necessarily welcome, but which influence the choices I make, the interests I pursue, the people I love and the way I love them. I also accept Freud's contention that this hidden self makes itself known to us—or rather, we make ourselves known to ourselves or to others—through secret channels and unintended gestures. We glimpse it in dreams or express it, unwittingly, through our verbal slips and bodily processes, our flushing, our vague malaises and our inexplicable medical woes; we give it form in our art. British sculptor Henry Moore's famously gigantic tactile nudes are said to have had an umbilical connection to the fact that as a young boy he used to massage his mother. This reminds me of a set of post-it notes someone gave me one Christmas, with a picture of old Sigmund alongside the quote *When you mean one thing but say your mother.*

My mother, as it happens, is also an artist. For a long time she has explored in her prints and paintings the collision between native vegetation and human patterns. She views the earth from above as if through some high eye: huddles of remnant forest dissected by fields and fences and furrows; bald hills draped with fluid linear contours. Before and after. Wilderness and constraint. One of my favourite works is an etched landscape of neatly sectioned fields intersected with meandering creek lines and dark clotted pools. The fields are filled in from above in orderly rows that mark the lines of their plantings. And from beneath (a sepia stain) blooms of submerged water seep upwards and through.

My mother.

When I visited her in hospital a few nights after the surgery to remove her cancerous kidney my mother reported a dream she had had the night before. It was not like her other dreams.

Generally, she said, 'people tend to plod around in my dreams, looking for a door or a place or a toilet, and nothing much happens'. But in this dream she had discovered or been delivered a box of light bulbs. What interested her about the bulbs was that she knew with the logic of dreams that if she could work out how to turn them inside out she could transform them into Christmas decorations. This appealed to her immensely. But as she got to work, she realised that the light globes were multiplying. Faster than she could transform them, they began spreading around her. She woke into darkness and an unfamiliar unease. She climbed out of her bed and raised the blinds. Wrapping a blanket around her, she moved to the chair against the window and here she sat and waited for the sun to rise over the warehouses and terraces and sports grounds of East Melbourne.

The thought of my mother sitting there alone like that makes my heart hurt; an ache behind the breastbone that does not go away even when I rub at it. But as poignant as this story seems to me, at least my mother knew she had been asleep and was now awake. This is not the case for some people waking from anaesthetics. William Morton's historic public demonstration of surgical anaesthesia in the Ether Dome may have been the first record of anaesthetic awareness (his young patient having later admitted to being in pain during the procedure). But his rival for the title of founder of modern anaesthesia,

Horace Wells, had already beaten him to another dubious distinction, although he was not to know it: the first recorded case of hidden awareness in anaesthesia.

This contradictory notion loosely describes the experiences of people who can be shown to have taken in information during surgery but who later have no knowledge of it. While Wells' ill-fated attempt to publicly demonstrate surgical anaesthesia with laughing gas destroyed his career, the patient who had ruined his demonstration by crying out as Wells pulled his tooth later claimed to remember no pain. He was unaware of having been aware. By today's standards Wells would almost certainly have been deemed the more successful anaesthetist. (Plus, the drug he used for his demonstration was nitrous oxide, still the workhorse of many of today's anaesthetic mixes—unlike ether.)

If only Bernard Levinson been there on the day of Horace Wells' doomed demonstration. He might have hypnotised the young patient and taken him back to that moment when his tooth was drawn and he cried out, before forgetting what had happened. That said, hypnosis is, in its own weird way, as mysterious as anaesthesia, and considerably less reliable. Psychiatrists warn that in this vulnerable state patients may unwittingly confuse or even create events—'confabulating' memories, dreams and imaginings into some hybrid beast they might wrongly believe to be real.

o

Among the papers in my study is a precious and fading fax, sent to me by Bernard Levinson, with the notes he wrote after that flawed and fascinating 1965 study. Here is twenty-two-year-old motor mechanic Mr R. Under hypnosis a month after his dental surgery, Mr R also reported memories of the procedure, but in his case the mock crisis appears to have been largely overshadowed by a real drama. Just

before the anaesthetist interrupted the operation, the surgeons accidentally cut an artery in the man's mouth. Now Mr R appeared to be
reliving the hitherto forgotten episode in Bernard Levinson's rooms.

Mr R: My gum feels like it's being cut. It feels like they're
breaking my tooth: with a hammer and chisel, or something—and they're picking out the pieces. I can taste blood.

BL: You can taste blood?

Mr R: Ya. I can taste blood—and they're pulling now.
Cutting and having trouble I think. Pulling out bits on this
side. Little bits here and moving something. Uh...uh...my
hands are being held.

BL: How do you mean, your hands are being held?

Mr R: I don't know. I've just got that sensation. My hands are
held fast to my side.

BL: Anything else? Anything being said?'

Mr R: Some people are speaking over there. Something about
a dental artery. My mouth is full of blood. It feels like it's
bleeding a lot.

BL: What's he saying?

Mr R: Got to cut deeper—or something like that. Someone's
saying there's a nerve there.

[*A little later in the interview, Mr R has mentioned the anaesthetist, and Levinson asks if he recalls Viljoen saying anything
during the surgery.*]

BL: Can you go back now and try and hear what that voice
which you described to me was saying?

Mr R: He's saying it's all right. Yes, it's all right now, they can
finish the job.

So what just happened? And what are we to make of it?
Levinson believes that the mechanic was retrieving an unconscious
memory formed under deep anaesthesia. ('I kept on saying to the
anaesthetist, you've got to go deeper, and I will signal to you when

the electroencephalogram is flat, and he had never taken his patients to that level of anaesthesia.'). Others have suggested that Mr R and the others who reported similar experiences after the mock crisis might not have been as unconscious as Levinson liked to think: perhaps the anaesthetic (an ether-based cocktail also including nitrous oxide) had left them awake enough to register parts of the procedure before forgetting again. Perhaps these were not memories at all: perhaps the patients were merely responding to cues Levinson himself had accidentally given when he hypnotised the ten after— or even before—their operations. It is impossible to know. And of course, all this happened a long time ago. By the 1970s ether had largely fallen out of favour in Western nations—not only did it smell bad and induce an unbearable sense of suffocation, it was highly flammable (even the carcasses of animals euthanised with ether are potentially explosive). In most parts of the world it has long been superseded by other inhalable anaesthetics. In the operating theatres of the new millennium, with their panoply of drugs and monitors, their sophisticated anaesthetic cocktails, few anaesthetists would seriously entertain the possibility that experiences such as recounted by Levinson or Cheek could happen today, if ever they did.

But suppose for a moment that Levinson is right. What if something about the effects of ether—or even of that particular cocktail on that particular day—means that those memories were both unconscious and real? I can't help wondering about the patients who became agitated when later questioned under hypnosis—and about the two who claimed to remember nothing at all. Levinson has no idea what became of them. Maybe they walked out of his rooms and that was the end of it. But there must still be tens of thousands of other people walking around today who have had ether anaesthesia. Might some of them still be carrying fragments of their surgeries around inside them?

There was a strange case, reported in the mid-1980s by Australian psychologist Julius Howard, of a twenty-nine-year-old woman who had suffered chronic insomnia following a hysterectomy three years earlier. The patient, said Howard, 'had been aware vaguely of some fearful anxiety which had kept her awake, but had no idea of its real meaning or cause'. Under hypnosis, however, she remembered the anaesthetist saying she would 'sleep the sleep of death'—a claim the anaesthetist later confirmed. The next time Howard saw her, he said, at a follow-up three years later, the insomnia and anxiety had disappeared. Howard referred to another patient who had become suicidal after a minor operation. Under hypnosis, she later reported hearing the surgeon say, 'She is fat, isn't she?'

Again, such scenarios can't be scientifically replicated. Hospitals have ethics committees to make sure of that. But nor can they be dismissed out of hand.

An 'adequately' anaesthetised patient will feel, see, smell and taste nothing until they regain consciousness. But they may still hear—unlike the other sensory systems, the brain's auditory pathways resist to some extent the depressive effect of the drugs, meaning that hearing is often the last sense to fade under anaesthetic. And they may still form memories—even without knowing it. While Bernard Levinson's study lives on today largely as a curiosity, there is plenty of evidence that information can still enter and be processed within an anaesthetised brain.

Shortly after my first meeting with Kate Leslie in her tiny office at the Royal Melbourne Hospital, she faxed me details of an experiment reported by New York anaesthetist David Adams in the late 1990s. Adams and his team had taken twenty-five unconscious heart- surgery patients and played them audio tapes of paired words: boy/girl, bitter/sweet, ocean/water…About four days after the operation, the team had each person listen to a list of single words—some of which had been among the word pairs played while they were unconscious—and asked them to free-associate, or respond to each with the first word that came into their minds. The patients were significantly better at free-associating the word pairs they had already encountered than those they hadn't. Not only had they heard the information, they had, without knowing it, remembered it. Ocean water. Bitter sweet.

Admittedly this is nowhere near as interesting or complex as announcing that the patient is turning blue. But it does suggest that while only a small fraction of patients have conscious memories of their experiences on the operating table, many more of us may have unconscious traces—things we don't even know we know that may nevertheless affect how we will later behave.

Most of life is like this. I remember the moment (sitting in my car in my early forties, the recently single mother of a young son) when I realised that the place I had arrived at in life was exactly where I had always imagined myself being. Not a place that I had planned. Nor a place that my younger self might have selected had she been offered a menu of options. But the place that I had dreamed myself towards. Blindly, diligently. Repeatedly. As if I had a map that was secret even to myself, but that I had followed all the same, slipping in and out of relationships, jobs, predicaments: unsure for the most part how I came to be where I was. And without ever realising that I had drawn the map myself.

It was, at least in part, unconscious forces that propelled me as a younger woman, some years before the Adams study was published, to Darwin in Australia's tropical north. I had left Melbourne after a failed relationship in pursuit of a newer, I hoped less fallible, one. I moved into a tiny sweatbox above a fish and chip shop with the man I had recently fallen in love with. It was a deep, rectangular space with no hot water in the shower and with one long wall looking onto the neighbouring brick wall about a metre away. It was very dark and very hot. The cockroaches were the size of jam-jar lids, and they flew. A large rat used to climb the outside guttering and walk across the windowsill. But the place had been imparted a reckless sort of charm by the addition of textiles, floor rugs and Aboriginal artworks, and by the colour scheme, which included rooms of aqua and tangerine. It was like living inside a Rubik's cube. Outside, on the streets, everything was so bright I could scarcely drag my gaze to the horizontal. Mangoes rotted on the pavements and I would swerve to miss them as I rode my bike slowly to the Parap pool and back. In summer the sea was unswimmable, taken over by swarms of deadly box jellyfish. Even in winter the water felt as if you were plunging into your own urine, and there was always the chance of crocodiles.

During the days my partner would go to his air-conditioned office and I would stay at home and try to make a living as a freelance journalist, hoping the sweat from my fingers would not short-circuit my laptop. Sometimes I would go down to the supermarket and wander around the freezer aisle where it was cool and I could pretend I was doing something useful. Often I would simply lie on my back watching the ceiling fan go around.

From time to time I would be sent to do a story fifteen hundred kilometres to the south in the desert country around Alice Springs. Stepping out of the plane into the exact moistureless heat I would feel myself start to wake up, a blip of excitement deep in my stomach, the dog smell of dust and temperatures that plunged wildly at night. In Darwin the towels went mouldy and I felt that I was enveloped in a viscous haze. My partner was away a lot, during which time I felt disconnected and lonely. When he was in town we would drink and smoke too many cigarettes. When he was away, I would drink and smoke too many cigarettes. I used to joke to long-distance phone friends that living in Darwin was like finding myself on a package tour, sharing a room with someone I couldn't stand: myself.

A year or so into my time in Darwin I went to see a counsellor, a kind man with strong calves who wore long shorts to work. Among the things I remember saying to him, which mostly centred around a muffled, corrosive unease about my relationship with the man I had followed across Australia, was that I felt that the centre of my chest was rigid and heavy, as if I was carrying something inside me, a black box, and that sometimes I had trouble breathing.

o

The idea that there may be two types of knowing—one you know about and one you don't—first began to take hold in the late nineteenth century. But unlike the psychoanalytic unconscious later postulated by Freud—brimming with memories and desires, lost (temporarily or forever) to the conscious self—these early experiments hinted at something in a sense more mundane, a perceptual unconscious mediated through senses such as sight and sound.

In 1898, US psychologist Boris Sidis undertook a study in which he asked people to look from a distance at letters and numbers on cards and report what they saw.

> [T]he subjects often complained that they could not see anything at all; that even the black, blurred, dim spot often disappeared from their field of vision; that it was mere 'guessing'; that they might as well shut their eyes and guess. How surprised were they when, after the experiments were over, I showed them how many characters they guessed correctly...

They had taken in more than they knew and their behaviour showed it even when they denied it. How much subjective reports such as these can tell us about the existence or otherwise of unconscious perception is arguable, but Sidis thought his findings adverted to 'the presence within us of a secondary subwaking self that perceives things which the primary waking self is unable to get at'. This, he believed, was evidence of a mysterious hidden force at the heart of each of us. 'The life of the waking self-consciousness flows within the larger life of the subwaking self like a warm equatorial current within the cold bosom of the ocean.'

Similar sorts of experiments cropped up over the next half-century, but were generally met with scepticism from a populace not yet shaped by Freud, Jung and their successors, and who (like me) did not much like the idea that people could be pushed and pulled by inner forces beyond their control. It wasn't until the late 1960s and early '70s that scientists got serious about investigating this intriguing but elusive form of perception. They took patients with damage to the visual centre in one hemisphere of the brain (rather than in the eye itself), and who could therefore make out objects clearly through one eye and not at all through the other, and presented shapes or patterns to the so-called blind eye. The subjects—while protesting they could see nothing—would most often be able to correctly 'guess' what they had seen. These experiments in 'blindsight' have been followed up with other studies showing the same can happen with hearing, touch and smell. Other experiments famously showed that patients whose short-term memory had been destroyed through disease or brain damage could nevertheless be shown to have 'remembered' people and information without knowing it.

Researchers these days distinguish between explicit memories (those you can remember having) and implicit, or hidden, memories which are inaccessible to their owners but can be identified by changes in performance or behaviour—the process known as priming. New brain imaging technology is beginning to show which parts of the brain light up during such unconscious learning. But at this stage, scientists remain uncertain whether they are looking at two or more distinct or perhaps overlapping memory systems, or one that perhaps expresses itself in different ways.

It took until the mid-eighties for researchers to start testing in a systematic way whether similar processes might be at work in anaesthetised patients.

In 1985 a team led by US psychologist Henry Bennett—this was the same edgy, fast-talking Hank Bennett I met in Hull—randomly assigned thirty-three patients in hospital for hernia or gall bladder or spinal surgery to two groups. During surgery all patients wore headphones. Patients in the larger, control, group had the sounds from the operating theatre relayed back to them through the headset. The remaining eleven were played a pre-recorded tape interspersing suggestions about how well they would heal, with songs and music. Five minutes before doctors reversed the anaesthesia at the end of the operation, each of these patients was also delivered a personal message through their headphones. The pleasant recorded voice of Bennett, whom the patients had already met, talked about the patient's postoperative recovery and goals, and then made an extra suggestion about something the patient should do during an interview scheduled for two days later. 'When I come to talk with you, you will pull on your ear. Your ear might itch a little and you will need to pull on it, or you might just know to pull on your ear. That way I will know you have heard this.'

At the subsequent interviews none of the patients reported any memory of the surgery. Nor did the study report any differences in recovery between the groups. But it did show that patients who had been played Bennett's message were around twice as likely to touch their ears as those from the control group. They also touched their ears more often—a total of sixty-six touches compared with eighteen.

Even when the patients were hypnotised and 'regressed' back to the time of the operation, none remembered the ear-pulling suggestions. But the fact that nine of the eleven nonetheless pulled, two of them repeatedly, suggested, said Bennett, a failure of memory retrieval rather than one of memory formation: the memories were there, but unavailable to the conscious mind—or even perhaps to language. The patients' bodies did the talking.

There was another interesting aside to the study. When Bennett hypnotised them after the surgery, two patients did turn out to have some memories. One young man remembered hearing music, a familiar tune that he liked to hum to himself, by jazz great Chuck Mangione. The other was a thirty-five-year-old woman, not from the experimental group but from the control group who had had the sounds of the operating theatre played through her headphones while doctors tried to perform a graft onto her thigh bone. Under hypnosis the woman said she remembered something being wrong—'...my leg, it's not going to work right. The doctor said it wasn't going to work the way it should'.

When researchers listened to the recording made of the surgery, they found that forty minutes into the operation her surgeon had said this: 'We've got this all goof-balled here, didn't we...this is going to be a terrible bone graft. It's going to be the worst bone graft ever...this is going to be awful.'

The woman took longer to recover than anyone else in the study, and needed twice as many pain medications as the next-highest user. Whether her pain could be explained in part by the surgeon's lurid prognosis, or whether this was the inevitable result of a 'terrible' bone graft, the researchers did not speculate.

Weird science

The first anaesthesia conference I attended was the annual scientific meeting of the Australia New Zealand College of Anaesthetists in 2000. I was working on a feature story on anaesthetic awareness (the sort you know you're having). I had arrived, notebook in hand, at the Crown Towers hotel on the banks of the Yarra River to find suited waiters serving tea and coffee from white-draped trestle tables. It was a Saturday afternoon and the gathered delegates, many in jumpers and slacks, were mingling and chatting in a soothing, businesslike sort of way. The industry display was in an adjoining room and here, along with more tables bearing bite-sized pastries, medical manufacturers and retailers had assembled the latest anaesthetic equipment and drugs, among which small groups browsed. It was a very smart-looking display—the first impression was of the cosmetics section of a plush department store, except that men seemed to outnumber women. The booths were brightly coloured, with posters and displays and a feeling of polished chrome: bright, efficient, slightly unsettling. Several of the booths featured elaborate displays with what looked like shop dummies lying on trolleys, being subjected to various unpleasant procedures. On one there was a disembodied moulded head, neck arched back, mouth open and grimacing around a gag-like apparatus through which a tube protruded. The promotional material told me this was a new intubation device to let anaesthetists pump air into the lungs of paralysed patients.

There were pharmaceutical reps spruiking products I had never heard of. *Mesmerising price* said one poster. There were snatches of conversation. 'They'd rather not be sick,' one man told another over tea in white cups. 'They'd rather tolerate a little pain and not be nauseated.' Most of the conference I found incomprehensible. There were sessions with titles such as *Advances in the Management of Thromboembolism and Thromboprophylaxis*; *Reduced Neuropsychological Dysfunction Using Epiaortic Echocardiography and the Exclusive Y graft*; or *The In-vitro Effect of Sevoflurane on Gravid Human Myometrium*. I chose only those with titles I could pronounce or that had been recommended to me as good general topics. Even then I found myself sitting through talk after talk in which the language and concepts were almost completely impenetrable. People chuckled at jokes I hadn't seen coming. I sat with my tape on, taking intermittent notes, trying to follow the new strands of meaning and waiting. Beyond a few passing references and one lunchtime discussion group, the question of patient awareness during general anaesthesia seemed to go unnoticed.

But every now and then, someone would say something that would wake me up.

The conference was divided into three streams—anaesthesia, intensive care and pain medicine. At 11.15 on the Sunday morning, Melbourne psychiatrist Professor Graham Burrows was in Palladium C, delivering a talk on Novel Psychoactive Agents in Pain Management. Much of the talk, according to the scant notes I took, was about the relationship between pain and depression and the role of psychiatry and drugs in treating chronic pain. Right at the start of the session, however, was one throwaway line that I marked with two heavy black biro lines. 'Years ago I learned that you could take people who had been anaesthetised and hypnotise them, and some of them I could get to recall what the surgeons and anaesthetists were talking about during their anaesthetic procedure, and it taught me very quickly that you have to be very careful what you say when you're doing...anaesthesia.'

Several weeks later I walked late one afternoon down the drab corridors of Melbourne's Austin Hospital, past a sign that read *Chaplains Dial 9* to Burrows' office. Burrows, a man I guessed then to be in his sixties, divided his time between teaching and practice. He was, as I would discover, formidable: medical director, professor of psychiatry, promoter of numerous committees and causes, advocate, author, workaholic. Officer of the Order of Australia. Chairman of the Australian Society of Hypnosis. More.

His office, in a windy tower atop the hospital, was furnished with three grey leather armchairs, two televisions and, on the walls, pictures of tigers, seals, a lynx and an owl. Burrows himself reminded me of a beaver—small, alert, busy—or perhaps a fox: reddish hair and a quick, impatient intelligence. He didn't exactly bark, but he talked quickly, without waiting for my responses. His manner was that of a man used to being heard, helpful and slightly brusque.

Burrows was interested in anaesthesia, he said, partly because his wife was an anaesthetist (she tried to keep people asleep, he had joked at the conference, while he tried to keep them awake), and partly because, as a psychiatrist, he was aware 'that many things that occur in our life we register without necessarily consciously knowing them'. Sometimes, for instance, in his clinical work the police sent him clients who might have witnessed crimes. 'We've used hypnosis in clinical cases where the person while hypnotised is able to describe the car, the numberplate, although in their conscious state they weren't aware that they knew.'

Sometimes, he said again, you could do the same with surgical patients. 'You can hypnotise some people and they will recall things that happened in surgery, which they didn't know that they knew.' Most likely, he said, the memories would have been formed as someone was going into or coming out of the anaesthetic—half-asleep, half-awake—although sometimes the patient might believe they had been awake throughout. The point, he said, was that it was not always easy to tell how deeply unconscious a patient was. 'It's fair to say that most modern anaesthetists are very much aware of the need to be alert to the fact that the person can be hearing things. So you don't tell smutty jokes, if you like. Or make rude personal comments about the person. I'm sure there's an exception every so often, and people will recount that.'

Beyond that, he did not have a lot to say on the topic. He did, however, have plenty to offer on the effect of general anaesthetics on the brain. The thing to remember, he said, was that anaesthetics were very powerful drugs. Anaesthesia, like hypnosis, altered consciousness. And, as with hypnosis, it was hard to predict how those alterations might affect different people. 'Now, the psychological impact of surgical anaesthesia on patients can be very positive and it can also be negative.' Anaesthesia was, after all, a chemical process that changed the neurochemistry of the brain. Different drugs did slightly different things to different brains. 'I won't get too high-powered on the influence, but that influence can have quite a lasting, telling effect on them.' You might, for instance, wake up looking and feeling normal but be unable to perform simple mathematical tasks you'd carried out with ease only hours before. You might no longer be safe behind the wheel of a car. These effects could last twenty-four hours or more.

A small proportion of patients, he said, had quite strange reactions. Some became very anxious, some had panic attacks, some felt indecisive. Others experienced what psychiatrists call 'depersonalisation'. 'They feel that their body is altered in some way, that their hand's too big or too small, that their tongue is too big or too small, or their abdomen and so on.' Some anaesthetics could cause what he described as marked depersonalisation. 'I remember seeing one patient who thought she was a fibreglass ski-board. She was really quite bizarrely affected.' Others might have a sense of 'derealisation', in which it was the world around them that distorted, 'so the table's smaller or bigger, or the door's further away, or the foot doesn't quite touch the accelerator pedal, and so on'.

It was all very Lewis Carroll.

o

Early morning. Screams from the garden. Our daughter, curled on the ground near the rabbit hutch, clutching her foot. She has impaled herself on a rusty nail, which is in turn attached to a lump of wood. I give it a tentative tug. More screams. We have never got through the emergency department faster. There is no blood, but the sight of a ten-year-old nailed to a fence paling seems to galvanise the staff. In a curtained-off room beyond reception, the doctor regards my daughter's dramatic footwear. I get the sense that left to his own devices he might simply have given the plank a short sharp tug. But no, we'll give her some ketamine, he says. Ketamine is one of those dissociative anaesthetic drugs that Graham Burrows talked about.

Minutes later my daughter slumps back on the bed looking dazed, then, as the doctor gives a hearty yank, lets out an extended yowl before subsiding back. She looks up at us blearily, then with incredulity. 'Hey-ee. You've got three eyes,' she says as I move towards her. 'That's so weird. Wow.' She looks at her father. 'Ooh, Daddy, you've got four eyes! Woah, everything's moving.' Then to both of us, and perhaps the doctor and nurse also: 'I love you! I love you! Wow. Your faces are so big. You look so weird.'

I think of a T-shirt I saw years ago with three words on the front, one beneath the other: the first, clear black print; the second, wavering; the third almost indecipherable. *Drink. Drank. Drunk.* I thought it was pretty funny at the time.

Drink Drank Dru

Blink Blank Blun

She won't remember any of this, I decide, as my daughter beams up at us, cross-eyed. But she does. She remembers a dream she had before she woke up to find us all morphed into many-eyed Cheshire cats. 'There were streamers falling from the ceiling,' she tells us later, 'made of film reels from old movies. They were just hanging and falling, and Daddy and you and [*her brother*] and Boingo [*the rabbit*] were all in different corners of the room, and I knew I had to rescue you all, but I didn't know who to rescue first.'

So here we are in the depths of my determined daughter's psyche. And what does she want? She wants to save us.

Not so blank then.

o

Graham Burrows again: odd anaesthetic reactions could take place in 'so-called normal people' he said, depending upon the anaesthetic agent. There were others, too, who following a general anaesthetic could even become psychotic; sometimes the drugs could precipitate an underlying condition, or reactivate a previous disorder. Then there was a group—probably larger than many realised—who went on to become depressed after an anaesthetic. 'Most of it's transient, and short-lived, but the tearfulness, the abreaction as we call it, the emotional outpouring that occurs, is quite common.'

Psychiatrists sometimes even used anaesthetic agents deliberately to trigger such responses in patients, though not so much these days.

In the end, he implied, it was not always, or even often, possible to administer hypnotic drugs with any certainty as to their effects. 'In short, the person undergoing the anaesthetic from a psychiatric or psychological point of view can have very positive results because their lump or their pain or whatever it is, is taken away. But it can also be negative if they have both their own personal fragility or vulnerability, and also because of the chemical processes of the anaesthesia on their particular brain, at that point in time.' Good anaesthetists knew to thoroughly assess their patients after surgery. They knew to look for emotion. Not that anaesthesia was traumatic for most people. It wasn't. 'But for some people it's very traumatic—'

'Which I presume relates to some of what you were saying—?'

'With hypnosis,' Burrows cut in. 'It was. The abreactive sort of stuff. What I was really saying,' he continued, 'is, um, do you know what you got for your fourth birthday?'

'No.'

'No. But if you were a good hypnotic subject I could find it out, OK, because everything that's actually occurred to you is registered up there. Do you know that?'

o

Weird hypnosis fact #1

No one really knows what hypnosis is.

Weird hypnosis fact #2

Hypnosis can change our perception of pain.

Weird hypnosis fact #3

It can also change how and what we remember.

Hypnosis is a curiously liquid phenomenon. A naturally occurring trance state of the kind you might enter while reading a good novel, in the hands of a skilled (or in some cases unskilled) hypnotherapist or hypnotist it may be used to achieve ends that range from the therapeutic to the bizarre. Other than that, definitions lap and overlap, encompassing a seemingly eccentric array of behaviours and experiences. But there is broad agreement that at its heart lies a condition of inner absorption and focused attention that can leave you more than usually receptive to suggestion (your own and other people's), more than usually able to tolerate internal contradictions, and in which you can experience disturbances in perception (the way things feel, look, sound or taste) and memory. We do it all the time. Daydreaming, gazing out of the train window, listening to music. Hypnosis works very well with ten to fifteen per cent of people (these types tend to lose themselves in a task or activity: the sort who can keep reading as the house burns down around them); and poorly with ten to fifteen per cent. Most of us are somewhere in between.

Sadly there was no time for me to find out from Graham Burrows what I might have got for my fourth birthday, but even if I had come up with something under hypnosis, there would be little chance of knowing for sure if the memory was accurate. There are some fairly major problems with using hypnosis to measure the experiences of unconscious patients. Not only do we not know what we are measuring, we don't know what we are measuring it with. And hypnosis, while fabulously intriguing, is notably unreliable as a means of tracking down uncooperative memories, particularly in the absence of corroborating evidence. There is also a growing consensus that the role of memory is less to capture accurate representations of the past than to build dynamic models to help us navigate the future. Memories, rather than solid and unchanging, are fluid and mutable. A shifting amalgam of sensory input, emotion and imagining, laid down, organised and later retrieved through complex overlapping brain and body systems. Each time we replay a memory—even the memory of a dream—it changes, sometimes melding with other memories and mental images to form a new composite. What we end up with may include 'real' information, but may not tell an accurate story. Or vice versa.

Yet anaesthetists and hypnotists have more in common than most doctors might like to think. More than sixty years before Horace Wells first wondered about the pain-relieving potential of ether, German physician Anton Mesmer began employing a form of hypnosis (though that term had not yet been invented) to cure an array of odd, sometimes painful, and hitherto intractable ailments. Mesmer's elaborate treatments relied on props that reportedly included iron rods, glass shards and sometimes the accompaniment of a glass harmonica, and were underpinned by his conviction that he was channelling a sort of magnetic energy—'animal magnetism'—that ran between and through people. Unsurprisingly, he eventually fell foul of the medical establishment, and retired hurt. But mesmerism outlived him. By the 1830s, doctors in France and England had been documented performing major surgical procedures, including in at least one instance a mastectomy, apparently painlessly, using only hypnosis. A decade later, Scottish physician James Esdaile reported having carried out around three hundred such operations in India in the six years from 1845 (the year before Ether Day). His list of 73 'painless Surgical Operations' performed at Hooghly in West Bengal over an eight-month period in 1845 included the following: arm amputated (1); breast amputated (1); penis amputated (2); contracted knees straightened (3); ditto arms (3); and the removal of 17 scrotal tumours weighing from eight to eighty pounds.

Such techniques did not work with everybody (although Esdaile noted that Indians by and large were more responsive to his techniques than people back home) but his success rate was startling. At a time when around forty per cent of surgical patients could expect to die during or as a result of the procedure, the attrition rate among Esdaile's patients was reportedly closer to five per cent.

For those who respond, hypnosis can be a powerful tool. Neuro-imaging studies show that hypnosis appears to alter activity in parts of the brain that respond emotionally to pain—the message gets to the brain, but the brain doesn't care as much as it would otherwise. There is also evidence that hypnosis might disrupt the pain relays travelling along the spinal cord—perhaps blocking or limiting the information that gets to the brain in the first place. Animal magnetism it is not: but had brain imaging technology been available back in Mesmer's day, he might well have been vindicated. By the 1950s, the British Medical Association had recognised a place for hypnotism 'in the production of anaesthesia or analgesia for surgery and dental operations', as well as in childbirth. The American Medical Association endorsed the use of hypnotism for doctors three years later. Back in 1846, however, public interest in such strange and imprecise magic was all but obliterated with the advent of ether and nitrous oxide, and the surgical proliferation that followed. But if you look, you can still find evidence of such practices quietly continuing in pockets today.

o

Not far from where I live in Melbourne is a genteel row of faux-Georgian terraces that used to house the Victorian branch of the Australian Society of Hypnosis. Some years ago I collected from this office a videotape the society sometimes used in training. On the tape, punctuated by some unfortunate B-movie music, is a clip of a woman having abdominal surgery with no anaesthetic beyond the calm voice of her hypnotherapist. For an hour, as her surgeon (who later admits to having been more stressed than his patient) cuts and stitches, 'Bev' lies quietly on the operating table, imagining herself at a family picnic.

'Open your eyes just as soon as you are ready,' says the hypnotherapist after the surgeon has finished stitching Bev up, 'and you can be wide awake and fully alert and feeling just fine. Are you happy now?'

B: [*laughing*] Yes.

H: Did you feel anything?

B: No, just a bit of a [*inaudible*] in the belly, that's all. I'm feeling really good, it is like I have a handbag sitting on it, sort of heavy, but not painful at all. I was aware of what was happening. Cutting didn't worry me at all and the stitching didn't worry me at all.

Quite what enables someone like Bev to cheerfully undergo an ordeal that for others would be life-threatening remains, like so much in this conversation, deeply mysterious. Some researchers believe it might be a genetic trait. They point to the fact that your capacity to be hypnotised remains stable throughout life. One study found there were differences between the corpus callosums (the bundled fibres that bridge the brain's two hemispheres) of the people who were most and least easily hypnotised. Whether this might also help explain the strange reports of patients, including those in Levinson's study, being able to access under hypnosis memories apparently laid down under surgical anaesthesia, no one knows. Memory is weird.

Moonless nights

As part of my continuing rehabilitation after my back surgery, I have begun swimming regularly at a local pool. It is not a beautiful pool, at least not underwater. Standing in the shallow end, I can look out across the water's glittering surface to enormous windows through which gum trees reflect passing time in the shadows on their trunks. But underwater it is a different story. Cracked white tiles with darkening grout, filaments of hair, wayward bandaids, mucous trails that spiral downwards or hang, mid-water, like fish roe. It doesn't really bear thinking about. And so I don't.

First is the retreat into body, the expansion of muscles, the engine of breath, tightening discomfort in my legs and shoulders, a niggling irritation, and somewhere along the way, hopefully, release. At some point I realise I am no longer thinking. I am moving through dapples of light. Of course, the moment I have this realisation, everything changes and I am back to tiles. So I say to myself the word 'dappling' and repeat it up and down, up and down. After a while I allow myself to start thinking again, but now it is different. Instead of chasing small tight thoughts, I find myself observing, almost as if from above, the pattern of the thoughts and how they fit together. I can travel to a section of manuscript that has been troubling me and move it elsewhere, understanding without interrogation why it belongs here and not there. Then I finish my swim, get out of the pool and generally forget. I retain scraps: signposts, sometimes. But the big picture, the three-dimensional knowing, is gone until next time my head is underwater.

How, then, can we hope to track down memories that are hidden even to their owners? Particularly if their owners were not even conscious when the events occurred?

In the wake of Hank Bennett's ear-pulling experiment, a small cohort of studies emerged, seeking evidence that people might take in information during anaesthesia, even unawares. Some researchers played patients encouraging messages or soothing music during surgery, to see if it helped reduce recovery time, nausea or post-operative pain. Others further investigated the possibility of priming patients to learn words or change their behaviour as a result of suggestions made while they were unconscious.

But you can't study memories like these directly. You can't, for instance, walk up to someone sitting in their hospital bed and say, 'Is there anything you know that you didn't know before but don't know that you know that might be affecting you now?' It would be a bit like asking me if my unexpected interest in anaesthesia—a topic in which I had no interest whatsoever before meeting Rachel Benmayor—might have anything to do with submerged unconscious processes of my own. It is a good question but I can't, by definition, give you a good answer.

I have wondered the same about the doctors and researchers I've spoken with while working on this book. 'So, did you have any anaesthetics as a child?' I would ask casually towards the end of an interview. And yes, quite a few of them had, some of them very unpleasant. 'It was perfectly legitimate to put someone through the really terrifying experience of having an anaesthetic induced with ethyl chloride and ether,' recalled a quietly spoken Sydney surgeon and ethicist, Miles Little. He had vivid recollections of three anaesthetics he was given as a child. 'Having had one of those anaesthetics I can tell you that it really is a quite shattering experience...the sense of impending death. You feel that you can't breathe, that you can't control anything, and people are making only token efforts to communicate with you, they're physically holding you down while you struggle. Yes, it was an absolute nightmare...I have nightmares about it still.'

Not that this would qualify as an unconscious memory. But might it have influenced his decision to become a surgeon, without his having known it? It is possible, in any case, to know something and to not know it at the same time. I do it all the time. One me will arrange to have coffee with a friend on Thursday, while a different me, or a different part of the same me, will meanwhile make an appointment with a physiotherapist for the same time. Many of my friends have started complaining about their memories recently—it's as if having finally wrestled their lives into some sort of shape, they now start forgetting it. But the appointment thing isn't really, or is not only, forgetfulness. I haven't forgotten either plan. I have simply stored them in separate sections of myself and failed to sync the information. This process might be underpinned in the ways memories are manufactured in the first place. Rats, at any rate, have been shown to process a single fleeting memory in several distinct areas of the brain. In my case, the bits of data (friend, physio) are all there and separately available to me, they just don't join up.

Hank Bennett remembers a childhood anaesthetic. 'Well, I had ether anaesthesia when I was a boy, but there is little memory there...I just remember being far away and fingers down my throat and people talking...yeah, kind of scary.'

It didn't sound very momentous, but then again how would you know? How would he know? It was possible, I thought, that it was because of that very experience that Hank had gone on to become a psychologist who specialised in anaesthesia. Maybe it explained all that nervous energy. Perhaps if Hank were to be hypnotised, he might even discover some more visceral memory of what had happened. Or not.

In the end, testing for memories hidden even to their owners is like trying to find clouds on a moonless night. You can't see the cloud, but you might be able to make out where it has blocked the stars. Researchers trying to track these wraiths tend to sidle up, dissimulate, pretend to be looking for something else. Among surgical patients, the most common techniques include word-stem completion tests, such as that used by the Adams team in New York (boy/girl, bitter/sweet, ocean/water) and others in which an unconscious patient might, for instance, be read the words *pear, banana* and *pineapple*, and then asked on awakening to say the first three fruits that come to mind. The results have been infuriatingly inconclusive. Potentially important studies including Levinson's fake crisis and Bennett's ear-touching instruction have not been replicated, or not consistently. Many have been criticised for their methodology. Others show effects too small to be statistically significant. The study designs vary wildly. Even the same researchers using almost identical study designs get different results.

This failure to replicate is not a new theme in science. We are in the middle of a so called replication crisis, with multiple studies— some quite famous—proving difficult or impossible to restage with the same results. This has been particularly true of psychology and clinical medicine. The causes are varied and may derive in part from pressures to publish and failings in quality control in a competitive working environment. The result: shaky, sometimes shoddy, science. But it is also true that some fields—particularly those lacking the sort of strong theoretical basis that underpins the study of, say, physics— are simply much harder to investigate. Cancer, for example. Or consciousness. Or the study of memory—especially if those memories are supposedly laid down while the memory holder is in a chemical coma.

To start with, an operating theatre is a terrible environment for doing controlled experiments—that is, experiments designed to exclude all but the particular influences being studied. More like controlled chaos. Patients of different constitutions and body types are wheeled in for different procedures and anaesthetised for different lengths of time at different depths. Trying to replicate or compare studies is even trickier. Different anaesthetists use different drugs. Different drugs alter patients—and their memories—differently.

Some researchers have tried to smooth such logistical wrinkles by experimenting with volunteers whom they anaesthetise but don't operate upon. This means they can control much better for the type of drug used and how long the person is unconscious. The problem is that doing such tests without surgery is a bit like testing your wind- screen wipers without rain: your results may not tell you anything very useful. A surgical incision has a galvanising effect even on an anaesthetised patient: as the scalpel enters, her heart beats faster, her blood pressure rises, sometimes she jerks. She might edge closer to consciousness.

It may also be that surgery by its nature imprints itself into her brain's more primitive emotional memory centres, and that this may happen even when she is, in surgical terms, adequately anaesthetised. Psychologists have long known that memory is modulated by the circumstances in which it is laid down. We remember things that mean something to us: conversations about our health, for instance;

or the shape of our bodies. In particular we remember events that are frightening or threatening—even when we don't want to. Fear is a powerful teacher. Neurobiologist James McGaugh writes that in medieval times, before written record-keeping, a young child might be asked to witness an important event or exchange before being summarily thrown into a river. 'In this way, it was said, the memory of the event would be impressed on the child and the record of the event maintained for the child's lifetime.' Under stress the body releases hormones that interact with the amygdala, the small structure tucked into each of the brain's temporal lobes which is involved in modulating the storage of fearful and emotional memories. (People with damage to their amygdalae appear not to experience fear in the way the rest of us do.) In its extreme form this fixing of fearful images may congeal into the nightmares and flashbacks of PTSD. One theory is that, under anaesthesia, the stress hormones that surge into the bloodstream when a doctor cuts us might activate the amygdala and increase our chances of learning information, albeit without knowing it. At least one study has shown that anaesthetised patients are more likely to learn words during 'surgical stimulation' than before the knife goes in.

The problem is that most of these studies involve small numbers of patients—often fewer than one hundred. Even today this sort of research takes place at the outer reaches of medical science, where medicine merges into psychology, neurology and sometimes philosophy. What Kate Leslie described to me as 'spooky little studies'. Few practising anaesthetists would know they existed.

And even when patients do seem to have taken in information, albeit unwittingly, the memories (or, at least, the evidence of them) are often fleeting. One of the best ways to locate elusive memories is to do so in an environment or state similar to that in which you laid them down. Here I am in the kitchen dourly scrubbing grease off an old frypan when I think of something I want to get from the lounge room. I set out to fetch it, but by the time I get there (along the way having picked up a discarded towel and wrested a toilet roll from a dog) I have no idea why I am here. I know that I have come to get something, I can feel the fact of the memory, but I can no longer remember what it is. The more I think the less I know. Frustrated, I return to the kitchen and the pan; hands back in the tepid, soapy water. And immediately I remember what it was that I wanted—music.

Some researchers have speculated that one reason patients tested soon after an operation show the most evidence of memories is that the sounds and smells of the recovery room where they are tested would be similar to those in the operating theatre—as would their physiological state, still adrift on the residue of the anaesthetic drugs (the information bracketed by time and place). Some suggest this may also explain reports of patients heading home after surgery, minds soothingly marinated in nothing-muchness, until they return to hospital for a visit or another procedure and find themselves overwhelmed by anxiety or flashbacks.

This is also one of the reasons proposed for why 'memories' of surgery not available to our conscious minds might turn up later under hypnosis—the hypnotic trance somehow echoing the anaesthetic stupor.

One of my favourite studies, mainly because they actually went to the trouble of doing it, took place at the Scottish seaside in the mid-seventies. Researchers approached a group of divers in Oban on the west coast and asked if they would help them with a study on 'context-dependent memory'. Once the obliging divers were in wetsuits the scientists had them learn lists of words either on the beach or six metres underwater. Afterwards they tested them to see how much they remembered. It was cold and wet and the logistics were challenging, but what they found was that it didn't much matter where the divers did their learning: on dry land or the ocean floor. What did matter was where they were tested. Those who had listened to words underwater could remember far more when tested underwater than they could on land, and vice versa.

Many years after I had heard him speak in Hull, I came across a written account by US anaesthetist Anthony Messina of that traumatic experience of childhood surgery—memories that had stayed hidden until he was an adult, but that resurfaced dramatically one day early in his medical career.

> During the first few months of my residency, while attending a lecture on muscle relaxants, I read a case report written by an anesthesiologist in 1948 describing his experience of self-injection of curare. I had an uncomfortable feeling, like the topic was familiar to me. A week later, I anaesthetised my first child [*using an inhaled anaesthetic and a paralysing muscle relaxant*]. Suddenly, I became very upset and had a flashback. The nightmare that I had experienced for years as a child had actually happened. Once I had the flashback to my childhood experience, I concluded that I must have been drawn to the field by some unconscious process. And that my purpose was to prevent other people from becoming victims of what I went through as a child.

Of course there may have been other reasons Anthony Messina went on to become an anaesthetist, but there is little doubt that the experience has shaped his adult life. As a cardiac anaesthetist he advocated the use of techniques that allow surgeons to operate without paralysing patients. He recently completed a high-level review of data spanning from 1950 to 2016 on ways to reduce awareness during surgery.

..

Another reason why people might not retain information delivered to them during surgery for long, if at all, is that most of it is really boring. Boy/girl, bitter/sweet, blah/blah. Once again, we can blame Levinson. The emphatic emotional reactions of some of the patients subjected to his famous mock crisis ('I don't like the patient's colour!') mean that today's researchers must make do with blander fare. They usually try to prime patients with lists of 'neutral' words—peach, grape, melon—unlikely to be either meaningful or memorable. Others have tried to prime for more complex tasks by playing anaesthetised patients tapes of obscure factoids and then testing them later to see if they get the answer correct.

But as Bernard Levinson himself has pointed out, if you were in surgery and your brain was indeed able to take in some of what was going on around you, perhaps this is not the information you would fix on either. 'I am walking across a suspension bridge,' he told an audience of anaesthetists at the first MAA conference in Glasgow 1989. 'It is only ropes and a few slats of wood. Thousands of feet below me is a raging, rock-strewn river...My whole being is focused on getting to the other side. Behind me, someone is saying...orange... pigeon...what is the blood pressure of the octopus...?'

Lost days

I kept thinking about what Melbourne psychiatrist Graham Burrows had said. About my fourth birthday and all the other lost days sequestered inside my head ('…because everything that's actually occurred to you is registered up there. Do you know that?').

Did I? Not really. But I wanted to.

It took me four months to arrange a preliminary appointment with Graham Burrows. This was mid-2005, four years after our initial interview. His secretary was helpful and harried. Dr Burrows was very busy. Could I send an email? I sent two, both saying more or less the same thing. I was working on a book, I was interested in implicit learning during anaesthesia. I was interested in clinical hypnosis. I was interested in the relationship between the two. 'On a more personal note—but also something I would like to write about in the book—I am hoping that you (or if you think it more appropriate someone else) could do some hypnosis work with me, partly to demonstrate the process, but also to help me try to understand my preoccupation with this topic.'

Burrows' secretary emailed me: 'Sorry to take so long in getting back to you—Professor Burrows' answer is yes.'

I spied him outside in the corridor, a smallish, reddish figure, carrying a plate that held four party pies with sauce. He ate as he walked. Inside he got straight to the point. The book, what was it about? Who was funding me? What did I want from him? All the things he wanted to know made sense but he seemed to want to know them all at once, all in his determined staccato. It was unnerving. I stumbled my way through a partial explanation: Rachel Benmayor's birth story, my interest in the philosophical and psychological dimensions of anaesthesia, other stuff. I trailed off. Was this helping? In a way, he said, but it all sounded a bit gobbledegook. He said this not unkindly, and I found myself agreeing. 'And I'm not certain,' he added, 'whether you're trying to sort yourself out, or whether you're trying to sort out other things.'

The meeting went on for half an hour and for much of it I felt that I was running to catch a bus that had left the stop ahead of me. I had brought with me to his rooms a sheet of paper on which I had written out my questions for him, and these I shouted as I ran. From the back of the bus (one of the open-backed red buses of my London childhood), Burrows hurled his answers. Eventually, halfway through our meeting, he simply reached across and took the sheet from me. Pre-empting my flailing interjections, he started asking and answering my questions himself, speaking in concise, precise nuggets. The complexities of memory, the limitations of hypnosis, the difference between the conscious and unconscious minds (to start with, these were processes, not places, and secondly, 'Well that's very complex, that would take a whole book to answer.') Always that intense categorical focus. He had discovered hypnosis when studying science and had begun with chickens and snakes before moving across to medicine, then psychiatry and eventually starting the Australian Society of Hypnosis. The thing was, he said when I finally managed to ask, that hypnosis was not something you dabbled in. You did it properly. It was not an entertainment. Also, it could be completely unreliable, 'particularly if the technique used is poor'. Besides, he didn't have time.

But, he said finally, if I was wanting to understand myself, if I was willing to enter a genuine psychotherapeutic relationship with him, then that would be different. He could see me as a client. He sent me away with a copy of his textbook on hypnosis, instructions to see my doctor, get a blood test, complete a detailed form about myself, keep a diary and fill in a daily mood chart. Three months later, just after Christmas, I returned and we embarked on a process compromised throughout by the fact that we wanted completely different things. He wanted to diagnose and treat me; I wanted to get hypnotised.

In the end, we lasted six sessions. From the outset I felt we were engaged in some sort of struggle. Each week I would go away and fill in the mood charts and the diary and the dreary, detailed summary of my life so far. Each time I returned he would reach for and scrutinise them at speed, all the time catapulting questions. ('Don't worry,' he said once, 'I can do both.') We talked about my moods, my relationships, the sagging sack of my inner life. We talked about my health and about hypnosis and my ambivalence about committing to this therapy. We talked about his practice; he mentioned murderers he had interviewed (he was sometimes called as an expert witness in court cases), and other journalists he knew ('you'd be surprised'). He told me that he used to demonstrate the power of hypnosis on medical students by having them close their eyes and feel that a hand had gone numb, before he pushed a sterilised needle into their palm. We talked about the place of drugs in psychiatric treatment. I found this last conversation disconcerting.

Early on, he arrived at an appointment with his left arm in plaster. He said he had broken his wrist skiing in Canada, knocked

over from behind by an out-of-control snowboarder. Burrows had
bound the arm himself, he said, using self-hypnosis, and had skied
with it like this for several days before eventually getting it plastered,
at his convenience, at the end of the holiday. Now, he said, the cast
was letting him get on with his day to day life. It might be a bit
annoying, but it supported the arm while it healed. By analogy, he
said, the plaster might be like medication.

I wasn't sure I liked where this was going. Medication? I'd
tried anti-depressant medication once before and had not much liked
anything about it. I had not persevered, as advised, or given it a
chance, but had taken myself off it after a few months and felt neither
better nor worse as a result. Now I felt obscurely like the character
in a comedy who hops on a gurney to hide from the villains, only to
find himself in theatre about to have his leg amputated. (This is an
exaggeration.)

Finally, however—the hypnosis. A relaxation exercise. Burrows
asked me to sit back in my chair and imagine myself on a comfortable couch in a room where I felt safe and relaxed, a secret, stress-free
room. Following his instructions, I moved my attention through
my body, progressively loosening each limb, letting numbness move
through my body, feeling warmth spread up into my chest. It felt a
bit awkward, but fine; a feeling of heaviness. 'And when you want to
wake yourself up you can, easily, by counting backwards from three.'
Later, he said: 'At least we know you can be hypnotised,' And he
gave me a tape of the exercise to take home and play to myself in the
evening, or whenever I needed to relax.

I took it home and played it. Diligently. The problem was
that much as I wanted to let go, sink down, find my secret room, I
found that every time I turned on the tape, part of me was resisting.
The more Burrows told me to let my body go loose and floppy, the
more my body stayed stiff and hot. The more Burrows told me that

my shoulders, my arms, my hands were going numb, the more I imagined him sticking a needle into me. At our final session, he looked at my mood chart with its erratic undulations, announced that I had a depressive disorder and said I should consider prescription drugs. His tone seemed brusque. I should go away and think about it. Normal people didn't have a graph that looked like this.

That was the last time I saw him.

In the years since, when I have glanced back at those encounters it has been with mild embarrassment—a little mind gap that when I push against it opens to reveal something closer to judgment, aimed both at myself and at him. Me for being foolish, self-serving, impure of motive. Him for...What? His manner, his message? For telling me I might need drugs? And what had it all been for, anyway? Mainly I have avoided looking back at those sessions at all. Not long after the final one I realised I was not going to write about them. Not in this book. Not anywhere. Even thinking about them made me feel uncomfortable. Murky.

Recently, after I heard the news of Graham Burrows' death, I listened back to the relaxation tape he had made me: the non-relaxation tape, as I used to think of it. I had to find new batteries for my antiquated Sony Walkman, with its anti-rolling mechanism. The words, when they came, were slightly distorted. The tape sagging. What I heard was completely unexpected.

Burrows' voice: *Now stretch yourself out, close your eyes and let yourself relax.* But this wasn't the haranguing, robotic tone of my memory. He sounded calm and convincing. Kind, even. As I listened again to the tape, I found my breathing deepening, the muscles of my face and neck beginning to relax. If I had focused enough my hand might even have started to go numb. Most of all he sounded absolutely normal. I could not, and still cannot, reconcile the voice on the tape with the voice I had been imagining.

It occurred to me that I had been a terrible patient.

Then I looked for the first time in many years at the diary I had kept during the time I saw Burrows, the one that he had asked me to write.

> Hot. Too hot. I keep worrying about the weather. It feels apocalyptic. I keep thinking: this is how it's going to be, more and more heat, and I think about trees dying and rivers drying and air conditioning failing and all of us scratching around in this terrible heat till we die.

On it goes. I am sleepless, I am stressed, I am angry, I am guilty, I am afraid. I am driving through a sort of thick sadness. I worry that the bamboo we've planted down the side of the house will invade the neighbours' garden and destroy the fence. I worry about the algae in the kids' pool and the fact that the chlorine has not got rid of it. I wonder if the algae have mutated into super germs.

> Sleep poorly again—dream that in the bottom of the still-green paddling pool are three drowned puppies…I know I should get them out, but I can't bear the thought of having to pick up their cold wet bodies.

I am not a happy human. I am not even a healthy human. And then this:

> February 21, 2006
> We are in the grounds of what might be a school. Me, Pete and the kids. Some sort of carnival. People everywhere. And permeating the whole, a sticky, oozing dread. No one else seems to notice, all the heedless happy families, but I know what they don't. Beneath the school is a dungeon; and in the dungeon is a creature so malevolent, so evil, that if it gets out

it will kill us all. People keep taking it in turns to go down there and hurt it, mock it. Even from the playground, I can picture it—the squat muscular little troll's body, slashing at their arms through the metal bars. I have to get us away. I find the kids on the climbing frame. But now the dream morphs. I'm in the corner of its cell, flattened against the wall behind a wooden box or cabinet. There is a part of me that feels sorry for it, everyone laughing and taunting, but I know what will happen when it is unleashed. I can feel its terrible pitiless hatred. I also—and this, I understand later, is the true source of my terror—sense that even though it cannot see me, it knows I am here, it knows who I am. When I wake I can feel the feeling of the creature and my fear of it so vividly I am convinced it is real. That it can only be kept at bay by dint of constant vigilance. As soon as I start to think like this, I lurch towards a new terror. I will go mad. I get up, start to write and then stop. It is a long time before I can take myself back and know the thing I don't want to know. There is no escape. The rage is mine. The creature is me.

This was the dream I woke from on the morning of my second interview with Chris Thompson, the anaesthetist who sent me into a kind of trance, the one I came to think of as Mr Anaesthesia.

The most famous
anaesthetist in the world

The Medical Sciences Building of the University of California San Francisco is a sandy slab of around twelve storeys a short walk from Golden Gate Park. It has rectangular grids of municipal-style windows that proceed dourly across the building's otherwise bland facade. On the day I visited, many of the windows were obscured by curtains or drooping blinds or the backs of cupboards or cardboard boxes or just grime. It looked as if it had had a hard night.

The Anaesthesia Research Laboratories were on the fourth floor. From the main corridor, a small pink and green linoleum-tiled entrance hall sloped upwards rather quaintly as if towards a nursery, and then opened into a longer corridor, where, a few doors to the left, and behind a large metal knocker in the shape of a lion's head, was the office of the most famous anaesthetist in the world.

Arranging a time to meet with Edmond I. Eger II had been tricky. At seventy-seven, he still worked full-time and was away a lot travelling. To my emailed request for an interview he had first suggested that we speak by phone. When I persisted, he responded with an exuberant OKEEDOAKEE. Just before I was due to fly out of Australia, the interview was postponed a day. I persisted partly because Ted Eger knows more about anaesthetics than just about anyone else, partly because he does not believe that a properly anaesthetised patient can remember anything (consciously or otherwise) and mostly because, twelve years before, he had headed the team that set out to repeat the unrepeatable experiment and put Bernard Levinson's startling thesis to the test.

Now I was standing outside his office wondering what sort of person would decorate his door with a lion's head knocker, and what it might say about his inner drives. From around the corner a man appeared. He was small, almost elfin, with a thin face and a keen, speculative expression. He wore a blue and white striped shirt and a dark blue tie decorated with mauve and orange butterflies. His feet, rather disarmingly, were clad in open sandals through which his besocked toes poked blackly. We shook hands.

'They call this my den,' he said, gesturing fondly as he led me in.

The room was small, maybe three by four metres, and into it were crammed three desks and five chairs. The walls were covered in bookshelves and family snaps, kids' pictures, a huge blackboard, a wedding photo. Ted Eger sat on a swivel chair in front of his desk and I on a shabby office chair next to a small couch piled with paraphernalia including two pairs of shoes. A heap of brown cardboard boxes teetered nearby. On the desk beside him two computer monitors sat flanking each other, alongside several tins of McCann's oatmeal cookies. On another desk a laptop sat open. Here was a room so embedded with personality you could not imagine anyone else ever inhabiting it. There was even a pop-up toaster.

As a young man in the 1960s, around the time Bernard Levinson was staging his now famous mock crisis, Eger had set out to solve a problem so basic it seems astonishing that nobody had done it before. Through a series of painstaking—and, to an outsider, unsettling—studies he set out to measure the relative strengths of the various anaesthetic vapours then in use, and to calculate how much of each it would take to keep a patient unconscious. Eger and colleague Giles Merkel had been prompted by a mentor, John Severinghaus, who wanted them to investigate the properties of a newly discovered anaesthetic vapour. To do this they would need to be able to compare it with other vapours already in use, but the problem was no one had yet worked out a way of doing so.

Eger knew from recent studies that by measuring the concentration of the gas an anaesthetised patient breathed out of her lungs—the 'end tidal gas'—he could calculate the concentration of the drug in her brain. That was the easy part. What he needed, though, was an 'end-point', an unambiguous marker by which he could usefully compare the strength of any one vapour with another.

First, he and Merkel practised on dogs. Then, with another young colleague, Larry Saidman, Eger turned his attention to people. The pair arrived at the starkly simple idea of drugging patients until they no longer responded to commands ('Open your eyes'; 'Squeeze my hand'), and then having the surgeon cut them to see if they would move. If they did, Eger increased the concentration of the gas and asked the surgeon to try again and, if necessary, again, until, at the point where the person stopped moving, he recorded the concentration of end-tidal gas they were exhaling. Over the next few years, he and Saidman did this for hundreds of patients, of different ages, with different anaesthetics, in different combinations, individually and in small groups. Then, for each permutation, they took the highest concentration at which each patient had moved and the lowest concentration at which they hadn't; they found the midway point and called it MAC.

..

In the recondite world of surgical anaesthesia this concept made Eger a superstar. MAC—the initials stand for Minimum Alveolar Concentration—revolutionised anaesthesia and became the standard by which many anaesthetists still judge how much of a given drug to give a patient. Importantly, MAC is a measure not of anaesthetic depth but of drug potency. It tells doctors what the chances are that a surgical patient will remain safely unconscious at a given dosage of any anaesthetic vapour or gas. It also allows doctors to use drugs in precise combinations.

Some observers caution that MAC is only a measure of probability—it cannot tell for sure whether an individual patient is conscious or not—and it also changes with the patient's age, and depending on what other drugs it is mixed with. Nevertheless, for many doctors MAC remains anaesthesia's gold standard, and Eger, now in his mid-eighties, its standard bearer. He is a steadfast believer in its efficacy. 'Despite its imperfections and limitations, it remains the standard because nothing thus far invented is better.' As a unit of measurement, he points out with pride, MAC is to anaesthesia what centimetres are to distance and degrees Celsius to temperature.

And Eger believes in measurement. If you can't measure it, it doesn't exist. You might call him an anaesthetic rationalist. Certainly he was not in any way convinced by the odd claims being made by an unknown South African psychiatrist.

Then one day in the early 1990s, a quarter of a century or so after Bernard Levinson had published his study, Eger picked up the phone and on the other end was Hank Bennett, then still a young New York psychologist. This was some years after Bennett had successfully persuaded unwitting patients to touch their ears in a post-operative interview—and more than a decade before I met him in Hull. Bennett had never met Eger, but he knew him by reputation. Now he was calling from New York City with a proposition.

'He introduced himself,' recalled Eger, 'and said, "I understand from things you've written that you don't believe awareness occurs during an adequate level of anaesthesia."

'I said, "That's correct; awareness does not occur at an adequate level of anaesthesia, with inhaled anaesthetics."'

Then Bennett asked how he knew.

'And I said, "Well I just *know* these things."' Eger laughed. 'And it was displaying my usual arrogance. And he persisted, like a good scientist would. He said, "Doctor Eger, how do you know?"'

'And I finally...had to say, "Well I don't really know, I don't know for sure, but I can't believe that anyone remembers anything under anaesthesia; certainly at MAC, nobody remembers anything."

'He said, "Dr Eger," (in a very nice way; Hank is a very nice guy), "Dr Eger, prove it."'

Ted Eger has a reputation, depending on who you talk to, of being delightful and brilliant or arrogant and brilliant. Sometimes all three. In the early minutes of our interview, as I proceeded through a rambling explanation of my project, he leaned back in his chair with a small and not very comforting smile, as if sizing me up for sport. Later, in the middle of an entertaining and well polished life history, he announced that he had been for two years running the captain of his school's winning checkers team, and gleefully issued a challenge. The checkers triumph had been, in his telling, the high point in an otherwise unimpressive childhood and early academic career.

'My parents were affluent. I wanted for nothing. I graduated in the lower fifth of my high school class undistinguished in all ways except that I was the captain of the checker team which for two consecutive years won the all-Chicago championship, an accomplishment about which I am exceedingly vain—and,' he continued with slightly narrowed eyes, 'I can beat anyone in this room in checkers. Any time, any place. With my eyes closed, probably.'

From time to time as he talked he cupped his face in his hands and peered from between his palms, almost childlike, as if he were a small boy who had surprised himself by losing his hair and sprouting glasses.

As a bright but disengaged teenager, Eger had once taken a job selling shoes in one of the poorer areas of Chicago. He lasted a day. By the time he got home, he was more tired than he had ever been. It occurred to him that he didn't want to do this for the rest of his life. 'I think you call it an epiphany.' Instead, and inspired, he said, by the books of microbiologist Paul de Kruif, he decided to study medicine and become a country physician.

His second epiphany came the first time he anaesthetised a patient. He had just finished his first year in medical school and was on a summer placement with an anaesthetist. On his first day, the senior anaesthetist showed him what to do—how to start the drip that delivered drugs into the woman's bloodstream; how to adjust the dials that released the gases nitrous oxide and oxygen into her lungs; how to hold the mask over her face. He told Eger to watch the rebreathing bag that moved steadily in and out as the woman drew air from the anaesthetic machine and then breathed it out again. Then he left the room. Eger was in charge. He watched as the patient lost consciousness. Then he realised she had stopped breathing.

Horrified, he told the surgeon, who immediately began resuscitation. ('So the surgeon is squeezing on the chest of this woman who's having some minor procedure, and who I'm about to kill.') And then the bag began to move again. A nurse ran for the anaesthetist, who explained that all Eger needed to do if the bag stopped moving was to squeeze it, in and out, in and out; this way he could breathe for the patient.

'I finished that day I think more tired than I was trying to sell shoes. I was drained. And I finished, thinking that I had nearly killed a patient, I had nearly killed a human being. And that if I went into anaesthesia,' here Eger's voice dropped to a delighted, theatrical whisper, 'I could do that every day! Every day I could take a patient's life into my hands. Every day. I could do that!' He straightened and took a breath. 'Changed my life! The hell with Paul de Kruif, I'm going to be an anesthesiologist!'

In the decades since MAC, Eger has cemented his reputation investigating the pharmacology of the numerous vapours used in modern anaesthesia. He has made his life's work studying how they get into, move around and then leave the body, and documenting these processes in scientific papers and books that are still standard texts for anaesthetists the world over. He has also become a well known and often sceptical voice in the debate about awareness and memory in anaesthesia.

But Eger, not just a believer in science, is a man who likes a challenge. And Hank Bennett had just challenged him in terms he could not resist.

o

Not long after that phone call, Hank Bennett came to San Francisco, and in a series of carefully controlled experiments the men set out to resolve the matter. With a team of researchers, they played tapes to anaesthetised patients with messages such as 'yellow banana, green pear', or just white noise; then, when they woke, asked them to think of a colour or a fruit. All to no effect. (The patients who heard yellow and green were no more likely to name those colours than those who heard white noise.) Then they tried with Trivial Pursuit-style questions: what state has an elephant-leash law? (California, as it turns out); what state was Robert Redford born in? (again California);

what is the blood pressure of an octopus? (70 mm of mercury when underwater—same as you or me). Afterwards they tested the subjects with multiple-choice questions. Nothing.

'So now we are at odds,' recalled Eger, 'with those that have a belief—and it is almost like a religion for some of them—at odds with the group that says you can remember things, that you can recall things under anaesthesia.'

Finally they rang Bernard Levinson in Johannesburg.

You would be hard pressed to find two men less alike. Eger small and combative with his quick, hungry brain; Levinson tall and charismatic with that resonant, beguiling voice. Eger had heard him speak about his mock-crisis study not long before at a conference and had been impressed, despite himself. 'When he describes it, you just sit up and take notice; a) because it's a fascinating experiment; and b) because he is just *so* charismatic, a wonderfully charismatic guy who is honest as the day is long...So here we are, we've got *nothing*, and he's got *something*—that's impressive!'

But, he added, the experiment had needed bringing 'up to date'.

Eger leaned forwards as he talked, hands clasped between his knees. 'The study was *flawed*, fatally flawed. For one thing, Bernard knew what script the patients were getting, and for another, there wasn't a control.'

This time, he said, his team would do it, and do it right. 'We'll repair the flaws.'

The replication study was driven by Ted Eger with nine researchers, including Levinson, Bennett and a young man called Ben Chortkoff, Eger's fellow at the time. (He looked, Kate Leslie told me much later, 'a bit like John Kennedy junior, except less dead'.) It took place in a small operating theatre at the UCSF medical school and was conducted with what an observer described as military precision.

It found absolutely nothing.

Well, almost absolutely nothing.

Levinson, Bennett and Chortkoff interviewed one hundred young men, finally selecting the twenty-two they could most easily hypnotise. The men were put to sleep using modern drugs, not ether, and after fifteen minutes at a relatively light anaesthetic were given a paralysing drug. Then the anaesthetic was increased, though not to surgical levels, and breathing tubes inserted. This time none of the researchers who would later interview the subjects were in the room, nor would they find out until the end of the study what information the young men had been exposed to under anaesthetic.

They were an odd group. Eger the sceptic, Levinson the believer, Bennett, younger than both, excited and more than a little nervous. But they were all scientists, and emotional men, and a sort of love grew between them. In our interviews, Levinson and Bennett both described the time as a highlight of their careers. Chortkoff, too. Levinson for his part recalls one day looking up as he was hypnotising one of the subjects to see that Bennett, who was standing next to them, had also entered a deep trance. 'When he woke up he smiled, and I smiled and we just went on with it.'

At the heart of the study, as with the original, was a fake crisis, with the wording updated for a nineties audience: 'Oh shit, who turned off the oxygen? Who disconnected the cylinder? Damn it, he's turned blue. God, his lips are blue. Get that thing connected again. You got it? OK. I'm going to give him some more oxygen now. [*fifteen-second pause*]. Ho boy. OK. He looks better now. I think we can continue.'

Eger recorded the message in his own voice and it was played to the anaesthetised subjects on stereo earphones that also allowed in sounds from the operating theatre. Here, though, the study departed markedly from the original. Five days later, the men were anaesthetised again, this time using a different drug. The order in which they received the two drugs was randomised and balanced so that equal numbers received each drug on each occasion, without the interviewers knowing who got what when.

This time Eger delivered a quite different 'drama' through their headphones, varying the order in which the subjects heard the two scenarios. 'Hey, Ben, I think this study is going well. This is the best job we've done. I think the volunteer is going to be pleased. God, he's really doing great.' After a fifteen-second pause, Eger continued, laying it on thick: 'We're moving right along. I think we're going to do a record this time—it's moving so fast. Things are going so damned smooth. I don't think we've had a volunteer this good.'

The study that was published in 1995 went under the unwieldy title 'Subanaesthetic Concentrations of Desflurane and Propofol Suppress Recall of Emotionally Charged Information'. It failed to replicate Levinson's original findings and is generally interpreted as having invalidated the 1965 experiment. Even under hypnosis, none of the subjects remembered the fake crisis.

Eger, modest in victory, says the difference may have been in the drugs used or it may have been in the methodology. By exposing the young men to both threatening and banal dramas, and by ensuring the interviewers had no way of knowing which of these any participant had just experienced, the study design minimised the effects of chance or bias. 'And that's what science is,' says Eger now. 'It's the ability to replicate something. If you can't replicate something it's not real. I think things do happen by chance, but if you can't replicate it, if it isn't robust enough to replicate, it doesn't exist.'

There were, however, some other intriguing differences between the two studies. Perhaps the most critical of these was the drugs. Instead of ether, Eger's team alternated between the gas desflurane and the intravenous drug propofol. Given that ether was no longer in use, it made sense to update Levinson's study with the sorts of drugs that contemporary patients were likely to encounter, although it made it impossible to draw any direct conclusions about the experiences of Miss D, Mr R or any of the other patients who passed through that South African dental surgery that day in 1965.

Then there was the fact that the subjects were not surgical patients, but paid volunteers. This is the point that Bernard Levinson kept coming back to when I spoke with him in South Africa, and which, he argued, put them in a very different position from the ten men and women he used in 1965. Paid volunteers, he argued, might be prepared to endure without undue stress situations they would not put up with otherwise. Nor were they vulnerable in the way a patient is vulnerable. 'It is a very stressful thing,' said Levinson, 'entering into an operating theatre with some kind of problem: "What is going to happen to me now? Am I going to lose a limb? Maybe I am not going to wake up. Will I have pain when I wake up?" But paid volunteers enter with a whole different feel: "This is going to be a job at work, I'm going to be OK, they are not going to harm me, they *wouldn't* harm me, and this is what they are going to do because I read the consent form very carefully, and it is OK."'

Levinson's paperwork had been primitive by comparison. 'My consent forms were a sham. They consented to "having an operation"…that's all. It was just taken for granted that during anaesthetics we could expose them to all sorts of things, as long as we didn't wilfully or knowingly damage them.'

And it is this, argues Levinson that has made his classic experiment impossible to repeat. His study may have been flawed, he said, but so was Eger's. The young men in Eger's study knew beforehand that after they were unconscious, they might be presented with 'a drama similar to conversations that may occur at any time in an operating room during a real operation'.

'This is the flaw,' said Levinson from Johannesburg, 'this is the very flaw of that experiment that Ted Eger and I did. He is going to contest this, but it was a major flaw that every one of these volunteers knew exactly what we were going to do...We had *told* them—so in a real profound sense, they were not patients, they were very sophisticated guinea pigs.'

Eger and Chortkoff have mounted the opposite argument, that informed consent if anything increased the likelihood of the young men remembering the crisis, by alerting them to all the possible risks of anaesthesia, including death (information that might, arguably, heighten their anxiety and, with it, their resistance to the anaesthetic drugs).

'We repeated the experiment,' said Chortkoff with finality in response to my suggestion that Levinson's original study was unrepeatable. I had rung him in Salt Lake City, where he was a Professor of Anesthesiology at the University of Utah. As the first author on the report, it was Chortkoff's job to develop and manage the study and write it up. He is adamant that the replication 'drama' was every bit as convincing as the original. 'Ted's a phenomenal actor...It was quite frightening to listen to.'

There were other differences. For one, the volunteers were not cut—meaning their nervous systems were not subject to the galvanising effects of incision—making unconscious learning less likely. Offsetting this was the fact that the Eger study used lower concentrations of drugs than would usually be used for surgery, suggesting that the volunteers ('all lovely bright kids', said Levinson) were less heavily anaesthetised than the patients in the original experiment. Certainly that was the aim, said Chortkoff, who insists the team wanted to give the experiment every chance of working.

And, while Eger's subjects were not opened up, they were each subjected to a 'noxious stimulus'. About half an hour into the procedure, ten minutes before the staged 'drama' unfolded, anaesthetists inserted breathing tubes down their airways—an extremely uncomfortable process if you happen to be awake—and, like surgery, known sometimes to rouse patients. Interestingly, while none of the volunteers claimed when questioned after the anaesthetic to remember the tubes being put in, the report noted that, 'after at least one anaesthetic trial, half stated during hypnosis that they felt something in their throats, something that hurt'.

'Pressure...in my throat,' reported one young man, '...as if my tongue is being squeezed out of my mouth (and) something is being forced down there.'

There were various possible explanations, said the report, including that the volunteers had known beforehand they would be intubated, and also that they may have confused the experience with memories of the tubes being removed when they were waking.

There was also the fact that, apart from one young man who spontaneously described intubation under hypnosis, the others only professed memories after being prompted by team members. And hypnosis, as Eger was quick to remind me, has its own problems.

But there were other signs that some volunteers may have taken in more than just the anaesthetic drugs. One young man, immediately on awakening, said: 'I think people were nervous but I kept on breathing. Was there some kind of problem? I think you guys were getting scared...something was wrong.' Another said, 'I heard someone say the oxygen was off or something...but I couldn't talk.' Both had just emerged from the 'crisis drama'. Under hypnosis, each showed indications of having been aware. 'I felt panicked motions around me,' said the first. 'Something went wrong,' said the second. Both had had particularly low doses of the anaesthetics. After these two, the scientists increased the drug concentrations for the remaining subjects, though still not to surgical levels.

Yet, three other men went on to make similar comments, one upon awakening and two, volunteers 4 and 21, under hypnosis.

Interviewer: Has something gone wrong?

Volunteer 4: Yeah.

Interviewer: How do you feel?

Volunteer 4: Kind of nervous…It's something to do with death. I might die or something…they say they're going to do something to me…dangerous…I don't remember being told about this…I want to protect myself.

Volunteer 21: There's something wrong in the room or something…and with me. But it doesn't seem like a tape, it seems like everyone is rushing around or something…it's harder to breathe.

Oddly, both these accounts followed the upbeat drama, suggesting, said the study, 'that some spontaneous responses may reflect individual anxiety and/or fear associated with anaesthesia rather than the imposed crisis'. The study did not record whether volunteers 4 or 21 had previously received the 'crisis' drama, nor speculate on the possibility that, if so, they might have been remembering that earlier drama. Chortkoff said later that in the absence of the original study logs he could not rule out this possibility, but that it would have been unlikely. The report did, however acknowledge 'the intriguing possibility that some unique set of variables (which may not include anaesthetic concentration) result in awareness'.

Either way, intriguing. If the young men were not showing evidence of some sort of hidden learning, their fears certainly seemed to attest to the acute vulnerability of the patient facing general anaesthesia.

Eventually I asked Ted Eger about Bernard Levinson's assertion that the very fact that the volunteers had been told to expect some sort of crisis ('a traumatic suggestion' was how Levinson put it to me) under anaesthesia might have caused them to react differently than had they genuinely been undergoing surgery.

'The volunteers knew what was going to happen,' I said.

Eger looked aghast. 'No they did not, that's not true.'

I repeated my claim: 'He [*Levinson*] said to me that [*the volunteers knew*] there might be some kind of staged crisis.'

'No, no that would have been a mistake. If we'd told them that, then that would have skewed their perceptions. I don't believe that's correct. I think that we did not tell them, we may have told them that there would be messages that they would be sent, but there was no statement, let me see when did we publish that?'

I passed him the study, which mentioned the possibility of 'a drama'.

'Yeah,' he said after a moment, 'but that says nothing about a crisis.'

Eger remains convinced of his results—and certain that using his MAC formula the chances of awareness, remembered or otherwise, are 'vanishingly small'. That said, there have also been reports of awareness in patients on inhaled anaesthetics—even at MAC. And even under surgical levels of anaesthesia, the brain can process auditory signals. While some anaesthetics are good at suppressing sounds, others are less so.

'Have you had any anaesthetics?' I asked Eger later. And yes, he had. Twice as a child he had been put under with ether, once to remove his tonsils, once to fix his fractured nose. It was an event, he said, he would have avoided at almost any cost. 'It was an experience of breathing something that was terribly pungent, difficult breathing and a sensation of swirling down into a pool of darkness with sounds such as you might hear as you swam underwater in a swimming pool, a buzzing sound, and then you reappear and you are alive and nauseated and throwing up.'

Then he added that perhaps it wasn't, after all, his day spent selling cheap shoes as a Chicago teenager that had set him on the path to becoming an anaesthetist. 'Maybe I've wanted to go into anaesthesia so I could control that [I'd never] get one of those ether anaesthetics again. It was an awful experience.'

When I returned home, I rang Bernard Levinson and put to him Eger's distinction between 'drama' and 'crisis'. Levinson paused and then said, carefully: 'Ted Eger is a beautiful guy, he's a wonderful guy and unbelievably articulate, but he is, um, he is a believer in his anaesthetics and isn't comfortable seeing that they may be allowing thoughts to come through. You understand what I'm saying?'

As it turned out, there was one statistically significant finding reported in Ted Eger's replication study. As part of the study design the team decided to repeat the ear-touching test that psychologist Hank Bennett had devised all those years before to test for unconscious memories in surgical patients. Overall, Chortkoff and Eger found no evidence that volunteers who had been instructed to touch their nose or ears after waking up from surgery were more likely to do so than those who had not. But when the team separated out those young men who had been the most easily hypnotised beforehand, the results showed that, when interviewed later, this group were more likely to touch themselves as instructed. Not a great deal more likely, but more likely than chance.

'There was one statistically significant result,' conceded Eger, 'and Hank will point that out...[But] why the hell you'd remember someone telling you to pull your ear, I don't know.'

o

Can we ever know another human being?

Even the ones we love? We think we do; we learn to interpret, sometimes to rely, but in the end it's all circumstantial. Action, declaration, intimation. We create a working hypothesis we call husband/lover/child/mother, and we test it, through observation, information, sometimes provocation, a multitude of incremental, unrepeatable experiments, and in the end, if the membrane holds, if the sun continues to heave its way up and down and around, we agree to accept that it is so; we make each other solid.

'Consciousness is individual and subjective and it has therefore been held that it incapable [*sic*] of observation and description in a scientific manner. Against this contention there are certain arguments.'

These words I find among a fat wad of photocopied A5 pages that have lain for some years now in an improvised cardboard container in a shelf in my study (the same shelf where it turns out I have stored my itinerant X-rays). My mother's younger brother, Jim, sent it to me soon after my spinal surgery. I have known in the back of my mind that it was there, have perhaps even thumbed its pages before this week, although if so I don't remember. Blame the drugs (OxyContin, Endone—whatever it took in those submerged postoperative months). Nor do I know why I decide now is the time to open it. What I find when I do is a draft manuscript of a book, *Mechanics of Mind*, written in the years from 1942 to 1950 (there is a question mark after these dates) by H. R. Love: my grandfather.

What had I known about my mother's father before? That he was a doctor, that he had been in the war. That after his early death more than one older woman approached my not-yet-mother to tell her, 'I once danced with your father.'

That it was he who encouraged her to study art.

His obituary in the *Medical Journal of Australia* in 1956 shows a photograph of a pleasant-looking man in uniform, hair slicked over, head slightly forward; my mother's long face and steady, amused gaze. The article described his clever, penetrating mind, his early years studying medicine in Melbourne, his return to Brisbane to practise as an assistant to his uncle, his enlistment in 1939, his posting as an ambulance officer, first in England and then, in 1941, to Tobruk, 'where he served throughout the siege'.

These things I knew, a little.

What I hadn't known, or hadn't known I knew, was that after the war my dancing grandfather had slogged for nearly a decade over a manuscript on—what?—*consciousness*. With no less a goal than to articulate a scientific framework within which to reconcile the conflicting approaches to its study.

It is not that he believes science has all the answers. 'Practical human affairs are well served by the scientific approach as long as we never lose sight of the fact that it is not ultimate truth with which we are dealing.' But within these constraints, H. R. Love believes science to be 'the method, par excellence, for the practical conduct of human affairs and the advancement of human understanding'. Mind and matter are indivisible.

It is at times painful to read this unpublished opus: the effort of the gathering and referencing, the typed and scribbled-upon pages, the crossings-out and the writings-in, the arrows and underlinings; the assembling and corralling of sense and meaning.

The grandfather I never met is a reductionist, by and large.

In general terms it is believed that the brain is the physical organ of mind or consciousness. This belief rests upon certain self evident observations and propositions [*some crossings-out*]. The first simple and fundamental proposition is that consciousness can be consistently abolished for the time being by sleep, drugs and infection, trauma and metabolic upset. The evidence is of course indirect and depends on the inability of the individual to give any account of what has happened without or within himself during the period of unconsciousness. [*There follow a dozen or so more crossed out lines. Then, in his decisive doctor's handwriting:*] For practical purposes however consciousness and capacity for behaviours may be assumed to be lost during the action of these agents.

In my mother's studio upstairs at King William Street, she steps back from her easel. Attentive, poised, relaxed. This is her in her natural setting. Surrounded by canvases, brushes, rolls of wire, creased stubs of acrylic paint. We are talking about a painting. It could be one of a number of paintings. She is standing back, regarding an aerial landscape, its creeks and rivulets, its fences and windbreaks. She cups her hands on her hips. She talks about perspective and focus. About needing to pull this section forward or push that section back. The ways in which the frame alters the way you interpret the lines and planes within it. She moves forward and back, in and out, entire and of herself. Beloved. At times bewildering. My mother.

My grandfather's first argument is language. His second is art.

While 'the data of consciousness can only be individually described', he says, it can be pooled though language and other symbols to establish 'a department of common knowledge'. Further (and following some discussion about the ways in which our shared physiology and 'sympathy' make it likely that our subjective experiences are essentially comparable), he says this data can be channelled, through the making of art in all its forms, to express emotions, ideas and states of mind. 'Art is to subjective experience what mathematics and science are to the universe of common knowledge.'

Can we ever know another human being? I don't believe so. Not fully. But rifling through my grandfather's typewritten pages, I experience within my own body, within my subjective self, a flare of recognition.

ADRIFT

The island

The year after Ted Eger and Hank Bennett tried and failed to replicate Bernard Levinson's fake-crisis study, Canadian psychologists Phil Merikle and Meredyth Daneman set out to clarify the 'confusing picture of significant and non-significant results' from tests for unconscious perception during anaesthesia. Their 1996 review, which analysed the data for more than forty experiments involving 2,517 patients, concluded that simply saying nice things or suggesting positive outcomes to patients during surgery had little or no effect on their recovery—although it might possibly help reduce their pain. Merikle and Daneman did, however, find 'considerable' evidence that specific information presented during surgery was both perceived and remembered—as long as patients were tested as soon as possible after surgery (within thirty-six hours). After that the effect seemed to disappear. Even so, the authors speculated that patients might sometimes hold onto unconsciously perceived information for considerably longer.

But so what? If you imagine memory as an interconnected network of traffic lights that co-ordinate the flow of traffic in all directions across a suburb or even a city, the sort of learning we are talking about here might represent the brief illumination of a single traffic light—one connected to an older, more primitive grid. This is what is known as perceptual, rather than conceptual, priming. It registers things rather than concepts, words rather than ideas. It springboards off old memories rather than laying down new ones. Information (a word, a silence) is processed to some degree by the nervous system, but not interpreted or articulated in relation to all the other things we know.

In fact, Merikle and Daneman later went on to argue that it may, in the end, be impossible to 'prove' once and for all the existence of unconscious perception, even in fully conscious people. A more useful approach, they said, might be to ask simply does it matter? If these shadowy perceptual processes exist, do they differ importantly from their more forthright cousins? Are there differences in the types of information perceived, or the ways in which it is interpreted? Might it, in the end, make a difference to you or me as the owner of the memory?

Well, yes, it might.

Consider the work of American researchers Sheila Murphy and Robert Zajonc, who in the early 1990s divided volunteers into groups and showed them a series of clearly visible Chinese written symbols—ideographs—which they then asked the participants to rank according to whether each might represent a 'good' or 'bad' concept. The volunteers had no idea what the symbols meant. But what one half knew and the other did not was that, just before the researchers presented each symbol, they flashed up an image of a human face—either smiling or scowling. The researchers did this to everyone, but while the people in one group saw the images for long enough to consciously register them, the others saw the faces so quickly that none reported having noticed them at all. The group who knew what they had seen were told to ignore the faces and to get on with the job of ranking the symbols from one to five, which they did. Intriguingly it was the other group—those who were unaware they had even seen those fleeting expressions—whose rankings were most likely to be affected by them. A smile was more likely to produce a 'good' ranking, a frown, bad. Those who were aware of the facial expressions seemed able to quarantine themselves from their influence. The others weren't. People's feelings were more strongly affected by the things they didn't know they knew than by the things they did.

The ideograph experiment was one of a number of studies that Merikle and Daneman went on to examine in a paper exploring the impact of unconscious perception on conscious volunteers. 'Taken together,' they concluded, 'the results of these studies provide rather compelling evidence for the importance of unconscious perceptual processes.'

Scoot ahead a decade or so and a different group of researchers are experimenting with a different type of (pre-)emoji. This time they have substituted the smiling and scowling faces with fearful ones—a universal signal of danger—while hooking up their volunteers to state of the art neuroimaging machines. Scientists at Columbia University Medical Centre did this in 2004 and found that if you show someone a fleeting image of a fearful face, their amygdala—that almond-shaped bundle in the centre of each brain hemisphere that helps process emotional memories—lights up, even when the owners of the amygdalae deny having seen anything untoward; and particularly if they already have an anxious personality. Again, when the fearful faces were shown for long enough for the volunteers to know they had seen them, things changed. In this case they processed the information in a completely different part of the brain, suggesting, said one team member, 'a very important role for unconscious emotions in anxiety'.

In fact, studies of conscious volunteers suggest that unconscious or implicit perceptions can affect not just our feelings but our moods, our judgment, our physiology, even perhaps our behaviour. All without our knowing it—or being able to control it. Early in my research an Australian anaesthetist alerted me to a study by New York psychologist John Bargh.

It was already accepted that unconsciously perceived information could have a powerful effect on how people interpreted the world. Experiments on racial prejudice in the US in the 1980s had shown that people could be primed to view others in a positive or negative light simply by first showing them subliminal images of an African American face. But the scientists investigating such disturbing patterns still believed that while people might not have much control over the way they *felt* about things—or people—they did have some degree of choice about how they *behaved*.

Not necessarily, warned Bargh. In a series of classic experiments, he and his team showed that people could be unwittingly primed to butt into a conversation simply by first getting them to rearrange sentences that included words such as 'rude', 'obnoxious' and 'bold'. In another study, people exposed to words such as 'old', 'lonely' and 'bingo' were timed walking away from the experiment more slowly than their fellow participants. In another, non-African American students shown subliminal images of African American faces went on to behave more aggressively towards experimenters than those who had been primed with Caucasian faces. All without the participants having any idea that they were being manipulated. Again, the results have been inconsistent. Several well-publicised studies early this decade failed to replicate various of Bargh's findings on behaviour priming. But a 2016 meta-analysis of the literature in the prestigious *Psychological Bulletin* confirmed a small but robust effect—particularly when the behaviour or goal was important to the person being primed. It also pointed to 'potential real-world implications' of such priming.

..

The real world, of course, is even more slippery than the (relatively) controlled confines of the testing laboratory.

I met Kathryn Hall, like several of the people who wander in and out of these pages, at a writers centre outside Sydney. She was taking time away from her daytime jobs as a graphic artist and mother to work on a book for teenagers. A few years before, Kathryn had gone to hospital for an operation on her sinuses. For some reason I have always imagined a sinus as a body part, like a small bit of spiral-shaped pasta tucked somewhere up the nasal passage, but it turns out to be more of an absence: a cavity in the bone. Kathryn, in any case, remembers nothing apart from waking congested and in pain. And feeling a bit odd. 'This kind of peculiar feeling,' she said. 'I had this shaky sensation. Like my body was on edge. A shaky sensation under my skin. I just put it down to the anaesthetic.'

But almost a month later she was still having that sensation: 'Like I was on edge all the time, and the anxiety thing creeping in, and starting to be worried. Just feeling like something was wrong with me.' She felt that she was going to die.

The feeling escalated over three or four days. At first, she said, 'it was more a sense of feeling out of control, something happening in my body. Shortness of breath, couldn't breathe properly, and just that shaky feeling, but much, much more intense.' By the fourth day she was in a strange doctor's surgery, her heart doing a drum solo. 'I had pain in my neck. I couldn't breathe. It was absolutely terrifying.' The doctor examined her and told her quietly that she was having a panic attack.

Although Kathryn had dealt with anxiety before, triggered in part by a serious car accident she had been in as a younger woman, she said she had never experienced anything like these attacks. Kathryn went to her own GP and told her she suspected that the feeling was linked somehow to the operation. She had a vague memory of something her anaesthetist had mentioned when he came and saw her afterwards. About her blood pressure having plummeted during the surgery—the fact that it had been tricky to get it back up. 'It was just a very passing comment. It stuck with me, but I never really thought about it.' Her GP was unconvinced; she felt Kathryn was suffering from an unrelated depression as well as anxiety, and recommended drugs and counselling. Kathryn duly began seeing a counsellor. The process has been helping somewhat. Her psychologist believes the anaesthetic might have reopened a door to traumatic events in Kathryn's earlier life. She hasn't had any more panic attacks. 'But I still do have this very base concern that I'm dying, that there's something wrong.'

She just doesn't know what it is.

Three things we know, and one we don't:

1. We know that the brain's auditory pathways can continue to process sound after we are unconscious.
2. We know that implicit memory or priming can continue in anaesthetised surgical patients to the same degree as in conscious volunteers.
3. We know too that, at light doses of some anaesthetic drugs, while patients quickly lose the ability to form conscious memories of disturbing images, the threat-detecting amygdala can keep pinging away behind the scenes.
4. What we don't know is what any of this might mean for a real person having real surgery in a real operating theatre.

All of which helps explain the continuing allure of an odd and inventive German study from more than twenty years back. In the mid-nineties, a team led by anaesthetist Dierk Schwender played tape recordings to forty-five people having heart surgery using one of three different anaesthetics. Some time between when their chests were sawn open and bypass surgery began, two-thirds of the patients were played a ten-minute message including an abridged version of Daniel Defoe's *Robinson Crusoe*—the story of a castaway who, shipwrecked and alone on an inhospitable island, eventually learns to survive and flourish with the help and companionship of Man Friday. 'The story was meant to be a parable for the patients to cope with their current difficult situation and facilitate post-operative recovery,' explained the authors. Three to five days later they interviewed the patients. First they asked each if they remembered anything of the surgery. None did. Then they asked them to say the first word that came to mind when they heard the word 'Friday'.

'Last working day of the week,' said one. 'Fish for lunch and dinner,' said another.

But other patients went on to make a different connection.

'When you say Friday, I think of an island and the story of Robinson Crusoe,' said one, 'but I think this has nothing to do with your question.'

'When you say Friday,' said another, 'I remember that when I was a child we used to play on a little island in a river near my parents' home. We called that place Robinson island.'

None of the fifteen patients in the control group—those who had not been played the story tape—linked the word 'Friday' to Robinson Crusoe. Nearly a quarter of the remaining thirty did: seven people, five of them with one particular anaesthetic.

Schwender and his team had used an EEG to monitor the transmission of electrical impulses from each patient's ear to the part of the brain responsible for processing sound. Some patients' EEG readings showed little or no activity in the primary auditory cortex during the time when the messages were delivered; and those subjects showed no evidence of hidden memory. But the patients who mentioned Robinson Crusoe were all among those in whom these auditory signals (known as 'auditory evoked potentials') had continued. In other words, their brains were still processing the words, at least partially.

The Robinson Crusoe study has been something of a Rorschach's test for those interested in how much patients can take in when unconscious. Different researchers have seen different things in the study's blurred outline. To Schwender it suggested a measurement tool (auditory evoked potentials) that might be used by anaesthetists to prevent surgical patients forming not only conscious but unconscious memories. To others its message was that different anaesthetics provided differing levels of protection against memory formation. For some its main lesson was that patients do not form memories at deeper levels of anaesthesia; for others that even an adequately anaesthetised patient can take in information.

To British psychologist Michael Wang, however, it was the story at the centre of the study—of a man alone on an island—that provided its force. For Wang, it was the emotional correspondence between Crusoe's predicament and the patients' own experiences that most resonated. This study, he argued at the time, hinted at something deeper than mere word association. It suggested an emotional learning more resistant than verbal memory or language to the effects of some drugs: an inarticulate feeling network that could be activated unconsciously and that might then translate into actions and behaviours that could affect our lives in all sorts of ways we couldn't imagine. Abracadabra. *As I say it so it will be.*

It's an appealing story. Rich, resonant. Allusive.

Except that many years later, not long before he retired, Wang would attempt a replication of the Man Friday study, this time with intensive care patients. The result? Nothing. There were differences in the staging of the experiment (they waited longer before interviewing the patients). But none that even Wang felt could account for the result. It was, he acknowledged, disappointing.

So there we are. Again.

Now you see it, now you don't.

o

There is something very reassuring about talking with British psychologist Jackie Andrade. I don't know what she does after hours when she is not teaching and researching and speaking to people like me. Maybe she behaves erratically. Maybe she makes wild unsubstantiated claims or stands too close to strangers. But I don't think so. She has a soft Devon accent and a calm and straightforward way of explaining her work that, each time I have heard her speak, has left me feeling, I suppose, that I am in good hands. The first time she heard claims that people could form hidden memories while anaesthetised, she was incredulous. Even after she was persuaded by colleagues in the mid-nineties to carry out a review of the available literature, she remained underwhelmed at the evidence. The issue, she felt certain, was in the study designs or anaesthetic techniques. 'I was the biggest sceptic of the lot.' This was not to say she was convinced by Ted Eger's 1995 rerun of Bernard Levinson's fake crisis. ('I think it would have been very interesting had it worked...I think it's less interesting that it didn't replicate it.') In the end, however, like Eger, she determined to let science decide.

After a preliminary study led by one of her PhD students, Catherine Deeprose, the pair set out, like Eger and Bennett a decade earlier, to settle the matter. Working with surgical patients drugged with the intravenous anaesthetic propofol and nitrous oxide, and using the BIS monitor, they mounted a painstaking study designed to confirm whether memories could really be awakened and reactivated during deep anaesthesia. 'I was convinced,' said Andrade years later from Devon, where she is now professor of psychology at Plymouth University, 'that if you did the tests properly and used a good measure of depth of anaesthesia, to ensure patients were truly unconscious, there would be no memory.'

But there was.

'And we *did* do them properly!'

How big was the effect? Not big. Pretty small in fact. Presenting words to anaesthetised patients improved their chances of later selecting those words in a word-stem completion test by thirty-three per cent, but it still only amounted to a 'quite small' figure, said Andrade. On average patients remembered half a word out of a set of seven. Nor was this new information they were learning—simply existing memories being jogged.

Even so.

'Having said it's small, the reason I think it could be really important—and this is speculative—is that for ethical reasons we've only done studies with neutral words that people are very familiar with already—words like table and automobile, things like that.'

Andrade then went on to hypothesise (as Levinson had suggested about Ted Eger's replication of his own fake-crisis study) that the reason the experimental effect was so small was because the words did not matter enough for the patient to process them. Offer the anaesthetised you or me something we care about—our name, for instance, or the name of our illness; or a prognosis—and we need less mental juice to process that information than for something irrelevant. It's a bit like suddenly hearing ourselves mentioned across a crowded room despite all the competing chatter. Basically, we have had so much practice over a lifetime of recognising that (very particular) word that it skates nimbly along its own well-worn brain pathways with minimal effort on the part of our already overloaded neurons. Andrade makes a parallel with anaesthesia. 'Even if there's very little activity left in your auditory cortex, this information can get through better than irrelevant information.'

The other reason she believes her study is important is that, while the memories being created in her team's experiments are single words that piggyback on knowledge the patient already has, each word can trigger a network of associations.

> So if you're self-conscious about your body, for instance, and you overhear somebody saying 'fat' and you interpret that as applied to you, that won't just activate the word 'fat', it will activate all your anxieties about your weight and how you look and those sorts of things. I'm picking this example because this is something that anaesthetists *do* say about their patients, because it's harder to anaesthetise somebody who's obese, so they're very likely to comment on their weight because it's important for them in deciding how to do the anaesthetic.

Andrade's research raises the possibility that, in this instance, the patient's brain could still react to those comments even while she or he was anaesthetised. Again, she said, all speculative—and likely to stay that way. Even if, ethically, researchers could go around saying alarming or insulting things to unconscious surgical patients, it would be very difficult to attribute any changes in the patients' behaviour solely to hidden memories of the event. There are all sorts of reasons why people feel odd or upset after surgery: pain, sleeplessness, anxiety, changes to body image. And of course many—most—people seem to leave hospital feeling relatively sanguine. But this did not have to mean the issue was trivial, Andrade said. 'Because of course, in the course of doing their work, surgeons and anaesthetists and theatre staff can say things that are much more profound from the patient's point of view than we could ever do as experimenters.'

Dreams

One day early in my research, I rang my father and told him I was writing about anaesthesia.

'Oh,' he said, 'fancy that. I had one of my ether dreams just the other day.'

My father, like many in his generation, had his tonsils taken out when he was around ten years old. This would have been in the late 1940s. He does not know what anaesthetic he was given, though he remembers clearly something being held against his face. Fear. A sense of suffocation. A bad smell. Probably ether; maybe another early anaesthetic, chloroform. As he went under, he had a vision or dream. In the dream, he said, he was sitting in the sky with his legs straight out in front of him. As he sat, feeling quite relaxed, he saw in the distance a cloud moving towards him, a large white cloud, 'which came inexorably closer and closer'. The closer the cloud came, the more uneasy my father became, until it slowly enveloped him, first the toes, then the thighs, 'then the lot'. In the years since, he had experienced a recurring nightmare in which this vision, or variations on it, was repeated. There he would be sitting in the sky, legs stuck out in front of him, and then there in the distance, moving towards him, was the cloud.

What was the feeling? I asked him.
'Oh,' he said. 'Oh. Absolute terror.'

Dreams occupy an amorphous space in anaesthesia theory and practice. Patients often wake from surgery and report having dreamed (recent studies suggest somewhere between twenty and fifty per cent of patients might do it) and traditionally doctors have paid little attention to these reports. Most doctors see dreams as curiosities, or perhaps as a sort of psychic static—like 'noise' in digital photography; an artefact or drug-induced hallucination. Certainly they have been happening for as long as people have been being anaesthetised.

Not long after William Morton's miraculous 1846 demonstration of ether anaesthesia, a surgeon called Henry Bigelow visited Morton's rooms to witness the dentist at work with his new technique. Bigelow had already had some experience with ether, as with nitrous oxide—though not in a surgical context. 'In my own former experience,' he noted of ether, 'the exhilaration has been quite as great, though perhaps less pleasurable, than that of this gas [*nitrous oxide*], or of the Egyptian haschish.' He watched, fascinated, as Morton moved through his list of patients. One, 'A boy of sixteen, of medium stature and strength', inhaled for some time and eventually passed out for three minutes, during which time Morton extracted a troublesome molar. 'At the moment of extraction the features assumed an expression of pain, and the hand was raised. Upon coming to himself he said he had felt no pain but had had a 'first rate dream—very quiet [...] and had dreamed of Napoleon...''

Another patient, wrote Bigelow,

> was a healthy-looking, middle-aged woman, who inhaled the vapour for four minutes; in the course of the next two minutes a back tooth was extracted, and the patient continued smiling

in her sleep for three minutes more. Pulse 120, not affected at the moment of the operation, but smaller during sleep. Upon coming to herself, she exclaimed that 'it was beautiful—she dreamed of being at home—it seemed as if she had been gone a month'.

These results, said Bigelow, were typical of ether: 'Dr. Morton states that in upwards of two hundred patients, similar effects have been produced.'

> The character of the lethargic state, which follows this inhalation, is peculiar. The patient loses his individuality and awakes after a certain period, either entirely unconscious of what has taken place, or retaining only a faint recollection of it. Severe pain is sometimes remembered as being of a dull character; sometimes the operation is supposed by the patient to be performed upon somebody else.

From time to time, in fact, the dreams were so enjoyable that doctors were shocked. American anaesthetists Robert Strickland and John Butterworth noted a decade ago that within a few years of Ether Day reports had started appearing in journals of patients, mainly women, waking from anaesthesia in a state of high arousal, some reporting erotic dreams, some using obscene language. New England physician Moreton Stille cited a report in the 1850s of a woman in Germany emerging from an ether anaesthetic 'in a highly excited state...her eyes sparkled and a certain erotic excitation was very observable'. In a case mentioned by a Professor Dubois, a Parisian prostitute having vaginal surgery later reported erotic dreams. In another of Dubois' cases, 'The woman drew an attendant towards her to kiss, as she was lapsing into insensibility, and this woman afterwards confessed to dreaming of coitus with her husband while she lay etherised.'

Such cases, while striking, were unusual. But Strickland and Butterworth note that some of today's commonly used anaesthetic drugs can elicit similar responses in modern patients. Indeed, they said, '[t]he authors have encountered the problem of sexual ideations or dreams in sedated or anaesthetised patients in their own anaesthesia practices...' One of the anaesthetists I spoke with in the process of researching this book told me about a patient who had awoken from surgery looking very pleased with herself and immediately asked what drug she had been on. He told her he had been using propofol—an increasingly popular intravenous drug favoured by anaesthetists for its ease of use and patient satisfaction.

Why, he asked?

'You won't believe this, but I've just had a half-hour orgasm!'

Anaesthetics are well known to have a disinhibiting effect, particularly in the second stage—the evocatively named plane of delirium, or excitation. Like alcohol, they can suppress our polite selves. It is not unusual for patients, just before passing out, to tell surgical staff how attractive they are, to invite them on dates or even to bed. Perhaps such recklessness flows through into dreams.

But while dreams are by their nature ephemeral, they can create some very tangible problems for patients and for surgical staff. In the years following Morton's successful demonstration of surgical ether, several cases were reported of women claiming to have been sexually assaulted after having been anaesthetised by their dentist or doctor. In the first of these cases to go to court, a Parisian dentist was accused in 1847 of abusing two girls he had etherised. One later said she had been aware of him touching her but that she felt unable to move or fight him off. The dentist was convicted, despite his denials. Some years later, however, the medical journal *The Lancet* published an article outlining various cases in which doctors or dentists had been wrongly accused by women under the influence of ether or chloroform. One woman woke after childbirth convinced her doctor had molested her, even though her husband had been there beside her the whole time.

It is hard to know what to make of these stories. On the one hand there is the extreme vulnerability of the women (and nearly all the early reports were from women), unconscious and open to attack from opportunistic medical practitioners. On the other are the mind-altering effects of drugs such as ether. Either way, the distress for the dreamer or supposed dreamer was real, and perhaps lasting. Stille was convinced that ether and chloroform could produce vivid dreams or 'memories' of events that had never happened or were 'real occurrences perverted from their actual nature'. What was striking he said, apart from their unreliability, was their tenacity—there was, he wrote, 'reason to believe that the impression left by the dreams occasioned by ether, may remain permanently fixed in the memory with all the vividness of real events.'

('Oh,' said my father. 'Oh. Absolute terror.')

In the years after Ether Day, the main lesson for the (exclusively male) surgeons and dentists of the day was to make sure they were never alone with unconscious—or seemingly unconscious—patients, particularly women. The other, related, lesson was that patients emerging from anaesthetics were not to be trusted. 'It is our decided opinion, that the evidence of even a partially etherised person should not be received as valid, without corroboration,' the *Boston Medical and Surgical Journal* said in an editorial of 1854. It is not surprising, in this light, that doctors tend now, as then, to dismiss patients' claims of anaesthetic awareness, and not just the erotic ones, as dreams or hallucinations.

In July 2009, amid emotional courtroom scenes, a Pittsburgh dentist was acquitted of multiple counts of sexual assault brought against him by seventeen former patients. Despite saying he found the women's accounts 'compelling and disturbing', and that he was confident that they genuinely believed they had been assaulted, Judge Mariani cited defence testimony that the women had been under the influence of powerful drugs designed 'to take away memory and take away perception'. Things ended very differently in 2014 for a Canadian anaesthetist who was convicted of sexually assaulting twenty-one sedated women during surgeries and sentenced to ten years in prison.

At the very least, what such experiences make clear is that the line between anaesthesia, dreams and reality is indistinct and some-times permeable.

o

> The dream which I had during anaesthesia came to mind. I was surrounded by sounding-depth made of paper-pulp with many fishes and basketfuls of bread. I dreamed I heard your [*the anaesthetist's*] voice which made me feel relaxed but I don't remember what you said.

This patient had been played the story of the miracle of loaves and fishes during anaesthesia.

I am the sort of person who likes dreams, my own and other people's. Not that I like all the dreams, or even many of the dreams, that I have, but I like the fact of them. I like the sense that somewhere beneath the thoughts and plans and entanglements with which I map each burdened day, there is another, wilder, me. One who is accountable only to herself. For many years I used to dream that I was about to go skiing. These dreams started in my teens, before I had ever put on skis. The dreams would be filled with a sense of enormous anticipation and pleasure, as I prepared myself for the descent. Inevi-tably, however, I would be unable to find my skis or the snow would have melted; or I would find myself not at the top of a brilliant alpine slope, but poised on the edge of what looked like an illustration in a cheap children's book—two-dimensional and badly drawn, a shabby theatrical backdrop.

These dreams always let me down—or I them—and yet what I remember most vividly now is the exquisite sense of possibility they engendered: that the slope existed; and one day I might ski down it. Perhaps they say something about my need for control. Perhaps if my waking life were less thought out, my dreams would not need to be as intrusive. As it is, there are dreams I remember more clearly than whole years of my waking life. My memory for events, places, sometimes even people, is intermittent at best. There are decades, almost, of life from which I retain only scraps. But there are dreams that even now, years later, seem more essential, more alive, than anything that might have been happening in my day to day life.

Dream theory is as fraught and tangled as the dreams it attempts to understand. At one end of the spectrum are those who argue that dreams are simply the mental detritus generated by the night-time firing of synapses as they replenish and reorganise the brain. At the other, with the mighty shadows of Freud and Jung looming over them, are those who treat dreams as meaningful and often symbolic representations of conscious or unconscious memories or conflicts. A way of processing and resolving day-time fears. Coded messages from the self to the self. Either way, various researchers have pointed out that dreaming is in itself a form of consciousness, albeit one disconnected from the external world.

This fact alone, that I am the sort of person who dreams and remembers my dreams, also means I am statistically more likely to dream when under anaesthesia—or at least to remember any dreams I might have had. Not that I have any such memories from any of my brief early anaesthetic experiences. Each remains a void.

Yet something was happening to my dream life during the writing of this book.

> June 2005. Wake early from what feels like transient preoccu-
> pied sleep, thinking about structure and organising the book.
> Body tense, unrefreshed, it occurs to me that I have been
> thinking in order not to dream. Then suddenly clear as day,
> as if it has been lying alongside but in a separate container,
> comes the dream. Strange gothic tale. I am in a space that
> feels almost cave-like but is part of some big house—a cellar?
> In the dream there is a book and in the book is a story about
> something that happened here in another room, in the past.
> It happened to a man. What happened was so horrible
> that no one fully explains it. It is written up in this big old
> book, but the script is archaic, mediaeval perhaps, and most
> of the words I can barely recognise; enough however to get
> the sense that there had been some elaborate torture here,
> involving him being perhaps castrated. I am very aware of
> the horror of what happened to him. I identify quite strongly
> with him. All that remains, however, apart from the book,
> is a dried-out piece of skin or flesh. There is a little hair
> attached, which was what they cut off him. It is bigger than
> I had imagined, an irregular circular sort of shape, dried
> and blackened. I have to wipe it down carefully with a damp
> cloth. I am afraid it will fall apart with the pressure or the
> moisture, but it doesn't. Later I walk down a long corridor to
> find my son.

Back in the early noughties, Kate Leslie, the Melbourne anaesthetist who, with Paul Myles, shot to prominence through the B-Aware
study of the BIS depth of anaesthesia monitor, started thinking a lot
about dreams. Not the sort you or I have during the night. As part
of the post-operative interviews during the BIS study, she and Myles

had asked surgical patients if they remembered dreaming during the anaesthetic.

'I dreamed that I saw my daughter, who was pregnant, having a caesarean section,' said one woman.

'I had vivid dreams about rescuing a pup from a tunnel, flying a plane, swimming and being stuck in a boat,' said another. 'I felt restricted in my movements and felt I was gagging.'

Another dreamed he was fishing in a boat that sank in a storm.

Given that using the BIS monitor dramatically reduced the chances of a patient waking during surgery, Leslie wondered whether dreams, or at least some dreams, might indicate more than just psychic static—whether they might instead represent moments of awareness or 'near-miss awareness', in which surgical patients had not in fact been disconnected—or entirely disconnected—from the external world. This idea was given weight by the fact that dreamers tended to wake more quickly after surgery and be less satisfied overall with their anaesthetic experience.

Certainly, some of the dreams reported by patients in the trial seemed uncannily reminiscent of the experiences they had just been through in the operating theatre. 'I dreamed that I was having a conversation with my anaesthetist about the research trial. The dream was interrupted by the anaesthetist's voice trying to wake me up.'

Another possibility that Leslie was investigating, however, was that dreamers were in fact describing drug-induced hallucinations.

It was an almost direct reprise of the debate 150 years before, minus the sex.

But this time Leslie had a crucial advantage. Use of the BIS monitor had halved the rate of patients who reported dreaming during the B-Aware study. With the BIS she had a tool that could, she was confident, accurately measure how deeply anaesthetised a patient was. In a new study she and her colleagues monitored the

BIS values of three hundred patients undergoing elective surgery. They interviewed them immediately upon waking, and again two to four hours later, and then correlated these responses with the BIS measurements. Close to a quarter reported dreaming at one or both interviews. 'There's lots of dreams,' confirmed Leslie in 2006 shortly before the study was released, 'there's some great ones.'

And while many appeared not to be related to surgery, a few clearly were. She recounted one dream that suggested the patient had been awake.

> This woman was having something under my care—division of adhesions, that's right, in the tummy, so it was quite a stimulating operation—and towards the end of the operation she moved quite a lot, so I said, 'Don't worry, everything's all right, we're giving you more medicine,' (which is what I do, and everyone thinks I'm mad, but, you know...) and I put her back to sleep. Immediately post-op she said she had a dream that she was in a car, it could have been an ambulance, and it went down a big black hole in the road and it was falling down and she couldn't move but she heard a doctor say 'everything's all right'...Two or three hours later she couldn't remember very much about it at all.

Leslie reported this with good humour and a certain relish. She too loves dreams, though probably not in the way that I do: Leslie is a scientist.

In the end the team concluded that the vast majority of dreamers did so regardless of how deeply anaesthetised they had been. Most of the dreams were pleasant and many involved family or friends in familiar places. The reason for this, Leslie believes, is that most dreams do not happen during surgery, but later in the recovery room, either the legacy of the hypnotic drugs, or as the patient tips into normal sleep before they wake properly.

Anaesthesia, she stresses, is not sleep.

This is not to say it does not have similarities. Researchers have reported that some anaesthetics appear to recruit the brain's sleep circuitry. But it also has critical differences. For one, sleep can't kill you, as the drug propofol did the singer Michael Jackson. For another, if, while you are sleeping, someone sticks a small sharp knife into your leg or your abdomen or your eye, you will wake up. In any case, Leslie is now confident that, while intriguing, dreams reported by people waking from anaesthetics are largely irrelevant.

And yet.

She mentioned another patient she had met early in her research, a man who had had knee surgery, who had dreamed he had an Aldi supermarket inside his knee. There were lots of trolleys in the store, but not many people. He felt alone. The Aldi dream, said Leslie, had all the characteristics of a drug-induced hallucination. 'You know, it's the sort of thing you'd think about if you were taking mushrooms or something...'

I couldn't quite agree with her. I thought it was the sort of thing you might well dream about if you were having surgery on your knee: the metallic clanking; the sense of isolation. To me the dream seemed laden with allusion. I wondered if Leslie had ever shopped in an Aldi store. ('That would be a no,' she said later.)

'So symbolism's not necessarily important?' I asked.

'The only symbolism that's meaningful from my perspective is whether they're using information they obtained during anaesthesia to formulate the dream or not.'

I think about my father and his ether dream, and wonder if that would qualify as 'information obtained during anaesthesia', or whether that image of the cloud was formed on his way into or out of anaesthesia. It occurs to me that from the patient's perspective it is irrelevant at which stage of the process the information was obtained. What is relevant is that they now carry it with them.

I should state now that, like Ted Eger, I am a believer in science. I come from a family that favours it. My mother chose to practise art but her father was a doctor. My father, like me, has made a career trying to balancing the chaos of lived life within the constraints of journalism. When the 2004 film *What the Bleep Do We Know?* came out on DVD I watched it at the behest of friends and cringed: the tone, the broad vague assertions, the hokey music and graphics.

That said, I did later travel to Tucson to interview one of the scientists who appeared in that film. His name was Stuart Hameroff and he was a respected anaesthetist. He believed that consciousness was a quantum process arising through the interplay of tiny assemblies of proteins known as microtubules that organised activities within the neurons of the brain. He had previously teamed up with famed British physicist Roger Penrose to suggest that it (consciousness) existed in spacetime geometry (what Hameroff described as 'the fine scale structure of the universe') and was connected to the brain through the strange things happening in the microtubules. Hameroff was fascinating and might for all I know have been a genius. I didn't understand most of what he said. We didn't talk much about hidden unconscious processes or about what Bernard Levinson has described as the 'flamboyant charade' of dreams—though Hameroff did speculate that dreams might follow quantum logic, 'with bizarre multiple co-existing possibilities and deep hidden connections'.

None of this is quite what I was getting at, but, thinking about Bernard Levinson now, one of the things I realise I loved about reading and speaking with him was the way he talked about things. The raging, rock-strewn river; the current of anxiety flowing between the surgeon and himself; the layering and linking of things.

These are the tools of storytelling. Models of quantum computation, by contrast; the statistical analysis of dreams—these are the instruments of science: the systematic attempt, through precise and rigorous measurement, to know the world not as we feel it to be but as we can prove it to be. Or not to be. There can be few more necessary endeavours. But—and this might be what I was trying to say to Kate Leslie that day—I can't help knowing that between science and lived experience is a gap that wavers and widens depending on which bit of the world we are in the process of observing or testing, and that it is here, in this uncertain space, that many of the processes that make us most particularly human take place.

It is intriguing at any rate to look at the sorts of things people did remember dreaming. Of the forty-seven dreams detailed in Kate Leslie's 2007 study, five (a little over ten per cent) involved water or fishing.

'Camping on beach, went for a walk, saw a dam on the river high above the river. Was checking out the dams because the river was dammed up. It was still beautiful and he was with nice people.'

'Dreamed about a fish in a tank and seaweed surrounding her. Splashing around and the colour blue.' (This was from a patient suspected of having been aware.)

Several dreamed about work, and others also reported holidays: a school trip to the beach ('lots of fun').

But the most commonly reported dreams, by far, were ones involving family and friends. A third of dreamers conjured parents, children, siblings or partners. Occasionally these dreams were troubling ('Dreamed of his girlfriend. He had lost her and was trying to find her...').

But many were comforting.

'Dreamed that her boyfriend was by her side talking to her.'

'Dreamed that her family was surrounding her and supporting her.'

'Remembers being outside in a garden by herself. Remembers a swing and her sister being there. She hasn't seen her sister in 9 yr.'

'Dreaming a game of cricket. Was playing with her three children and four grandchildren…It was a beautiful day…'

Five or six patients reported unpleasant dreams.

'Dreamed about teaching. She was teaching a junior class and she was in pain and wanted her mother.'

'A tiger was chasing me. I was in a glass room and felt scared. Every glass door I went through, the tiger was there. It kept roaring and chasing me. I was running.'

And oddly, several dreams involved food. 'Dreamed about having a barbecue with lots of sausages. But she hates sausages. But she was really hungry.'

I am reminded of the nurse during the heart surgery I watched with Paul Myles who confessed that the smell of cauterised flesh could be distracting. 'Sometimes, if we're working before lunch, it makes me hungry.'

'What about people dreaming about barbecues and meat?' I asked Leslie.

As far as she could now recall, none of the patients she had dealt with had reported 'olfactory dreams'. Social dreams, yes; meat dreams, no.

But what about that one…?

Leslie spoke calmly. 'You're trying to draw an analogy between burning flesh and—I won't support that.'

I persisted. What about other reports from other researchers, in which people did occasionally mention, you know, meat?

Leslie paused for a very small moment and then continued as if the barbecue conversation had not happened. 'So, I mean I quite like my dreaming research, because I find it fascinating, it's my—you know, you have to find your own little, your own niche, and many think it's frivolous, but I think it's something that twenty-five per cent of people do—so I really enjoy exploring it further.

'In one way it would have been fantastic to find some spectacular connection between dreaming and being awake. But in fact the conclusion I've come to based on the research I've done is that it's a harmless peripheral phenomenon of anaesthesia.'

So that's the science.

But people do have some striking dreams after surgical anaesthesia. I met one woman, a screenwriter named Deborah Klika who, in the months after surgery, had a series of episodic dreams about driving a red car. In the first, she was at the bottom of a mountain; she was behind the wheel and with her in the car was the surgeon who had operated on her. In episode two, the two of them were driving up the mountain. In the final dream she was alone at the top of the mountain. The surgeon had gone. Her most powerful memory was of feeling abandoned.

Not long after my mother's return home after having her cancerous kidney removed, she had another dream. In recent years she had become intrigued by floating grids, which she superimposed over her aerial landscapes to disconcerting effect. The grid lines hover over the land like some suspended equation whose answer is implicit in its form. Mostly I find these works harder to love than her more organic work. I am not sure why. Perhaps it is that it feels a little as if I am viewing it all through an intricate rifle sight, or from a prison cell. Perhaps it is simply that they feel cooler and more cerebral without the welling water of the earlier paintings. Anyway, in this dream my mother was working on a painting, or trying to, except that the painting had been taken over by a grid, which had imposed upon both the dream and the dreamer its own precise rules. It needed to be filled in a particular way, my mother said, and would only let her move her hand across from one square to another when she had fulfilled its requirements. She didn't like it.

The first time my mother told me about this dream, this was pretty much all she said. The grid, the constraint, the unease. A month or so later, however, when we discussed it again, she remembered something else: on the other side of the grid was a group of men, watching her and smiling in a friendly way ('very benign'). Men in suits.

This conversation took place in my car on the way to find an upholsterer in Brunswick to refurbish two chairs that had been left to her by her own mother. Years before, when my mother's Aunt Nance was dying, she asked Mum to have some chairs reupholstered for her. At the time, said Mum, it seemed ridiculous. But now, here she was, doing the same, and somehow it made sense. She wanted them in good shape for whatever came next. I was driving and Mum was talking in the dreamy way you do when you are being driven and are able to look outward and inward at the same time. Then she remembered another dream she had had sixty years before, as a girl at boarding school. ('I did have a men-in-suits dream *years* ago.')

In this dream the suited men were in one of the school's courtyards. The grass in the centre was ringed by a brick walkway and the men were walking around it, sticking obediently to the path. In fact, Mum said, they probably hadn't even noticed the grass. 'They would have been absorbed in conversations that men in suits have.' My mother's feelings about the men were mixed. 'I actually saw myself as being in a much better position to the men in their suits because I could walk on the grass. And they wouldn't be game...'

'It was very strange,' she said.

She paused, before adding: 'But, then, my father always wore a suit.'

o

'Harold Love had at times what almost amounted to a phase of lethargy; but this was soon over, and normally his very considerable output of effective work was achieved with no apparent effort or hurry.' Obituary of Harold Russell Love, *Medical Journal of Australia*, September 1, 1956.

In his unfinished manuscript, my grandfather discusses the patterns of association and inhibition that compete for expression first within the nervous system and later the psyche. These latter inhibitions he calls 'thwartings'. Irritability, depression, physical malaise: these are some of the costs of thwarting. 'The reactive disturbances to which normal people are subject may be profound and incapacitating.' A response perhaps to a failure of the normal person to adapt to an unfamiliar or inhospitable environment; or to a mismatch between the demands of that environment and their ability to meet them; or between what they desire and what they can actually have. Or between two equal but opposing circumstances or demands. Such as might be presented in army service.

My grandfather saw the results of such thwartings close up during the 241 days in 1941 in which he was under siege with a garrison of Allied troops in the Libyan city of Tobruk: the soldier in action who starts 'running around wildly under fire'; the general who in a crisis remains 'passive, inhibited and incapable of action'.

My grandfather did not remain passive: 'Placed in charge of a large ward of physically exhausted and badly shaken men, his staunch outlook and vigorous personality restored their confidence and morale to such an extent that the great majority of them were soon back with their units.' Obituary of Harold Russell Love.

Perhaps this success in itself was a kind of thwarting. My grandfather doesn't say. But, as he makes clear, you don't have to go to war, or send others back into it, to be thwarted:

> The civilised social structure imposes many such thwartings upon the human organism and not the least important quality of man as a social animal is his ability to repress or sublimate his thwartings. At all points his desires are hedged about with restrictions, and his sexual, economic, aggressive, and flight reactions, even his laughter and tears, are subject to extraneous inhibitions reinforced by threat of social and other penalties.

Of his own thwartings my grandfather did not write, although the besieged months in Tobruk and later his own failing health must have qualified. From my mother I had the impression that the comfortable conservatism of Brisbane society could be burdensome. Gregarious, inquisitive, a lover of company, conversation and the arts, my grandfather, she said, liked to drink at the less salubrious hotels where the journalists drank.

In between it all, he wrestled with the book.

o

I dream, or realise upon waking from a dream, that I understand the purpose and function of dreams. They are not neural static (or dark matter or junk DNA). Nor are they simply the random off-cuts of our waking lives; they have a purpose. The function of dreams (I understand in my dreamlike state) is to recruit and recycle the detritus and props of our day to day life to illuminate something enormous, much more than the individual unconsciousness. Something true. I feel very certain of this, without knowing how or why or what it even means.

Altered states

One day as I reluctantly pushed myself into my study, it occurred to me I had been working on the same chapter for more than a year. Every time I sat down I seemed to disappear. It was like being in one of those dreams in which you are trying to run but can only move in slow motion. Each thought seemed to take an infinity. Each connection felt like the forcing together of negative poles. My brain was cheesecake. 'What you're describing,' said a friend, 'is resistance.' This resistance manifested in multiple ways: in walking, in talking, in shopping, in sleeping, in eating, in drinking, in a tight inky feeling in my chest. It manifested most vehemently and truculently in the endless heaving manuscript I was dragging around with me.

One day, I might, for instance, write this:

Australian philosopher David Chalmers has argued that a robust theory of consciousness will have to address two fundamental types of problem: the easy ones and the hard one. The 'easy' problems, he says with deliberate understatement, concern the precise mechanisms by which the human brain, with its billions of neurons connected by trillions of synapses, produces conscious awareness. The hard problem is to explain how this infinitely complex machinery gives rise to subjective experience, what Chalmers calls 'qualia': the felt experience of the colour blue, the precise ache of a Bach cello solo, or the cool suction of wet sand underfoot. While some scientists seem to be making progress on the first problem (identifying various brain sites and processes necessary for consciousness), Chalmers argues that a purely mechanistic model is unlikely to provide useful answers to the second question.

Then, alongside it, I might find myself writing something like this:

In my dream I am walking towards a cat in a basket at the base of a hill. As I get closer I become aware of a terrible smell and I think that the cat has gangrene. I know I should help it but I am repulsed by the stench. Then I realise it is not the cat that is smelling but an unhatched egg next to its basket. The egg has a tiny hole pecked through it, as if by something trying to get out, but the egg has gone putrid. Foul smelling stuff is bubbling around the hole. I notice now that the cat is in water, that it is almost submerged inside its basket. Suddenly, it gets up. It is big and black and supple. Without a glance it moves past me and swiftly away.

And there they would sit, two embattled thoughts, estranged from each other, and from me, until eventually I would move one, or both, and start again. This went on for years.

In the meantime, and with apologies to Chalmers, I wonder if his problems might usefully be hijacked to help examine unconsciousness—specifically the anaesthetic unconsciousness. The easy problem in this context would be to establish how anaesthetic agents interact with the human brain to bring about unconsciousness deep enough to enable a doctor to, for example, remove and replace your heart without your knowing about it. The hard question might be: what is the subjective experience of this unconsciousness? What, if anything, does anaesthesia feel like for you, the person being anaesthetised?

In Boston's Countway Library of Medicine is a slender volume with faded blue fabric cover and thin gold lettering. *The Anaesthetic Revelation and the Gist of Philosophy* published in 1874. In it, Benjamin Paul Blood, a sometime philosopher, poet and mystic fashioned a manifesto from the ephemeral insights gleaned through his experience with early anaesthetic drugs.

> After experiments ranging over nearly fourteen years I affirm—what any man may prove at will—that there is an invariable and reliable condition (or uncondition) ensuing about the instant of recall from anaesthetic stupor to sensible observation, or 'coming to,' in which the genius of being is revealed; but because it cannot be remembered in the normal condition it is lost altogether through the infrequency of anaesthetic treatment in any individual's case ordinarily, and buried, amid the hum of returning common sense...

Sarah Schmidt was thirty-two when she went to hospital to have surgery on an errant ovary. She felt unsettled right from the start, she told me, vulnerable and intensely exposed: 'I remember saying to them, please don't look at my body, don't look at my body.'

The anaesthetist tried to reassure her. 'It's OK, we're professionals.'

Sarah was not convinced, although when she woke, the operation over, she felt strangely calm. A couple of days later, however, back at home, she began to have the feeling that her surgical experience was insinuating its way into her waking life. First she started having fragmentary images. 'Just little spurts of memory.' Doctors talking. Then came a different and unexpected sensation. 'I had memories of coming out of my body—not having an overview of things, but just being in and out of my body the whole time while the operation was happening…I felt like I could just walk in and out of my body. Walking in and out. Like—it's a body, it's open for business [*she laughed*], you can just walk in and out of it.'

'You know when you get deja vu?' she said. 'You get that kind of unsettling rattling in your body—it was like that. That was the actual physical feeling. And if I thought about it a little more, it felt like I was just like a moveable person, I could be taken in and out of situations that I'd have no control over. Does that make sense? There's no other way to describe it.'

It wasn't disturbing at the time, she said, but the experience did disturb her now. Mainly because it kept coming back. The last time it had happened was a few months before we spoke. 'I was lying in bed and I got these really sharp pains in my ovaries and it just triggered off this thing, at night, and I had this, almost like being on a ride—whoa, I'm coming out, and then coming back in again. It was very strange.'

Anaesthetic drugs *are* very strange.

'Truth lies open to the view in depth beneath depth of almost blinding evidence,' wrote William James, American philosopher and psychologist, who was inspired by Benjamin Blood to experiment with nitrous oxide (still among the most widespread anaesthetic drugs in use today). He too wrote of the fleeting but vivid insights—'an intense metaphysical illumination'—that followed.

> The mind sees all logical relations of being with an apparent subtlety and instantaneity to which its normal consciousness offers no parallel; only as sobriety returns, the feeling of insight fades, and one is left staring vacantly at a few disjointed words and phrases, as one stares at a cadaverous-looking snow peak from which sunset glow has just fled, or at a black cinder left by an extinguished brand.

These days anaesthetic drugs are administered in combinations and quantities that ensure experiences such as James's are rarely if ever reported in the anaesthetic literature—although if you search 'laughing gas' on YouTube you will find plenty of very high dental patients.

But hallucinations *after* surgery, sometimes benign, sometimes terrifying, are remarkably common, particularly in older patients. My former French lecturer Colin Nettelbeck told me shortly after he retired about the day, several years before, when he nearly died of meningococcal disease. He fell ill just after dinner and deteriorated rapidly. By the time he got to hospital next morning he needed a wheelchair. He recalls a doctor asking his name; his own unsuccessful attempt to reply; the aching head—'Almost as if it had been laminated into different layers of pain.' He woke the next day in intensive care with a tube down his windpipe.

A few days later, in another section of the hospital, he became delirious. In this peculiar state, he felt vividly that he was doing battle with weird humanoid figures, and that he was losing strength. ('The space was how you might imagine Dante's circles of hell.') In another scenario he was on a beach defending a family who were being attacked by hoons with baseball bats. 'My own weapon was a pickaxe.' The dream/visions morphed, mutated and sometimes repeated. 'I'm wearing my long blue London Fog raincoat and I'm on the beach…and I'm very, very tired. I can barely walk…I'm looking for help from the people around me but they're all terribly feral and ugly people. They're looking at me scornfully.'

The causes of such hallucinations are unclear. Some researchers point to an inflammatory response that can affect the brain, particularly in older and less robust surgical patients. But while anaesthetic and pain drugs are among the likely triggers, the experiences seem to involve a melding of circumstances that surround our experience of surgery: events in the recovery room; our level of pain and anxiety; interactions with staff; as well as whatever it is we bring with us, the prisms and perspectives through which we experience our own worlds. It is a process that involves both the medical procedure and the person to whom the procedure is happening. The lines are blurred.

Which brings us back in a roundabout way to Rachel Benmayor, the woman who woke on the operating table feeling her child being cut out of her but unable to call for help. What happened to Rachel that day—the consciousness, the paralysis, the terrible pain—was just the beginning.

And then I realised that I was in a really amazing place. And I realised that I was very close to dying.

It was at this point that she shouldered through the flimsy threshold that marks the furthest reaches of science, and entered another realm altogether. I have no idea what to make of her experience. I can only tell you what she told me. Her story is neither reliable nor valid nor repeatable. Here, while she could still feel everything happening in her body, she was also distracted from it. She found herself in a vast room. A library.

It was like I was in the presence of everything that has been ever known by man and everything that ever will be. All things that could be known or understood were there, whether man had ever known or understood them. It was like there was this huge, huge vast presence and intelligence.

And in its presence, she said, she felt minute, fragmentary.

I had this feeling that I had seen something that no human being could ever, in a conscious state, be present to and be whole. That it was so vast that the consciousness of human beings—the little consciousness of human beings—unless it was under extraordinary circumstances, shouldn't or couldn't be privy to it. It was actually too big, too immense and I felt that I'd been forced there, and I had to survive it.

It sounds oddly like the experiences described by Jesse Watkins in R. D. Laing's 1967 classic *The Politics of Experience*, in which Watkins, following his own general anaesthetic, enters a sort of existential psychosis. 'I had a feeling at times of an enormous journey in front, quite, er, a fantastic journey, and…I had come to the conclusion, with all the feelings that I had at the time, that I was more—more than I had always imagined myself,' he told Laing, 'not just existing now, but I had existed since the very beginning, from the lowest form of life to the present time…and that what I was doing was experiencing them again.'

Ahead of him, he said, lay the most horrific journey. '[T]he only way I can describe it is a journey to the final sort of business of being aware of all—everything. It was such a horrifying experience to suddenly feel, that I immediately shut myself off from it because I couldn't contemplate it, because it sort of shivered me up—I was unable to take it…'

For Rachel Benmayor, for Jesse Watkins, these experiences (hallucinatory? visionary?)—one during an anaesthetic that failed, the other following one that had apparently worked—would vividly inhabit them for decades.

It was the same for a J. A. Symonds whose own experience following an operation under ether he recounted to William James:

A great Being or Power was travelling through the sky, his foot was on a kind of lightning as a wheel is on a rail, it was his pathway. The lightning was made entirely of the spirits of innumerable people close to one another, and I was one of them. He moved in a straight line, and each part of the streak or flash came into its short conscious existence only that he might travel. I seemed to be directly under the foot of God, and I thought he was grinding his own life up out of my pain. Then I saw that what he had been trying with all his might to do was to change his course, to bend the line of lightning to which he was tied, in the direction in which he wanted to go. I felt my flexibility and helplessness, and knew that he would succeed. He bended me, turning his corner by means of my hurt, hurting me more than I had ever been hurt in my life, and at the acutest point of this, as he passed, I saw. I understood for a moment things that I have now forgotten, things that no one could remember while retaining sanity.

Looking back on his own nitrous oxide adventures, James commented in *The Varieties of Religious Experience* on the persistence and authority of those visions, despite the near impossibility of knowing what to make of them.

One conclusion was forced upon my mind at that time, and my impression of its truth has ever since remained unshaken. It is that our normal waking consciousness, rational consciousness as we call it, is but one special type of consciousness, whilst all about it, parted from it by the filmiest of screens, there lie potential forms of consciousness entirely different.

And so it was for Rachel Benmayor, that day in the hospital as she gave birth to her daughter. In the vast space in which Rachel now found herself, the library—or perhaps something in the library, or something in Rachel—spoke to her. The things it said related directly to what was happening to her on the operating table, but were also universal—except for one that was just for her.

'So, the first thing that I was told was that life is breath. Life is Breath. Those three words. And what I understood from this was that breathing is the fundamental basis of life, and is our connection to life, and if we're not in that connection deeply, if we're not in that deep connection, then we're dying, we're dead.'

Her second message was more of a riddle—the sort of potted paradox with which rabbis and rinpoches tease the minds of young seekers. 'Everything is important, and nothing is important.' (She sighed as she said it). 'And that left me feeling in despair, as well as quite uplifted. It was such a dichotomy.

'The next one,' Rachel said steadily, 'was this: the reason why human beings don't like to feel pain is because, underneath all pain, physical and emotional, is the truth. Pain hides truth. So the truth is hard to find because it's underneath things that are not pleasant. But truth is not found in the pleasant. And when people move through pain, they find the truth. It's kind of a feeling of needing to accept the pain more, or to explore it more, or to be with it more, and to not be afraid of it.'

Was there a sense, I asked, that we tended to avoid pain because, frankly, the truth could be too much to bear?

'Yes, absolutely. Absolutely.'

So, here we have entered a realm where the strangest things can happen. Where a woman being cut open on a steel table can simultaneously be in an enormous library, hearing enormous messages. Where a fully conscious brain, apparently unimpeded by anaesthetic drugs, can manifest from the same set of neurons two overlapping incompatible realities, the one superimposed upon the other. *Look, look, it's a baby girl / The reason why human beings don't like to feel pain is because underneath all pain, physical and emotional, is the truth.*

It blows my mind. It blew her doctors' minds. And it very nearly blew hers away completely.

Rachel's next message was a personal one, relating to her

relationship with her husband. Then there was one final message. And this, she told me, was the one she had struggled with the most. 'That our life's purpose as a human being was to procreate. That having children was our primary focus as human beings.' This was not something Rachel had ever believed or wanted to. 'And I still don't want to believe it. I wanted my reason for being to be something a lot more elevated than having children…[But] there was this steady strong feeling…that that was true.' Whether that meant attaining a level of consciousness through her children, or continuing the human race, she did not know.

Rachel does not know if the words came from within or beyond her. Nor of course do I. But what her story did tell me was that within the reductive dualism of much Western scientific thought and language—conscious/unconscious, sleep/wake—here was something unaccountable. And while neurologists and psychologists could speculate about oxygen deprivation, hormone-induced hallucinations and electrical brain surges, what they could not account for was what was going on in Rachel's mind. The membrane, the messages. The otherness of it all.

I believed her account entirely. There is nothing I have observed in Rachel Benmayor that would make me feel otherwise. But the truth was that I had no idea what to do with her messages. I felt even that I had wanted something more from them—something that perhaps spoke more immediately to my own life. Some answer to a question I had not yet framed. The number 42. And where did they come from anyway?

Eventually I reasoned that the messages had (must have) erupted from within Rachel. Her own unconscious mind speaking at last—shrieking—to her conscious self: this is how it is; these are the things that matter. While most of the messages (except for the one about her husband) seemed universal, they did all relate directly to the awful situation in which she now found herself. For a long time I shuffled them around this manuscript, unable to decide where they belonged or what light they might shed on anyone but Rachel herself. Then I deleted them.

It would take me much longer to wonder if perhaps it was not, or not only, Rachel's unconscious—stripped back so brutally by the trauma of her daughter's birth—that was at play here, but my own.

Ghost stories

In the Blue Mountains west of Sydney there is a big yellow house filled with books. Varuna. These days it is a writers retreat. It was named by its original owners, the writer Eleanor Dark and her doctor husband, Eric, after the Hindu god of the oceans, and I don't think I have ever stayed there without the conversation drifting into talk of ghosts. One resident claimed to have looked out of her bedroom window on a moonlit evening to see a woman standing below in the garden looking back up at her. Another described a hand pressed against her shoulder. Midnight visitations, groaning bedsprings, baleful shapes in the corners. I stayed there with the American writer and teacher Robin Hemley, who reported seeing what appeared to be a sleeping form beneath the quilt in the Darks' marital bed. On another night, he woke in the same bed to see what looked like a figure standing against the curtains. He could not make out whether the figure was male or female but was convinced enough to ask out loud, 'Who are you?'

But in the main the ghosts are not of the house. They arrive with their owners and wait until these owners are soft and receptive before beginning to stir. Bottom dwellers compressed beneath the weight of unthought thoughts, they rise into the night like slow, flat fish. I experience at Varuna an unsettling sort of mingling, my days colonised by reveries and wavering absences; my nights swarming with half-thoughts and murky hallucinatory dreams. One night during the same week Robin Hemley saw shapes in his bedroom, another resident woke from a nightmare in which, through her mirror, she saw an old woman's corpse seize her from behind, wrapping pale powdery arms around her, locking them over her chest as she herself growled and sank her teeth into the sweet doughy flesh.

The house stands impervious; squaring its yellow stucco walls to the sun and the rain, holding calmly within it its cargo of unshelled creatures, mutant half forms, words. One morning I woke into the wash of dawn light and found waiting in the front of my mind the instruction, or statement: *permission to speak*.

But what to say? How do we speak the parts of ourselves that are not available to our own conscious inquiry? That we don't even know are there? And that may not, in any case, be available to language?

We can't march in with our big boots and kick down the doors (I have tried). We can't set traps for ourselves—we can see us coming. Sometimes we can create the conditions for those hidden parts to express themselves. We meditate or make art or do therapy or simply walk. But there are no guarantees. Consciousness is a small boat on an immense sea. We may learn to row, we may even rig up a sail, but we can't know what's beneath, let alone control it. Which means our conscious self can only ever tell us part of the story. The rest, that remnant topography, stays submerged beneath the surface of our daily life, creating its own currents and eddies and occasional whirlpools.

Sometimes it is left to our bodies to do the talking.

..

Around the time that David Adams published his study (ocean/ water) in the mid-nineties, I moved from Darwin to Sydney to write for the Australasian edition of *Time* magazine. The man I had gone to Darwin to be with had also moved down. For the last six months of our relationship we lived in separate apartments by the sea, unable to be together, unable to separate. I had three other close friends in Sydney at this time. Over a period of six months, one had a breakdown, one entered a deep depression and one began the final stages of his dying. In the early hours of each morning, as I lay frightened and sleepless in bed, I promised myself that today I would not drink and I would not smoke. Each night I came home from work, poured myself a glass of wine, lit up a cigarette, breathed in slowly and deeply, breathed out; made myself another promise. The friend I was living with was trying to lose weight and so kept the freezer filled with Lean Cuisine, which we ate two at a time, along with takeaway from the corner shop.

I had not been feeling particularly well for some time before I saw my doctor, but I felt that I was in better shape than most of those around me. My doctor looked at the results of the blood tests and told me I might recently have contracted the glandular fever virus and that my immune system might still be trying to combat its effects. 'Take a week off work,' she said. 'See how you feel.'

Walking away from the surgery, past the naval ships and ocean liners and crumpled grey waters of Woolloomooloo, I felt light and peaceful. I didn't believe I was ill, but I rolled the words around my mind. Glandular fever. Kissing disease. I rang work and went to bed.

Within three or four days I could barely walk. My legs, when I got up to go to the toilet or kitchen, felt light and shaky, far away from the rest of me. Alone in bed I felt neutral, dreamy, but as soon as I was required to do anything, I became teary, overwhelmed, exhausted. At the end of two weeks my flatmate put me on a plane to Canberra and my parents. There I stayed recovering for most of the following year.

For weeks, months, I lay in the bed that had been mine as a teenager, sleeping and staring at the walls. At mealtimes my mother brought me food, though I have no recollection of appetite. There were books by my bed which I did not, could not, read. Even speaking was too much. My words seemed pinned to the bottom of my jaw, and came out compressed and monosyllabic. I don't remember crying much, but there was a dampness, as if moisture were constantly seeping through my skin, and sinking. As if everything inside me had become viscous, liquid, beholden to gravity and I was draining always to the lowest point; the soles of my feet, my buttocks, my back.

Nobody knew what to call it—glandular fever, chronic fatigue—the labels drifted around but none seemed to stick. I don't remember any pain. I don't even remember depression, though it was there. What I recall is an exhaustion so utter that at the very centre of me I could only find cold.

My mother drove me down to the artificial lake around which the nation's capital is built. She parked in an alcove a couple of hundred metres from the water and we set off slowly together, my arm on hers, towards a wooden bench at the lake's edge. I walked like a very old woman, barely raising my feet from the ground. By the time we were halfway across I was spent—my body too heavy to drag, the rest of me insubstantial, as if I was spread so thin I would start to come apart, like clouds, and disappear. A thin, panicky feeling. We turned and shuffled back to the car.

And that was how it was. If I resisted it, pushed against the sickness, it would push straight back, a grey wash that could submerge me for days. I discovered that the things I had believed to be easy were often the most demanding. It was easier to move, to stand, to walk, than it was to think. It was easier to think than it was to listen. Easier to listen than to talk. As I began to get stronger I could measure my strength on any given day by my ability to communicate, my voice slow and flat, like a mop being dragged across a floor.

And then, beyond the outer layers of the illness (the weakness, the dullness of spirit, the incapacity), beyond too the concerns of others and the background guilt, was also a sort of luxury, a deep private pleasure in this passivity. I had given up: lain down. I was being looked after. My mother brought me soup in bed and my room was full of light and sweet Canberra air. Canberra has a reputation for being small and soulless, a suburb dressed up as a city, plonked in the middle of nowhere, three hours' drive from the ocean. But I loved it. It was a sanatorium. I liked its neutrality, its in-betweenness, its cafes and galleries. I forgave it its lack of a centre (even the large sign in its un-bustling main street, announcing 'city centre'). I came to love it less for what it was than where it was, six hundred metres above sea level in rolling high country, its air astringent, its streets lined with avenues of eucalypts. Somewhere buried among all these layers, too, unremarked on by myself or—in my presence at least—anyone else, was a profound sense of relief. Here, like this, no one could call me to account. I was a child.

This, then, is part of the story—the part that I know to tell. There is more to that story about illness. I feel sure of it. But how can I ever truly know?

Eventually I recovered. I resigned from my job and my relationship and moved to a seaside apartment in Sydney. In Bondi my bedroom window looked into the silvery yellow canopy of a huge old paperbark, and a five-minute walk away was the sea. On warm days I could wander barefoot with a towel over my shoulder to the beach and dive without thought into the crack of the waves. Everything was fresh and clean and salty. Most days I would pull on my walking boots and stride the two-and-a-half kilometres between the seaside villages of Bondi and Bronte. Along the ocean path cut into the sandstone cliffs, dropping down to cross pale sandy beaches and small rocky bays, then up again, taking the stone steps two at a time. Now and then, looking out across the ocean, I would watch pods of dolphins surfing the waves. Once, lying on my belly on a section of rocky overhang, I looked down and saw a solitary penguin in sharp muscular flight through the choppy swell.

But for all that I remember this re-entry into Sydney as a time of happiness and renewal, I had not managed to completely discard my old self. The stronger and healthier I felt, the more clearly I could see through the waters down to the rocks below.

Not long after I arrived I had an affair with a man who told me I was too nice for him. This was true, but when he dropped me I found myself retreating into a bleak, unedifying corner of myself. My doctor gave me the name of a woman in Paddington, a psychologist. She was a Buddhist, unnervingly beautiful with wavy dark hair and sometimes-fierce eyes. We did guided visualisations. She told me I needed to live less in my head and more in my body. When I felt anxious or uncomfortable, she said, the trick was not to avoid the feeling, but to observe it—size, shape, position, colour. She said the intellect was a tool and that I should not let it control me; that I should let myself be led by my unconscious. She suggested spontaneous acts such as driving home by a different and unplanned route, turning left or right on a whim. She had me sit with my eyes closed and follow the feeling of the breath as it entered and left my body. Even at the time I sometimes felt sorry for her. I talked around and around in circles. I talked about the man. I talked about other men. I talked I suppose about my family. Sometimes at the outer extremes of my awareness I could hear her trying to tell me things. But much of the time I did not, could not, listen.

Once or twice, though, things happened that I couldn't account for. One day as I was sitting on the couch in the room where she saw her clients I noticed a strange sensation. I was talking, I cannot recall what about. The memory is a feeling and an image: me talking, her listening, me talking and talking, and suddenly the sense that everything had shifted for a moment out of focus, as if sitting there in the room talking to my counsellor was not only me but, alongside, peeking out from behind, or from within, another me, a transparent glittering sphere that now slid across into the periphery of my vision. It was as if the self that had always seemed unavoidably, irretrievably set—gummed down and clogged up in an endless cycle of thoughts and words and stories—had quietly and unaccountably detached itself, and hung now alongside me, a momentary bubble upon whose gleaming skin my life, or the version I had been recounting, was reflected back for a few seconds in fleeting iridescent colours. Provisional. Passing.

It was not an idea or a metaphor. It was a feeling, almost a vision: very precise. I can no longer recall what became of the bubble, whether it burst or floated away or simply slid back inside, but as it all took place I tried haltingly to explain to my counsellor the feeling of what was happening ('Oh,' I think I said. 'Oh.') and when I looked back across at her I saw that she had tears on her face, which she wiped away with her hand, and I felt strange and light, as if nothing was solid.

It is hard to be certain, but sometimes I sense that my life is filled with such small slippages. And that what appears solid may simply be tiny islands of awareness surrounded by oceans of indeterminacy.

..

In any case, trying to interrogate even those parts of ourselves we are confident we *do* know is fraught. These days, the self that I know seems to me coherent, delineated. But in the end it is only the bits that are clear and delineated that make themselves available to be known—at least by the conscious me. In my life there are all sorts of gaps. In some of them I am sleeping, or on rare occasions fainting or even having an anaesthetic, but in others I am not. In some I am failing to appear at a party at which I was to have given a speech; or to make a phone call I have promised to make; or write a letter or an email to a friend, or commit to anything much at all. 'I know what you're like,' a friend once said, neither unkindly nor happily. I sort of knew what she meant. But what *was* I like? What am I like? What am I like when I am not here? Is that what I am like—sometimes here, sometimes not?

It is difficult to know what to do with these gaps. Perhaps the most peaceable strategy is to ignore them. Often I do. But sometimes the gaps spread and join and become presences. Like that strange ominous feeling that has travelled with me now for so long. And these are harder to overlook.

In an attempt to shift the feeling that threatened at times to submerge me, I began practising a Buddhist meditation technique called Tonglen. This was one in a big shapeless sack of strategies I rummaged through over the years (hypnosis, acupressure, herbs, talking therapy, walking therapy, white wine and red) to greater and lesser effect. Tonglen interested me in the ways in which it was similar to and different from anaesthesia. Unlike some other meditation techniques working with the breath, Tonglen did not involve the comforting idea of breathing in things you wanted (love, light, new shoes) and breathing out all the rest; it involved instead deliberately breathing in difficulty (yours or other people's: envy, pain, hunger, shit) and then breathing out something softer and lighter. It did not attempt to shift or excise, but rather to expand around hard things, and to bathe them in something like kindness.

Tonglen is the opposite of anaesthesia. It is a decision to move into discomfort, rather than away. It wakes you up and keeps you present. The in-breath is hard work—sometimes too hard. The out-breath can be too, but after a while, if things aligned, I found it softening the muscles and membranes of my chest, loosening the taut drum of my diaphragm, sending warmth spiralling down through my body to the pelvis and igniting its tiny pilot light, buzzing the soles of my feet. It is a natural muscle relaxant. I breathe in, I breathe out. I keep breathing. I come along for the ride.

I suppose, without knowing it, Rachel Benmayor might have been practising her own form of Tonglen when she turned around and burrowed into her pain that day on the operating table, until she pushed her way through and found herself in a vast space.

About halfway through the process of writing this book, I arrived for a two-week residency at Varuna, during which I had hoped to map out the structure of the book and work out exactly what it was I was trying to say. I knew I was writing a book about anaesthesia, but I didn't know why. Nor did I know why it mattered to me that I didn't know. Why does anyone do anything? What I was struggling with during my stay at the yellow house, however, was not simply why I was writing (and consequently, I felt, what I was really writing about), but who was doing the writing. There seemed to be two 'me's—each with their own agendas and itineraries and neither able or prepared to communicate with the other. Everything one wrote, the other rejected. One I will call the journalist—a pragmatic procedural self, this 'me' positioned myself as the objective observer reporting on what I found in my travels. The other I will call the dreamer. Not in the romantic sense, but the dreamer as fool, blundering around, kicking up fragments of a different story.

To the journalist this seemed highly suspect. It is one thing to have the 'I'—the so-called 'vertical pronoun'—writing itself into the story, offering opinions, musings and other such personal flourishes. But to have the 'I' as a subject of research—to take the vertical pronoun and lay it on the psychoanalyst's couch, or perhaps the surgeon's trolley (the pronoun now prone, horizontal)—seemed *improper*: self-regarding.

And yet every time I tried to harness my 'I' and wrest the book into a respectable journalistic narrative, it would thwart me. I would stand my pronoun ramrod straight, only to find it drooping and then subsiding wanly to the ground. Sometimes I would give in and decide to let it lie, only to be heckled by my conscious mind. *Do you really think anyone cares? Get up!* And so on. For several years already I had ricocheted between these two impulses, unable to reconcile them.

Finally, before this visit to the yellow house, I reached a decision that seemed firm. I would write a book about anaesthesia: its triumphs, its complexities and its perils. I would report in the first person—the pronoun standing duly to attention—about the people I had interviewed and about what I knew to be true. I would speculate modestly about the myriad uncertainties of a science that even practitioners agree is more of an art, and which involves the removal or alteration of an entity—consciousness—that we cannot yet define, let alone understand.

Above all, I would remain in control.

○

I am trying to find my dog, which is going to be put down. Not a dog I live with in my waking life, but another, a black Labrador.

The dog has already been taken away and is awaiting its death at a pound on the edge of town. This awful knowledge permeates my sleep. When I get there, however, my dog has gone. In its place, lying sick and exhausted on the concrete floor inside a large cage, is a young, very beautiful red setter. As I enter, the creature raises its head towards me and I see with slow shock that its muzzle has been sewn up with fishing line. The red dog pulls itself off the ground and limps towards me. Rising on its hind legs, it puts its forelegs on my shoulders, and rests its head against the left side of my neck. I can sense it begging me to save it. I feel great pity; I embrace and try to comfort it. But there is no sense that I can or will do anything to help it. The burden would be too great. Words come into my head. The dog's name: Gadget. (Why Gadget? I wonder, even in the dream.) Then the thought—with which I am already justifying my decision to abandon it—that red setters are not very intelligent dogs. I step away. The animal stands there, hopeless. I touch it on the back and I leave.

What to do with a dream like that?

Over time, various astute readers have suggested to me that this particular dream might not belong in this particular book, that it is a dream that emanates from somewhere else and that ought to be left there. Yet to me the dream—that image of the silent, silenced dog—seems not only a visceral evocation of the plight of a person who might be both anaesthetised and aware, but also to signify the chasm that exists between the conscious and unconscious minds: the one wordy, knowing, exclusive; the other voiceless, persistent, inclusive.

In the quiet after waking I lay curled on my side suffused with the knowledge of irrevocable loss. I had betrayed the red dog. And in doing so I understood that I had disavowed some helpless, voiceless part of me. The dream did not feel like a dream. The house was still and very dark. I did not know what the dog had been trying to say, but I could still feel almost physically the place above my left shoulder where it had nuzzled its head against my neck, and I accepted finally that I could not write this book without it.

SMALL BRIGHT FISH

General amnesia

June 2007. In a small room that leads into the operating theatre, a middle-aged woman lies on a metal trolley. Her hair has recently been tinted with a soft gold rinse and she makes small talk with the staff before she is wheeled in to the theatre. She is here for a hysterectomy, though no one mentions this, or the fact that she has cancer, which the doctors are hoping to contain by removing her womb. She has a cannula taped to the back of her left hand through which her anaesthetist—a craggy compact man, handsome, with dark hair greying at the temples and deep-set eyes—will shortly administer a milky drug called propofol.

The anaesthetist is Ian Russell. The woman, whom I will call Jenny, answers Russell's questions in bright monosyllables and rolls onto her side and bends her knees obligingly to her stomach, as instructed, for the trainee anaesthetist to insert first the injection of local anaesthetic to the skin and then the epidural cannula through which the nerve-blocking drug will be pumped to switch off sensation in her lower torso. The doctors give directions and make small, cheerful jokes. '[*This will be a*] little bit ticklish,' says Russell, as the needle is about to enter, and then when Jenny appears not to notice, 'Not ticklish. You're no fun!'

Jenny laughs thinly.

'Awrigh', nice and still then darlin',' says one of the assistants.

As he works, Russell issues instructions and explanations to the trainee anaesthetist who is still trying to insert between two vertebrae the implausibly large epidural needle. Then we move through the double doors into an operating theatre the size of a small classroom, with muted pink and blue linoleum tiles. ABBA on the radio: *SOS*. Machines bleat and instruments clatter as Russell and his trainee attach monitors: the pulse oximeter for measuring blood oxygen levels, the blood pressure cuff, the BIS monitor with its disposable electrode stuck like an oddly shaped bandaid on Jenny's forehead. Russell puts a long perpendicular strip of perspex under her body at shoulder height; on top of it is a black mould with a concave channel running its length. This supports Jenny's extended right arm. Then he attaches a black cuff around her forearm. It is made of some strong synthetic fabric and it reads *Lyall Willis & Co. Ltd. England latex free.* At her elbow he attaches two more leads that will allow him to send small electric shocks to the nerves which run down her forearm into her hand, to make sure that her nerves and hand muscles are still working when the cuff is inflated.

Russell gives the instruction to start the infusion pumps, which will push the anaesthetic into her bloodstream, and then puts a gas mask over her mouth and nose. 'Take a big deep breath.' Within seconds she is gone.

In 1993, as a little-known anaesthetist from the recursive Hull, Russell published a startling study. Using a technique almost primitive in its simplicity, he monitored thirty-two women undergoing major gynae-cological surgery at the Hull Royal Infirmary to assess their levels of consciousness. The results convinced him to stop the trial halfway through.

The women were put to sleep with a low-dose anaesthetic cocktail that had been recently lauded as providing protection against awareness. The main ingredients were the (then) relatively new drug midazolam, along with a painkiller and muscle relaxant. Before the women were anaesthetised, however, Russell attached what was essentially a blood-pressure cuff around each woman's forearm. The cuff was then tightened to act as a tourniquet that prevented the flow of blood, and therefore muscle relaxant, to the right hand. As a young intern Russell had learnt the method, known as the isolated forearm technique, from its inventor, anaesthetist Mike Tunstall. He had modified it himself to make it suitable for longer operations. By preventing the paralysing muscle relaxant from entering a patient's forearm, he hoped to leave open a simple but ingenious channel of communication—like a priority phone line—on the off-chance that anyone was there to answer him.

Once the women were unconscious Russell put headphones over their ears through which, throughout all but the final minutes of the operation, he played a pre-recorded one-minute continuous loop cassette. Each message would begin with Russell's voice repeating the patient's name twice. Then each woman would hear an identical message. 'This is Doctor Russell speaking. If you can hear me I would like you to open and close the fingers of your right hand, open and close the fingers of your right hand.'

Under the study design, if a patient appeared to move her hand in response to the taped command, Russell was to hold her hand, raise one of the earpieces and say her name, then deliver this instruction: 'If you can hear me squeeze my fingers.' If the woman responded, Russell would ask her to let him know, by squeezing again, if she was feeling any pain. In either of these scenarios, he would then administer a hypnotic drug to put her back to sleep. By the time he had tested thirty-two women, twenty-three had squeezed his hand when asked if they could hear. Twenty of them indicated they were in pain. At this point he stopped the study. 'My approval was to do a study of sixty patients altogether,' he recalled fourteen years later, 'but I couldn't really carry on, because they were all awake, nearly, you know.' When interviewed in the recovery room, none of the women claimed to remember anything, though three days later several showed some signs of recall. Two agreed after prompting that they had been asked to do something with their right hand. Neither of them could remember what it was, but while they were thinking about it, said Russell, both involuntarily opened and closed that hand. Fourteen of the patients who responded to Russell's question also showed some other signs of light anaesthesia (increased heart rate, blood-pressure changes, sweating, tears) during surgery, however ten did not. Overall, said Russell, such physical signs 'seemed of little value' in predicting intraoperative consciousness.

He concluded thus:

> If the aim of general anaesthesia is to ensure that a patient has no recognisable conscious recall of surgery, and views the perioperative period [*during the surgery*] as a 'positive' experience, then…[*this regimen*] may fulfil that requirement. However, the definition of general anaesthesia would normally include unconsciousness and freedom from pain during surgery—factors not guaranteed by this technique.

For most of the women in his study, he continued, the state of mind produced by the anaesthetic could not be viewed as general anaesthesia. Rather, he said, 'it should be regarded as general amnesia'.

The amnesic effects of hypnotic drugs are nothing new. The patient who, in 1845, ruined Horace Wells' demonstration by crying out as Wells pulled his tooth later claimed to remember no pain. In fact anaesthetists—and patients—have long relied upon the fact that, along with erasing consciousness, many hypnotic drugs prevent or disrupt memory. Amnesia—forgetting—is a useful and, many would argue, desirable side effect. For most of us it ensures that our first conscious memory after surgery will be of the recovery room or ward. It also means that if, as sometimes happens, a doctor deliberately wakes you during your spinal or brain surgery to check how you are going, you will probably answer her questions politely without recalling the conversation later. In recent years however there has been an increasing reliance on new short-acting intravenous anaesthetic drugs with powerful amnesic side effects. Sometimes they are used alone, sometimes in combination. One of the best known today is the sedative hypnotic midazolam—the drug that Russell was using on the women in the abandoned 1993 study. Another is propofol—the drug that he has just given Jenny to put her to sleep, and which today is probably the most popular intravenous anaesthetic in the world.

These drugs have many benefits in today's hospitals. They allow for a smoother slide into unconsciousness and, because they pass through the body relatively quickly, they allow doctors to give patients less anaesthetic—putting them at lower risk of drug-related harm and allowing them to wake up quicker, and with less nausea. Anaesthetists love them. And so do patients, on the whole.

What we as patients may not have considered, though, is that we are likely to start losing our memory for events well before we lose our consciousness of what is happening to us.

US anaesthetist Peter Sebel has described a disconcerting plane flight during which he ate a meal and made apparently coherent conversation with a fellow passenger, after which he went to sleep and woke up remembering nothing at all of the trip. Sebel, who later headed up a major US study into anaesthetic awareness, had taken a low dose of a drug known as a benzodiazepine (the best known are probably Xanax and Valium, but midazolam is another). He described the experience, or lack thereof, in a 1995 editorial, 'Memory during anaesthesia: Gone but not forgotten?':

> I was on an overnight transatlantic flight and said to my colleague, 'the dinner cart is one cabin ahead. I'm going to take a benzodiazepine so that I get a good night's sleep after dinner.' The following morning I awoke and said, 'That worked quickly; I was asleep before dinner,' to which he replied, 'No, you were not. You ate dinner and we talked all through the meal.'

Sebel had taken a 'sedative' dose of the drug—one that allowed him to function in a seemingly normal way, but which had profound effects on his brain nevertheless. At a higher dose, the drug would have knocked him out, at an even higher dose it might eventually have killed him. Benzodiazepines are a popular part of today's anaesthetic cocktails. Drugs such as midazolam are used to calm patients down before surgery as well as to put them to sleep, and then, generally in conjunction with anaesthetic gases, keep them that way. But before they have even knocked you out, they have knocked out your memory.

Sebel, in any case, had spent a chunk of his evening in a curious fugue state—fully conscious in the moment but unable to hold onto it in memory, or to know, except through the testimony of others, what had happened to him during that gap in time. It is a gap vaguely recognisable by anyone who has woken from an alcoholic stupor to find indefinite sections of the previous night missing. It is a gap also exploited by (mainly) men who covertly spike the drinks of (mainly) young women with a powerful drug called Rohypnol, once used as a pre-med in anaesthesia but now best known as the 'date rape' drug. It can render their prey groggy and compliant enough to allow themselves to be taken somewhere for sex, ('consensual' or otherwise), while leaving the victim with no memory of the attack, or even the attacker, and little recourse to justice.

More benignly, this gap is increasingly used by doctors for a growing subset of awkward medical procedures—ones that would once have been performed under general anaesthetic but can now take place in a state that anaesthetists sometimes call twilight sleep or, less poetically, conscious or procedural sedation. These include simple diagnostic tests such as colonoscopy (which involves navigating a very small camera on a long tube through your anus and around your large intestine) as well as major surgery such as some brain operations. It is an odd idea. Patients can sometimes obey instructions and talk with medical staff, but will later be able to recall nothing from the moments after the injection until 'waking' as if from sleep.

Another anaesthetic drug widely used for this purpose is propofol. Milk of anaesthesia. People sedated with propofol can hold onto old memories—who they are, why they are here, the capital of France—but lose track of new memories within seconds. The boundaries between consciousness, unconsciousness and whatever comes in between start to waver.

To anaesthetists it is all perfectly normal. On an anaesthesia discussion site I came across the following exchange.

Anaesthetist A: Conscious sedation can very well include conversation…even if the patient has no memory of it. Most often I spend the time at the end of conscious sedation cases answering the same questions over and over…they are sedated but have no recall but can converse.'
Anaesthetist B: Answering the same questions over and over has no relation to sedation. I do it with my wife all the time: 'Where were you?', 'Why are you late?', 'What were you

doing?', 'Why are you wearing golf shoes in the house?' On the other hand I might have been slightly sedated. :-)

Fifties humour aside, the advantages for both doctors and patients are clear. Sedated patients may be able to co-operate with staff, move when directed, cough on command and answer questions about their experiences. Smaller doses of drugs mean procedures that would once have required a night in hospital now take only hours. People 'wake' feeling sprightly, without the undertow of grogginess and nausea that might once have taken days to clear, or the risks of overdose. And, perhaps crucially, they are spared from remembering the indignity or discomfort of having a probe sent up their anus or down their gullet while in communion with a group of fully dressed doctors, nurses and other staff. It seems a convenient arrangement all around.

It is unsettling, though, to consider that at the heart of this altered state is an absence not necessarily of self but of memory— an oblivion at once retrospective and subjective. For the assembled doctors, nurses and anaesthetists, the working day is ticking by as predictably and incrementally as ever, as they delve into and perhaps chat with their seemingly cognisant charge. For the patient, time is being swallowed, or perhaps they are being swallowed by time, only to be spat out again later as if from a dreamless, unyielding sleep.

o

Back in the operating theatre, the overhead lights ignite and Jenny is bathed in a harsh whiteness that flattens her contours and leaches the colour from her soft body. Somebody pulls up her gown and fastens it so that it covers her breasts, leaving the rest of her exposed. There are eight or nine people now in the room. A young trainee anaesthetist with a round face tilts Jenny's face back and with the help of a metal implement inserts a long tube down her airway to help her breathe.

Ian Russell moves his face close to her ear. 'Jenny,' he says quite loudly, 'Squeeze my fingers with your right hand.' At first I think she has heard him. Her hand seems to close in a spasm around his. 'That's good, can you squeeze them again, Jenny?'

Then he says in the same clear voice, 'Jenny, can you let go of my fingers for a moment if you're awake? Let go.'

There is no movement. He prises his hand free. 'OK, so what we've got is a gripping,' he says to me conversationally. 'It's a reflex thing at the moment.'

This in fact is one of the grounds on which the technique is criticised—that it can be difficult to tell what is a purposeful movement and what is a twitch or spasm. Russell maintains that it is easy to know the difference if you take the time to check. The BIS monitor says 64—just above the recommended surgical range of 40 to 60. Staff paint brown antiseptic onto the woman's soft belly, then drape a blue cover over so that only the top of her face is clear.

Russell inserts two fingers again into Jenny's curled palm and speaks again into her ear. 'Jenny, squeeze my fingers.' Still the tightly curled grip. 'It's like a baby's grip, in a way,' he tells me, '…she wouldn't let go and she wouldn't squeeze.'

Russell now takes a pair of large black earphones and puts them over Jenny's ears. He turns on the tape that she will be played throughout surgery. Across the room the radio is warbling quietly. Classic hits. 'You Won't Find Another Fool Like Me.' The surgeons wear white gumboots and work quickly, hands dancing now inside her wide belly. A slight smell of burning. Staff talk quietly, intermittently. It is very matter of fact, although a tiny scrap of flesh sits disquietingly on her belly above the incision, like something left on the chopping board. Jenny is there but not. There is a sense more of vacancy than anything else—as if she has been deflated, and now she lies collapsed, waiting for someone to pump her up again.

A working hypothesis

The day before Jenny's surgery I had once again made the long train trip from London to Hull, past fields of lush flat green and blunt clumps of trees forming windbreaks: an efficient landscape, topped with low, textured clouds. Larkin country. I had learnt my lesson, and this time chose a small motel walking distance from the station, plain but inoffensive. That evening I met Ian Russell at a large, serviceable restaurant not far from the hospital. I had spoken to him previously by phone and found him helpful and frank. He had a daughter working in Australia and had trained there himself as a young anaesthetist. Over dinner we discussed swans, the isolated forearm technique and the permutations of consciousness. I had been prepared to find him a little intimidating. In print, he seemed more than usually forthright, at least for an anaesthetist. Instead he seemed relaxed and straightforward, although purposeful.

For anyone who has ever wondered about the point of international civic exchanges along the lines of 'sister city' relationships, Russell is proof of their efficacy. As a boy of eight growing up in Scotland, he was very taken when the nearby town of Perth received as a gift two black swans from the Western Australian city of the same name, and decided that when he grew up he would go to see some 'proper' ones. And so it was that his first job as a young anaesthetist was in Perth, Western Australia. On his first day in the operating theatre, he told me, he looked down at the paralysed patient and asked the question that had haunted him ever since. How could anyone be sure the patient was asleep?

The consultant anaesthetist, he said, had 'trundled out all the usual stuff about pulse rate, blood pressure, Guedel signs.' (Guedel was the guy who in 1937 mapped the planes of ether anaesthesia: *eyelid reflex abolished...paralysis of intercostal muscles* and so on.) The problem, said Russell, was that all of these signs were developed for ether, and depended on the patient's ability to move. Back home, at the Aberdeen Royal Infirmary, Russell continued to develop the work of his mentor Mike Tunstall who had first devised the isolated forearm technique to monitor women anaesthetised during caesarean births. For Russell, meeting Tunstall was life-changing. 'The answer I'd been looking for.' The two worked together closely and Tunstall encouraged the younger man to modify his technique for longer operations. Russell left Aberdeen in 1981 to take on the position of consultant anaesthetist at Hull. Shortly before changing jobs, he recalls walking unannounced into one of the theatres where a young woman was having her appendix removed. As he entered he overheard the scrub nurse telling the trainee anaesthetist that the patient was moving her left foot. He recounted the following exchange:

'What are you going to do?' Russell asked the young anaesthetist.

In answer, the young man picked up a syringe containing muscle relaxant and made as if to administer it.

Russell said, 'Let's just speak to her first.'

He asked the young woman to move her left foot again. Her left foot moved.

'Now what are you going to do?' he asked the anaesthetist.

'Give her more muscle relaxant,' repeated the trainee.

'Why?'

'Well she's moving her foot.'

'Yes, she's moving her foot, but why is she moving her foot?'

Silence. Russell spoke to the woman again, this time asking her to wriggle her toes. Which she did.

'She's moving her foot,' he told the trainee, 'because I asked her to. What does that mean?'

More silence.

'It means that she is awake,' said Russell.

'No, no, no, she can't possibly be awake! I'm giving her an anaesthetic.'

'No, you only think you're giving her an anaesthetic.'

Nine years after that encounter, in an arresting and provocative paper, American psychologists John Kihlstrom and Daniel Schacter observed that under hypnosis some people could be asked to study and learn a list of words which they were then instructed to forget upon emerging from hypnosis. When questioned, they would have no recall of the words they had learnt until the hypnotist gave a prearranged word or gesture, at which point the memory would return in full. 'By analogy,' they wrote:

> it may be that general anaesthesia leaves the patient's sensory and perceptual functions largely intact, but somehow impairs the formation of a permanent memory trace. From the standpoint of someone about to undergo surgery, this leaves open the horrible possibility that surgical patients are completely aware of what is happening to them during surgery, while the anaesthetic drugs produce an amnesia that effectively precludes postoperative recollection of their experiences.

Kihlstrom later said he had never seriously entertained this prospect: not in adequately anaesthetised patients. While it was possible in principle, he told me, he and Schacter had simply been comparing the effects on memory of general anaesthetics to those of other brain states in which one sort of memory (explicit) is impaired while another (implicit) might remain intact. 'All of this was mostly by way of laying out and analysing an issue that was sitting around.' The pair did go on to publish a study that found implicit memory in surgical patients. But this did not mean the patients were in any sense *conscious*, Kihlstrom stressed. 'Adequately anesthetised patients are unconscious by definition. The question then becomes: how much information-processing can be done by an unconscious person? The answer is: not much.'

What, then, to make of Ian Russell's patients squeezing his hand seemingly on command?

From where I now stand, Jenny's eye is half-open, like a child's in sleep, and I wonder briefly if she can see me. Russell puts out his hand and gently smooths it closed. Many doctors tape the eyes shut, he says, to protect them from injury—sometimes the surgical drape can rub against the eyeball, damaging the delicate surface—but he prefers not to. He says he once had a woman come to him after having been awake during her surgery. The only part of her body she could move, with enormous effort, was one eyelid. She described to him the struggle of forcing the eye open, and her desolation when the doctor simply closed it again. She tried again. This time someone shut her eye for her with tape.

The surgeons stand chatting intermittently, hands immersed in Jenny's belly. Theatre staff pass them slim silver instruments and white fabric swabs, which are wedged inside the flapping hole to help protect and hold her bowel out of the way. From where I stand near her head I can see a pinky-yellow rim of fat and pale flesh—it looks like pork—and the surgeons' latex-sheathed and red-streaked hands picking and probing with their clamps and scissors.

'You can have a look.' Russell gestures obligingly and, like an intruder, I creep a couple of steps closer. Inside the loose cavity of Jenny's abdomen, the doctors are snipping with their instruments around an irregular gleaming lump about the size of a plum. It looks terribly tender. As I watch, one of them dips in his hand and pulls from its dark, wet moorings the small purse of the womb. For a moment it rests there in his palm, glistening in its sheath, white-laced ovaries budding on either side. Then one of the blue-clad men leans across and puts the small bundle in a plastic kidney-shaped dish. 'So, that's what causes all the trouble,' says Russell philosophically, nodding at the dish and its contents. The wandering womb.

I notice a sharp line of pain across my chest. A rhythmic constriction. I remind myself to relax and breathe. In my mind I send some warm feeling towards Jenny.

o

In their 1996 analysis pulling together the numerous small studies into unconscious memory during anaesthesia, Canadians Philip Merikle and Meredyth Daneman posed the following question:

> Is it possible that general anaesthesia does not cause patients to become unconscious of all external events and that memory for events during anaesthesia actually indicates that patients experience fleeting moments of awareness during surgery?
>
> Given that the depth of anaesthesia fluctuates during surgery, it could be argued that any memory for information presented during anaesthesia may simply reflect brief periods of time during surgery when patients have some low level of awareness for external events. It is not possible to

give a definitive answer to this question because there is no
method available for continuously monitoring the depth of
anaesthesia…

Several of the anaesthetists I spoke with also speculated that
during anaesthesia, some patients might drift intermittently into
moments of wakefulness. Small bright fish that glint for a moment
and disappear. Again, much of what passes as evidence is circumstantial and often contradictory. Tests of hidden memories have trouble
distinguishing between those laid down without the conscious awareness of the memory holder, and those that might have been formed in
full or partial consciousness and then forgotten.

Researchers have tried to get around this wrinkle with a sleight
of mind called the process disassociation procedure. This relies on
the notion that the two different sorts of memory work not only in
different but opposite ways. An explicit memory, even forgotten, is
assumed to be under conscious control (though this too is debatable);
an implicit one, not. Thus a patient on awakening from anaesthesia
might be asked to complete word stems in two different ways: first,
by saying the first word that comes to mind, and, second by *not*
saying the first word that comes to mind, choosing instead a different
word with the same stem—a distinction apparently requiring more
conscious thought. My own brain boggles. Researchers then apply a
series of complex-looking equations to come up with a measure of the
relative contributions of conscious or unconscious brain processes to
any given answer.

But it is difficult to quarantine the two with any certainty.
Memories leak. And it is almost impossible to say for sure that a
memory now unavailable to its owner was formed consciously or
otherwise.

..

And what, *what*, *WHAT* is consciousness anyway? Neuroscientist Antonio Damasio thinks about this question a lot. One of his recent books begins in a plane. He has woken coming in to land, and now he contemplates what has just happened in his own mind. Not just the fact of the sights and sounds around him, but of his felt sense of himself at the centre of them, situated in space and time; coming home. He was asleep, now he is awake. But there is more to it than that: he is conscious.

For Damasio, consciousness is the end of a continuum of body-based experiences and mental states that start with the stirring of primordial feelings deep in the brain stem and culminate in you, wherever you are right now, reading this book and knowing you are doing so. You can be awake, says Damasio, without being conscious; you can have a mind that is active and forming images of the world around it—maybe even within it—without being conscious. You can have *experiences* without being conscious. It is the emergence of a sense of self as a protagonist of those felt experiences—'modestly at first, but quite robustly later'—that marks the beginning of consciousness. Mind with a twist, he calls it.

It's lovely stuff—Damasio writes gorgeously—but it's probably not much help to working anaesthetists: they tend to regard wakefulness as a bad thing. With or without an attendant self.

Some researchers have, nevertheless, hedged their bets and proposed a sort of almost-anaesthesia. A good-enough version, in which patients may be wakeful without being considered aware. Britain's Jaideep Pandit posits a state he calls 'dysanaesthesia'. ('Patients in this state can be aware of events but in a neutral way, not in pain, sometimes personally dissociated from the experiences.') Definitions waver and drift, although doctors who think about such things tend to link such experiences to lighter anaesthesia such as you might experience towards the end of surgery while being stitched up, or near the start when the breathing tube goes into your trachea.

In the end, however, the Canadians Merikle and Daneman concluded that despite the 'remote possibility' of some people experiencing moments of awareness during anaesthesia, it was reasonable to assume that patients were unconscious. 'It seems improbable that patients have experiences during anaesthesia that are similar in any way to the subjective experiences normally associated with conscious perception of external events. Thus a reasonable working hypothesis is that patients are unconscious during surgery.'

Ian Russell maintains the hypothesis is flawed.

In the absence of the isolated forearm technique, he argues, some of the studies supposedly demonstrating that people can form hidden memories while they are unconscious instead prove the opposite—that patients are frequently awake and sometimes in pain on the operating table but cannot remember later. He includes in this critique studies that have relied on EEG-based monitors to guide the anaesthesia. In mid-2006, to prove his point, he published a new study using the IFT in conjunction with a commercial depth of anaesthesia monitor, the Narcotrend, which, in addition to presenting the raw EEG, analyses brainwave activity and then converts the data into numbers and graphs representing the stages of anaesthesia. The study looked at twelve women having gynaecological surgery with muscle relaxants. Russell adjusted the amount of anaesthetic each woman received according to the feedback from the monitor. Once again he played each woman a tape that included his voice asking her at regular intervals to open and close the fingers of her right hand. Unlike the earlier experiment, all but one of the women had also been given an epidural nerve block to prevent pain. But the results were again startling. All twelve patients responded with their non-paralysed hand at some point during surgery despite the fact that on more than half these occasions the numeric readout either showed them to be at surgical levels of anaesthesia or was blank. Patients seemed to dip in and out of consciousness, sometimes responding in apparently deep anaesthesia but not at lighter levels. Again none of the women said they remembered the experience, though in interviews afterwards some recalled Russell's taped instructions.

More recently, Russell has staged similar experiments using the IFT alongside the BIS monitor. While the number of women who responded dropped to one-third when staff used an inhalation anaesthetic, another study using an intravenous drug showed that during BIS-guided surgery nearly three-quarters of patients still responded to command—half those responses within the manufacturer's recommended surgical range.

Russell is an admirer of the BIS, which he considers a useful tool, but his concern about brain monitors more generally is that the complex algorithms on which they are based tell the anaesthetist only the probability that a particular patient is asleep at any single point, and cannot account for the natural variability between patients.

Unsurprisingly, Russell has his own critics. Debate ricochets back and forth over the IFT's alleged technical limitations and what some see as its potential for distraction or even disruption during surgery. The manufacturers of the Narcotrend sent me a long and cordial defence of the monitor arguing among other things that Russell had used uneven and at times inadequate pain relief in the 2006 study—concerns that Russell has fiercely disputed but which were also raised about the studies using the BIS. Kate Leslie points out that Russell's studies are tiny compared with the BIS study she and Paul Myles carried out, meaning his results might have arisen by chance. In the BIS experiments above, she notes, surgery took place when patients were at the highest end of the recommended range (higher, she says, than is normal practice) and sometimes above it. Even many supporters see the IFT primarily as an experimental tool.

This is not to suggest Russell is alone in his findings. A 2012 literature review by a fellow Brit, Robert Sanders, showed thirty-seven per cent of anaesthetised patients responding to the IFT after 'noxious external stimuli'. That said, the review only included thirteen studies, most involving fewer than forty patients, and five carried out by Russell himself. There have been no large-scale clinical trials to assess the technique or determine its benefits or risks.

But the other intriguing thing about Russell's experiments with the Narcotrend and BIS monitors is the intravenous drug he chose to use: propofol. The same drug now coursing through Jenny's bloodstream as the surgeon plucks and snips at her abdomen. Russell loves propofol. It is fast and effective. His patients wake up happy and refreshed. He remembers one woman complaining when he woke her, saying he had interrupted a nice dream. Propofol is like a little holiday. Unlike many anaesthetists, Russell does not even combine it with a gas anaesthetic to give him more certainty. He says he already has certainty. The problem as he sees it is not with propofol, but with the doctors who use it, many of whom, he claims, do so too sparingly. 'Basically what is happening is you're tying the patients onto the operating table with your muscle relaxants, and they may be awake...'

The operation is nearly over. The doctors are stitching Jenny's abdomen. Russell starts to lighten the anaesthetic ('...just given her a bit more relaxant because she was wincing slightly; her hand had moved slightly and her eyebrows...a slight wiggle'.) Now the BIS has dropped again and she has stopped 'responding'.

'How did you know that was a relaxant thing and not an anaesthetic thing?' I ask.

'I didn't. I just thought she was, um, looking a little bit...' He glances at the woman on the table. 'Here we go,' he says, with interest, and moves across to take her hand.

'Jenny, squeeze my fingers with your right hand.'

And this is the moment.

From where I stand against the wall, level with her arm, I watch her hand close firmly and unambiguously over his.

'That's excellent. Wonderful. Now I want to know if you're comfortable Jenny. If you're comfortable, squeeze my hand twice.'

Her hand closes once more, clearly, purposefully. And again.

Like a message from a miner trapped far underground.

'That's fantastic,' Russell tells her, 'OK. Operation's nearly finished. Everything's going well.'

He moves away. The stitching continues. The BIS is back up to 64—above the ideal 40 to 60 range BIS manufacturers recommend for surgery, but within the accepted surgical range for these final stages of surgery, he says. He notes that under the protocol in Paul Myles' and Kate Leslie's B-Aware study, at this stage of the operation 'they were letting the BIS drift up to 75 for the last ten, fifteen minutes of the surgery' before giving a reversal drug to counter the paralysing drug. 'And they said the patients woke up very quickly. A lot of the patients were probably awake already...'

Jenny's BIS continues to hover around 65. Russell is relaxed. 'She gave a quite clear indication that she's comfortable.' Within a minute or so it is over. Jenny lies immobile on the trolley while staff pack up around her. The surgeon, a short pleasant man with a self-deprecating sense of humour, thanks the team. A few metres away, doctors discuss another case, a woman whose cancer has spread through her body. Any surgery, they say, would be palliative—to treat the pain, not the disease, which is now unstoppable. The doctors discuss logistics. There is some question about whether she is even fit for an anaesthetic. I look back across at Jenny lying silently in the centre of the room. I wonder if she too can hear what the doctors are saying, and if so what she might make of it.

The memory keepers

About three hours south of Sydney is a scoop of ocean called Jervis
Bay. We used to go there for summer holidays. I remember loping
down to the beach one Christmas morning with my sisters and Dad,
when he could still lope; topping the rise to see a pair of dolphins,
another; another; kinetic arches against the white blue. More recently
I have visited with a group of friends, one of whom has a house there.
Sometimes we drive around the corner from the main beach to a
smaller, quieter one, a vivid jag between two rocky outcrops. The
first time we went was the year of my back surgery. Everything hurt.
My body was foreign. I was afraid of movement, of jolting, of metal
snapping inside me and poking through. I moved like a stick figure,
step by stiff step, across the narrow beach and into the slot of the sea
until I was deep enough to sink. And then I let my legs loosen and
rise until I was floating. Head down (goggled, snorkelled) slow-flying
over the receding sandy floor, weightless, wantless, and all around me
twisting lozenges of light. Whiting.

Sometimes when I am in the unbeautiful pool, when I put my
head underwater and see darkening grout and nameless filaments, I
say the words to myself (dappling, dappling) and slowly, magically, it
is all there before me. Not the exact place, but an echo or overlay. A

feeling. All light and depth and splinters of silver. Whiting Bay.

In hospital, after her collapse, my mother woke morning after morning into a white room almost identical to the one in which she was actually lying. (Hooked to catheters and drips, a diffuse morphine wash.) This other hospital room looked the same but was, in some qualitative way, different. Mum was puzzled at how the same nurses appeared in both rooms. Narrowing her eyes. 'It's happening again'. Slippage. One night she dreamed of Brunswick Heads, a coastal town far from home. Had she ever been there, I asked, to the real Brunswick Heads? She could not recall. She thought she might have. Outside the wind thickened. In the night, she said, it sounded like the sea; perhaps that was why she was dreaming of the coast. 'I think a lot of my dreams come from the sounds around me.'

Another hospital. Sydney, 1997. My father, delirious. Flailing. The previous day he had been admitted to a private hospital in Sydney for heart surgery. My parents drove from Canberra and I from the Blue Mountains. Afterwards, my mother and I followed a nurse into the intensive care unit, where we found a row of four trolley beds lined up like prams against the far wall. On each one, motionless against the starched hospital pillows, a pale sunken head: balding, foetal and to me disconcertingly similar. At first I walked towards the wrong one. Mum called me back and for most of the rest of the day we sat or stood on either side of my father's bed as he made his ungainly, spasmodic journey towards consciousness. Like birth, like death, it took its time. Hauling himself out of his stupor, he appeared to recognise us and launched into a circular sort of conversation that was to continue for most of the afternoon. In between periods of mumbling and silence he would announce in tones of agitation that he needed to go to the toilet. One of us would explain to him gently and clearly what had happened, that he had had an operation, that the doctors had inserted a catheter so he could go whenever he wanted. Sometimes he would settle down for a minute, but at others would continue in increasing distress. 'This is awful. I want out, Bridgey,' —my mother's name, Brigid—'I want out!' And then again: 'I need to do a wee.' This went on for hours. Every few minutes one of us would explain again what was happening and he would subside. Minutes later it would begin the same refrain: 'Bridgey I want out; this is fucking awful.' A few times he reared up and made to pull the tubes out from his arm and get out of bed, and the ICU staff would hurry over and press him firmly down. Some were kind. Some less so. One nurse spoke to him loudly as if to a stupid child, and then to us: 'He's not making any sense.' My mother and I thought he was making pretty good sense. Once a male attendant muttered that if this had been the public system my father would have been properly 'restrained'.

Whether this would have been preferable to the practice, described in an 1834 edition of *The Lancet*, of treating post-operative delirium with a laudanum enema is hard to know. No one seemed particularly interested in why he was behaving as he was. His doctor told us my father had had a bad reaction to the anaesthetic. The next day, propped up in bed, frail but recognisable, he remembered none of it.

He went on to recover fast and fully, at least physically, although I felt it was a long time before he regained his buoyancy. Years later, however, comparing this experience with his childhood surgery, he was very clear which he preferred. Of the earlier anaesthetic he said:

There was a sense of suffocation. They put this thing, which presumably was soaked in the anaesthetic, they put this over your nose and mouth. This is my recollection. I'm not being unkind about it. I'm not saying there was anything brutal about the procedure, but that was the procedure. Certainly there was this sense of suffocation. You did *not* want this to happen.

It wasn't remotely like what happened to me last time [*with the heart surgery*]. *You* were all aware I wasn't having a nice time. *I* wasn't.

In the same edition of the *British Journal of Anaesthesia* in which Hull anaesthetist Ian Russell reported patients squeezing his hand during surgery even when brain monitors indicated they were unconscious, there was an accompanying editorial by New York anaesthetist Robert Veselis. I had first heard of Veselis through Melbourne's Kate Leslie. He was 'the memory guy', she said, adding that she had once had lunch with him in Paris. 'He's sort of kooky but really nice.' The next time I came across him was in this editorial, 'The remarkable memory effects of propofol', in which, after praising Russell's work, he went on to draw a completely different conclusion. What interested Veselis was not so much what the study said about the Narcotrend monitor—or indeed any other depth-of-anaesthesia monitor—but what it confirmed about the drug propofol, which he said must now be added to the list of 'prototypical amnesic drugs'—drugs that make you forget. Then, he went on to raise a rather startling question about the purpose of anaesthetic monitoring. '[T]he question is whether we want a monitor to detect unconsciousness or one that detects amnesia?' As long as anaesthetists could guarantee forgetting, he seemed to suggest, unconsciousness might be optional.

The article drew a swift response from Bristol anaesthetists Khaled Girgirah and Stephen Kinsella. 'It suits anaesthetists to tell patients that awareness is a rare complication, occurring in 1–2 per thousand,' they retorted in a letter to the journal. 'However, this figure relates to awareness with recall. We thought that it might be less reassuring to tell them that they have a 16 per cent chance of being awake during surgery, or even "you are sure to be awake for some of the time during surgery".' (They were referring to Ian Russell's studies using the isolated forearm technique.)

The pair then described a straw poll they had taken of sixty anaesthetists in their own hospital. The question was whether they, personally, would find it acceptable to be awake during surgery, 'even though you did not remember afterwards'. Three-quarters said no. What about being awake and paralysed, even without later recall? This time ninety-three per cent said no. Asked, finally, would they be up for the trifecta—awake, paralysed and in pain (albeit without any later memory of the experience)—the figure went up to ninety-seven per cent.

'We think that if most anaesthetists wish to be unconscious rather than amnesic during general anaesthesia,' Girgirah and Kinsella concluded, 'it will be a long time before it is possible to convince the public that this is acceptable or desirable.'

I phoned Veselis in his New York home, which he at that time shared with his wife, four kids, four rescue cats and two rescue dogs. He seemed easy to like. In practice, he said, he was not suggesting that it was all right for patients to be in pain even if they did not remember it. Pain during surgery could, after all, set patients up for chronic pain later. Like many of the surgical staff I spoke with, Veselis acknowledged it was not unusual for patients to wake during surgery. ('People wake up all the time,' one intensive care nurse told me, 'but we put them straight back again.') Ultimately, though, he said, for patients whose pain was well controlled, periods of wakefulness during surgery need not be a problem—as long as they didn't remember them.

'I think that most people seem to accept the fact that if the explicit memory has disappeared—or awareness has disappeared; you don't remember—there does not seem to be as much concern about that...'

The greater risk was posed by over-medication. His point, he said, had been that in their attempts to ensure that patients could not complain of having been aware, anaesthetists tended to give more anaesthetic than they needed to. In reality, and with today's clever drugs and monitors, it was no longer necessary—and could be dangerous—to keep patients that deeply drugged. 'Unconsciousness is a good starting point, but a more refined consideration is that actually what we want is amnesia—that is really what we want.'

In an eloquent response to his Bristol counterparts in *BJA*, Veselis argued that current practice was driven by anaesthetists' 'visceral fear of failure'. He recalled Horace Wells' disastrous 1845 demonstration. The screaming patient. The mocking onlookers. 'This untoward response to anaesthesia rests heavily on our collective consciousness, and is reinforced with every new case of awareness.'

The solution, he said, lay in understanding the complex systems involved, and making them reliable (which is perhaps a little like saying the solution lay in introducing the hydrogen economy or solving the mystery of consciousness). In practical terms, this meant understanding how each component of anaesthesia—particularly those elusive processes relating to consciousness, memory and pain—worked, and developing reliable monitors to measure them. Until then, he conceded, 'it is always safer and more reassuring to err on the side of over-medication'.

Towards the end of our conversation, I told him about my father and his ether dream. Veselis told me about one of the family's adopted dogs. This one had clearly been abused, he said, before coming to them. The animal would growl if anyone approached it from behind; and it was afraid of tall men. Veselis is a tall man. When we spoke, the dog had been with the family for fifteen years. It was still wary of Veselis, though not of his wife. It still growled if anyone came near its rump. 'It is fascinating how some memories stay there no matter what you do.'

Night football. Down at the oval, the girls' team is training. A little way back, a girl—dark glossy skin, dark glossy hair, maybe sixteen—watches with a small ambiguous smile as the dogs, blonde and black, lollop towards where she sits, legs crossed, on a wooden bench, watching. At first I think she is pleased (the smile keeps flickering across her face), but then I notice the small movements of her hands. (*Away. Away.*) I call the dogs, who oblige for now. The girl apologises. She's trying to get better, she says, with dogs. I apologise back. I ask if she was ever bitten. She says that no, but when she was a small child...So, where is she from? Sudan. (Oh, yes, of course, the dogs.) They used to run in packs, she says, around the streets. She left when she was four. A long time ago. But anyway. Now she is trying to train herself. The black dog, more than usually silly, snuffles once more towards her. Again the slight shrinking, the wavering smile.

Veselis has warned too against doctors relying on amnestic (forgetting) drugs to erase memories of events that have already taken place ('the much sought after retrograde memory effect'). 'Many practitioners remember an experience of a patient opening their eyes and looking at them when they should have been fully asleep!' he wrote in his *BJA* editorial on propofol. 'A typical response in such a situation is to give a sizeable dose of a readily available hypnotic/sedative drug. The nervous practitioner was [*sic*] then reassured when no memory of this event was present at the post-operative visit.' In reality, he said, any amnesia would have been due to drugs given *before* the event, not afterwards.

None of which would be news to Rolf Sandin, the Swedish anaesthetist whose team in 2000 showed that patients' ability to recall waking during surgery comes and goes depending on how long after the operation you speak with them. While benzodiazepines such as midazolam are useful for reducing anxiety, he wrote, their widespread use before surgery may have as much to do with their reputation for bringing about amnesia. This was a risky assumption, he said, given that the drug effects varied. 'More importantly, we believe that to carry out anaesthesia in a way that would require deliberate pre-emptive amnesia for intraoperative experiences is ethically unsound.'

One: it may not work. Two: it shouldn't have to.

As to how many people wake like this without later remembering; who knows? A new international study—the biggest so far—suggests that things may be quite a lot better than imagined. Or quite a lot worse. It depends on your perspective. After using the isolated forearm technique to test the responses of 260 surgical patients who had just been intubated under general anaesthesia, researchers found twelve people—4.6 per cent—who demonstrated what they called 'connected consciousness' (connected to the outside world, that is, rather than to their dreams or other internal states); five of whom indicated they were in pain; none of whom remembered later. This is a lot less than the previous estimate of thirty-seven per cent. But a lot more than the one or two in a thousand people who generally report having been awake in large-scale trials. Twenty to fifty times more. (And this isn't even counting the additional seven per cent who during the study moved a hand unbidden after having the tube put in, but before researchers popped the question.) Nor does it resolve the question of what it is exactly the researchers were measuring.

Ian Russell, for his part, remains convinced that a lot more patients are awake for part of their surgeries than they—or their doctors—know.

But so what?

'Robert Veselis says that might be part of adequate anaesthesia,' I suggested to Russell.

'I would say that it is probably possible that it is normal anaes-thesia, I wouldn't say that it was adequate anaesthesia.'

Again, so what? Despite some strongly held beliefs and a well-polished collection of odd anecdotes, there is little solid evidence for those who are convinced not only that many patients may be at least partially present during surgery but that this might matter later.

In Hull in 2004, on the second day of that perplexing memory and awareness conference, psychologist Michael Wang delivered a brief verbal report about a study he had carried out with Ian Russell and another researcher, looking at the mental state of eighty women in the three months after hysterectomy surgery. Based in part on the women's arm movements as measured by the isolated forearm tech-nique during their operations, the researchers divided the women into two groups deemed to have been lightly anaesthetised ('wakeful') or heavily anaesthetised ('non-wakeful'). None of the women reported any memories of the surgery, but psychological testing—one month and three months after surgery—showed 'a consistent pattern of higher mean levels of psychopathology in the "light" group in comparison with the "deep" group'. Basically, the lightly anaesthe-tised women were more anxious than the others.

On the same day in Hull, Wang and Russell presented another brief 'poster session'. This one related to a follow-up to Russell's disturbing 1993 study: the one he aborted after two-thirds of the supposedly unconscious women squeezed his hand to indicate that they were not only awake but in pain. Ten years later Russell, Wang and another researcher tracked down as many of the women as they could find and interviewed them about their mental health over the past decade. Although the numbers were too small for statistical analysis, the results were curious. Three patients in the group who had indicated during their surgeries that they were awake had suffered some sort of psychiatric disturbance since the operation. None of them had any previous psychiatric history. Nobody in the control group—those who had not responded to the command to squeeze Russell's hand during the operation—showed any evidence of distress.

Wang says he and Russell would have liked to expand the studies into larger trials that might provide some more definitive answers but lacked the resources to do so. Both remain concerned about what these experiences might mean for some patients' longer-term health.

Here is US medical psychiatrist Richard Blacher writing in 1984:

> It might behove us to rethink the routine use of amnestic drugs. While these have seemed to serve a most useful purpose in creating a calm aftermath to surgery, they mainly may, in reality, protect *us* from hearing upsetting details from patients, details that are now stored in the cerebral cortex but no longer recalled consciously...[T]he unconscious storing of a traumatic memory may well act as a chronic psychic irritant...

Not one of the anaesthetists I spoke with, apart from Ian Russell, supported this suggestion. Most argued in fact that it was immoral *not* to use amnestics, particularly if a patient was known to have been or suspected of having been awake, because traumatic memories could trigger post traumatic stress disorder. 'If someone woke up in the middle of one of my anaesthetics and I knew about it I would certainly give them an amnesic drug there and then,' one Australian anaesthetist told me. 'You might consider,' he continued, 'that if you could forget about it and don't remember it and don't go into any of the post traumatic stress disorder problems, that you've actually treated it.' German doctor and Nobel Laureate Albert Schweitzer might have been right when he said that happiness was nothing more than good health and a bad memory. (Schweitzer's wife, as it happens, was an anaesthetist.) Several anaesthetists I interviewed told me they had patients whose sole request before surgery was that they not remember anything of the operation.

I think of my son, now twenty, whom I recently retrieved after he had his wisdom teeth extracted under general anaesthesia. I found him sitting up in bed, grinning hugely and scooping enormous gobs of green into his bandaged face. The nurse regarded him wryly, gestured to me the flailing of arms. 'Most teenage boys wake up a bit feisty after dental surgery.' My son kept on beaming: 'Jelly and ice-cream! Best day ever!'

Even so, the patient may not be the only beneficiary of such oblivion.

Twenty years ago, if you were having your varicose veins treated you would have entered hospital the night before and been woken in the morning by a nurse to swallow your 'pre-med'—usually a powerful benzodiazepine sedative such as Valium—to make you sleepy and relaxed before going into theatre. You would have woken some time after the operation, probably feeling quite nauseated, and would have spent that night in the ward before going home the next day.

Today you are more likely to arrive at the hospital on the morning of the operation and go straight to theatre, where, as part of the anaesthetic brew, you will get a dose of a potent amnesic drug such as propofol. This allows doctors to use lower doses of the other anaesthetic agents, meaning you wake quicker, feeling better, and go home sooner. While this has benefits for you as a patient, including a lower risk of catching a hospital-borne infection, it also saves hospitals time and money. Occasionally a lot of money. People who wake up during operations—or at least people who remember waking up—sometimes sue. Traumatised patients in the US have reportedly been awarded damages in the hundreds of thousands of dollars. Others, including Carol Weihrer, have settled out of court.

○

New York psychiatrist David Forrest has a novel theory. He believes some patients might mistake surgical staff for aliens. Some years ago Forrest, a clinical professor of psychiatry at Columbia University, came across a book by Harvard postdoctoral psychology student Susan Clancy about people who believed they had been abducted by aliens. Clancy had noted that the abductees shared similarities including a history of sleep paralysis and the ability to be hypnotised: also, perhaps unsurprisingly, 'a preoccupation with the paranormal and extraterrestrial'.

Forrest went on to propose another possible link. Many of the reports of abduction, he said, bore 'more than a passing resemblance to medical–surgical procedures'. In a paper presented to the American Academy of Psychoanalysis and Dynamic Psychiatry in 2007, he went on to ask:

> Could dimly or subconsciously recalled memories of surgery play a part? One is in a state of altered consciousness (anaesthesia), surrounded by green figures (surgeons) whose eyes are more noticeable above their masks, in a high tech ambience with a round saucer-like bright object above (the OR light), and the body's boundaries are being breached by intubation, catheters, intravenous needles and the surgery itself. Perhaps surgery in childhood would be especially contributory...

He thought such forgotten memories might have been formed in the operating theatre before the patient passed out, or unconsciously during surgery. Like many of the stories of alien abduction, Forrest noted, surgery involved nakedness, pain and a loss of control—yet in both scenarios the probing figures were often felt to be benevolent. The similarities, he has since argued, are too great to ignore. He also suggests that physiological changes in the heart rate, blood pressure and muscle tone of self-professed abductees might be comparable to those found in surgical patients.

(I was excited to discover, after speaking with Forrest, that during the original B-Aware study of the BIS monitor, one patient did later report having dreamed about aliens, and thinking that 'aliens had taken over the operation'. It turned out, however, that theatre staff had been chatting about extraterrestrials during the procedure.)

Forrest admits that his hypothesis may be hard to test, partly because it is difficult to find authentic 'abductees' (as opposed to enthusiastic hoaxers) willing to participate in such formal investigations, but he says this doesn't mean it shouldn't be tested. If doctors are indeed causing such experiences 'in a small but vulnerable proportion of the population, which still might number in the millions,' he says, 'we should know about it'.

Aliens aside, this anaesthetic amnesia leaves us in the strange position of not being the keepers of our own memories. Instead the experience, or at least the recollection of the experience, is owned by other people: by doctors, nurses and other staff. By strangers. In some ways of course, this is true of much of life, and most particularly childhood. We forget what others remember. Strain as I might, I can only reconstitute at will a handful of memories before the age of about five. A concrete paddling pool in a park in Wimbledon, where I lived between the ages of one and three with my parents and later my infant sister, Sarah: me at one end of the pool all but submerged, eyes level with the dark glassy expanse of water, the late afternoon sun. Another afternoon in the kitchen at Box Hill, perhaps aged five; my baby sister

Jennet in the high chair; a knock at the door. Even these memories now exist more as markers, a reproduction of a memory that I used to have. Most of my early childhood exists, or can be narrated, only through the stories of my parents and to a lesser extent my sisters. And I in turn carry in my memory many of the remaining traces of my son's and daughter's early years. It seems to me a huge responsibility: to know so much more about a person than they can know about themselves. Or than they know that they know. ('Do you remember your fourth birthday?' asked psychiatrist Graeme Burrows. 'Because it's all inside you...')

o

I have found a new pool. A pool that is in reality two pools, in my mind superimposed one upon or within the other. Ringed by gum trees; ringed by apartment blocks and traffic. One is close to my house, one is a little further away. Both are long and lean and topped by sky and once my head is underwater they are the same. Dappling. Sometimes, like today, when the sun is out, the dappled shadows beneath me take the form of small three-dimensional structures that skate and warp along the tiled floor just ahead of me. Fluctuating versions of those 3D models of atoms or molecules or chemical compounds I sometimes come across in books on anaesthesia. Other days they stretch into an uneven whitish membrane more like the connective tissue you peel from the outside of lamb shanks. Or the shapes I see when I look into someone else's eye. I swim with goggles, and as I track up and down, up and down, I sometimes notice a small dark filament that floats in front of me within the pool of my own eye, keeping pace as I slide above the dapples.

Today I suddenly felt that the eye, my eye, was all around me and that I was the tiny speck hanging darkly before myself, a floating spindle around which the world and all its perspectives rushed.

The perfect anaesthetic

A while ago my father went into hospital again, as an outpatient, to have a colonoscopy. After the doctors had threaded a probe through the coils of his large intestine and found, or not found, what they were looking for, someone rang my mother. She returned to the hospital where she found my father lying in the recovery room, and asked, 'How did it go?' He looked at her with a weary disgruntled expression. 'I don't know. I'm still bloody waiting to go in!' This, from the point of view of Robert Veselis and almost every other anaesthetist in the world—not to mention my father—was the perfect anaesthetic.

Yet it is odd to think that my father may have been not only awake, but able to answer questions, follow instructions and perhaps even make conversation during all or part of the procedure. I picture him there in his indeterminate hospital gown, my private and dignified father, curled on his side, grunting in response to some probe or question. (Are you comfortable Mr Cole-Adams?) Actually, I don't want to picture it. But it is here, within a continuum of sedative states designed to ameliorate (and distract from) the discomfort of various minor but unpleasant medical procedures, that the largely ignored ethical conundrum posed by doctors' use of amnestic drugs is clearest. Exploiting the fact that under many anaesthetics, you or

I will start forgetting things well before we stop experiencing them, the practice allows doctors to place patients for a time in a sort of limbo—not quite here or there—washing around in a perceptual semi-present until the procedure is over.

When I first asked my friend who worked as a nurse in the endoscopy clinic if patients were ever awake during their procedures, she said that no, they were anaesthetised. When I asked if they sometimes woke up or talked during procedures, she said again that, no, she didn't think so. Then she thought a bit more, and said, 'Mind you, there was this man the other day...' The man had been having an endoscopy and what she had noticed first was the gagging sounds he made as staff pushed the tube down his airway. This was not all that unusual; the gag reflex can last well after a patient is unconscious. What caught her attention, however, was that the man was blinking his eyes rapidly open and shut, open and shut. He kept doing it until the anaesthetist gave him more propofol. Had he been awake? She didn't know. She hoped not. He didn't mention anything about it later.

Another day, she said, there was a minor emergency. A patient who was unconscious with a tube down his throat breathed fluid into his lungs. This is how people drown. The team immediately began suctioning the liquid out. During the drama the man woke, gasping, distressed. 'It's all right, everything's fine,' my friend heard staff tell him. 'You're just waking up in recovery. You've been having a dream.'

The man was all right, and everything did end up fine. But he had not been having a dream. Whether he remembered or later reported the 'dream' to staff, my friend did not find out.

Then there was the woman who screamed. This woman, my friend told me, had a condition affecting her blood vessels that made her particularly sensitive to pain. On the day of her colonoscopy, as the anaesthetist started pushing the anaesthetic into her arm, the woman began to scream. The anaesthetist gave her more of the drug. She screamed more. The screams were so loud that everyone in that surgery, including patients waiting to go in, could hear her. Eventually the anaesthetist pumped in enough of whatever drug he was giving her (probably propofol—it can sting) that she passed out completely. Afterwards she took a while to come around. My friend saw her in the recovery room, sitting in a reclining chair, woozily sipping her tea. The woman stayed there for some time, oblivious to the fact that every other person in that practice, staff and patients, had heard her cries of pain, and that she was the only one who didn't remember them. It wasn't until she was leaving that a staff member took her aside and told her some of what had happened—although in what detail my friend never found out. My friend was not critical of her colleagues, all of whom she said behaved in a manner that was professional. But she wondered sometimes about the woman. Should she have been moved into a more private space to recover? How much was she told? How much should she have been told?

o

Questions about the ethics of conscious sedation—'twilight sleep'— were raised more than twenty years ago by US law professor Maxwell Mehlman, bioethicist George Kanoti and paediatrician James Orlowski in an article subtitled 'What sound does a tree make in the forest when it falls on your head?' At the heart of the practice, they argued, was a trade-off between the safety benefits of using lower levels of anaesthetic drugs, and the risk of the patient suffering. Such trade-offs are not unheard of in medicine. The difference here, the authors argued, is that in the normal course of events, under the 'doctrine of informed consent', patients facing such a trade-off are entitled to a choice: more drugs, less pain; or less drugs, poten- tially more pain. But this suffering that patients don't remember feeling—is it still pain? And even if it is (or was) does it matter? The authors claimed that patients undergoing these procedures were not generally informed beforehand that they might be in pain, nor given the chance to request deeper anaesthesia or stronger painkillers. While this might be legal in most places, they concluded that it was not ethical.

They then drew a horrible parallel. Until relatively recently it was considered acceptable to operate on newborn babies without anaesthesia or pain relief. This was allowed on the grounds that they would have no conscious recollection of their experiences. These days, it would be unacceptable in all but extreme emergencies (for instance when anaesthetic drugs might themselves be life threatening).

Finally Mehlman compared conscious sedation with two other practices aligned to 'a small but intriguing class of deception-based medical practices' in which obtaining the patient's informed consent would eliminate the benefit from the medical practice itself. All three could be said to involve anaesthesia in one form or another. The first was the use of placebos—sugar pills—in place of pharmaceutical painkillers. By deceiving patients into believing they were taking drugs to reduce their pain, doctors could—through processes that remain deeply and wonderfully mysterious—convince them to convince their bodies that their pain had abated, thereby reducing their pain: the body fulfilling the mind's prophecy. The second example involved a different deception and a different pain. Mehlman mentioned a practice in which medical trainees in the US used to use newly dead patients to practise intubation—inserting a breathing tube down the patient's still warm airway—often without seeking the consent of the bereaved family.

In both these cases doctors could justify lying or withholding the truth by citing the greater good. The patient with a placebo achieved genuine relief without side effects. The trainee doctors learned a vital life-saving skill without inflicting further distress on grief-stricken kin. Can the routine use of amnestic drugs be justified in the same terms? The authors concluded not. They made a crucial distinction. In the first two cases, doctors were actually reducing or preventing suffering. But where amnestics are used in place of painkillers or full anaesthesia they are not preventing suffering, just the memory of it.

Occasionally not even that.

I am talking to writer Maree Kimberley, whose unconscious is a lush and slightly scary jungle. She has been creating feral gangs of futuristic young warriors who transplant eyes and feathers from living animals into their own flesh to help them fight. Right now, though, she is telling me about trying to climb off an operating table halfway through a colonoscopy. It was seventeen years ago, but, she says, 'I still bloody remember it.'

'They said I had to have this procedure and, "oh you might feel some mild discomfort". I don't know what they gave me. But I wasn't completely out of it. And all I really remember was just feeling this intense pain. I actually tried to climb off, literally tried to climb off the bed. And they had to hold me down, and I assume they gave me some more stuff, because then I sort of—I'm not sure how long it would have gone for, but probably at least thirty seconds, because they started to freak out. They're going, "calm down, calm down"— they're sort of trying to hold me. (Because obviously it's not good to move around when you've got something stuck up your bum.) I don't remember being frightened; I remember thinking, what the *fuck* are these people doing! I just wanted to get away.'

Then she passed out.

My family doctor has hinted more than once that googling is not a good way of making medical decisions. 'Kate, some of the people who write on those sites are a bit crazy.' Certainly in the lead-up to my back surgery, in the years I spent researching and resisting, I came across enough gothic horror to make me decide, ultimately, that the best medicine for me was simply not to look. Probably some of the people writing were a bit crazy. Mind you, if I'd been living in the sort of pain some of them seemed to have been enduring, I might be a bit crazy myself. And quite a few of them sounded reasonable and not mad or hysterical. Just scared, like me. When it comes to having a colonoscopy, a quick Google trawl will net enough stories of people being awake and unhappy during the procedure to make you, or at least me, think twice. In these instances you might argue that the problem lies not so much in the patients having been in pain but in them remembering being in pain.

But once again, pain may not be the worst of it. Robin Hemley is the US writer and teacher I met at the Varuna writers centre in the Blue Mountains—the one who saw a maybe-ghost in the room. Robin loves words. He grew up in a family of wordsmiths and has spent a lifetime juggling, weaving, collecting and, he freely acknowledges, stealing words. Back then he worked at the University of Iowa's renowned Writers' Workshop, teaching students how to find their own voices and tell their own stories. But for Robin, a dental procedure carried out under sedation became an unnerving experience of voicelessness. Beforehand the dentist had told him that although he would be conscious, he would remember nothing. Instead, Robin said, it was one of the most uncomfortable experiences of his life. The issue was not pain but—strangely—'a lingering legacy of shame'.

'I felt like a piece of furniture with just a slice of consciousness. I knew I was being manipulated. I could hear people and feel things, but I just felt utterly dead and stupid.'

Part of his terror, he said, arose from having lost control. 'You realise you're so vulnerable. Somehow it just feels like an insult. You feel as though other people are operating fully and that you're somehow at a lower level than they are. A lower life form.' He understood that this feeling was unwarranted. 'It doesn't make any sense at all. There is no reason for shame. But it feels as though you have somehow lost your status as a human being for a while. And you were in front of people in this state, so you're naked.'

Years later, a big British audit would confirm that Robin's experience was far from unique: one in five reports of accidental awareness had come from patients who had never been meant to have general anaesthesia in the first place, but had simply been sedated. Even so, their experiences—and the psychological impact—were 'similar in nature, though perhaps less in severity' than for patients reporting awareness during full anaesthesia.

In a 2014 editorial in Britain's *Anaesthesia* journal, following the release of the British audit, anaesthetists Michael Avidan and Jamie Sleigh would praise the project for its insights into patients' subjective experiences and interactions with staff. 'Unexpectedly,' they would write, 'sedation turned out to be a Bandersnatch'—the creature that bursts in towards the end of Lewis Carroll's 'The Hunting of the Snark', snapping its jaws, terrifying one member of the party to madness. The audit, they said, had highlighted gaping holes in patients' understanding of what sedation involved. 'Patients who are receiving sedation should be told unambiguously that general anaesthesia is not intended, awareness is common, and many patients retain memories despite receiving amnestic medications.'

Listening to Robin Hemley describe his dental sedation, I was struck again at the intensity of his reaction. What he was describing was not just an amusing anecdote, an oddity; it was a deeply felt experience of fear and powerlessness. Existential emptiness. Under sedation, his sense of self was not just altered but diminished. He became less. 'I always thought I'd like anaesthetics—like laughing gas. Now I think it's the last thing I'd possibly want.'

o

Needless to say I was less than happy when my doctor mounted what was to become a prolonged campaign to send me to a gastroenterologist for a colonoscopy. Eventually, nearly two years after her initial prompt, I turned up at an inner Melbourne clinic, tired and dehydrated after a day of fasting and a night of copious, saline-induced purging. After changing into a blue disposable robe, I was directed to a room containing a large grey recliner where I waited until the arrival of an anaesthetist called Alistair, who told me he would be giving me a combination of midazolam, propofol and a painkiller called fentanyl. I asked him to try to remember anything I might say during the procedure. 'Don't worry,' he said firmly. 'You won't be saying anything.'

I remember climbing onto the trolley in the small surgery, lying on my side, Alistair inserting the cannula in the back of my right hand, a nurse putting an oxygen mask over my nose and mouth while I continued trying to interrogate Alistair as to what drug was going in now. I felt completely alert. I woke forty minutes later in a different recliner, as if from a deep restful sleep. I felt no pain, just a languorous calm.

That said, even after I had stopped asking questions or responding to Alistair's, there is a chance I would still have been pretty interested in what was happening inside my own head. In a 2011 Finnish study sedated volunteers later reported a kaleidoscope of thoughts, sensations and experiences: hallucinatory, fragmentary and otherwise. One described a series of quick visions or dreams, including a football game. 'Suddenly [*after the football dream*] we were pirates, and at some point we went to swim'; 'When the drug started to work, my head came out of my body'.

So, again, that question. If under sedative levels of anaesthesia I find myself playing football or being a pirate, or my head comes out of my body, does it matter? Particularly if I don't remember any of it? Several studies have shown that following low doses of propofol, people who have lost all conscious recall of events may still show evidence of priming. When I asked Ben Chortkoff, the young anaesthetist involved in the repeat study that failed to replicate Bernard Levinson's 1965 experiment, he wrote back:

> The anaesthetic question I would most like to see addressed is the storage of memories in patients who have received benzodiazepines. A patient who has received midazolam can have a deep and meaningful conversation, demonstrating hearing intact, understanding intact, processing intact and functional on a level that allows humor etc., yet frequently, if asked a few hours later, the patient will report no memory of the conversation stating, 'wow, I've been totally asleep'.

But Chortkoff also wondered whether, rather than searching for unconscious memories for words or events after an anaesthetic, a more valuable line of research might be into the emotional impact of the experience of surgery, irrespective of whether the patient can be shown to have 'learnt' information during the operation. Such emotional memories might be inferred through mood changes, as well as the ususal physiological signs—heart rate, blood pressure, sweating.

Shortly after I interviewed Chortkoff in April 2010, he emailed me with a link to an NPR radio program. The story was based on a study that had recently appeared in the *Proceedings of the National Academy of Sciences* journal, looking at people whose ability to remember any new events (a family visit, the evening news) for more than a few minutes had been all but destroyed by damage to the hippocampus. The study's author, Justin Feinstein, then a graduate student in neuropsychology at the University of Iowa, told NPR that he often met families of Alzheimer's patients who were so disheartened by the belief that their loved ones would remember nothing of their visits once (or sometimes even before) they left that they couldn't see the point in visiting. Feinstein, however was not convinced that the encounters—or at least the emotions they evoked—were so quickly erased. To prove his point he assembled a group of people with hippocampal damage to watch scenes from shows such as Hollywood tear-jerker *Forrest Gump*—the one in which Forrest weeps at his wife's grave. Everyone was visibly moved, one woman to tears. And half an hour later none of the viewers could recall ever having seen the film. Then Feinstein asked the woman who had been weeping how she was feeling. 'Well,' he told NPR, 'it turns out she's still sad.' She was not the only one.

The story has a happy-ish ending. When Feinstein and his team then showed the same group happy clips—*When Harry Met Sally*, *America's Funniest Home Videos*—the emotion again outlasted the memory. They felt good, but again with no idea why. Feinstein hoped these results would encourage families and friends of people with severe Alzheimer's to keep visiting. Visits needn't even be long.

So what about you or me undergoing anaesthesia? Anaesthesia is not Alzheimer's. But might our feelings matter more than facts? 'I would like to see a study (like the Alzheimer's study but with patients who have had anaesthesia) that looked at emotion,' said Chortkoff in a follow-up email. 'I agree with you that this is a different category of implicit learning that would not likely be revealed by typical implicit learning tasks.'

o

In 2007, shortly after I returned from my research trip, New York surgeon Scott Haig published an eloquent and disturbing article in

Time magazine. Haig (a regular *Time* columnist) was writing about his experience with Ellen, a young mother and former cancer patient. She had come to him to have a biopsy on a growth near her collar-bone. Haig needed to remove a small portion of the lump for testing in the hospital's pathology lab, but Ellen was adamant that she did not want a general anaesthetic. She was afraid she might not wake up. Haig was clear about the statistical improbability of that happening. But he understood her desire for consciousness and agreed to do the potentially painful procedure under a local nerve block. He insisted, however, on having an anaesthetist at hand in case the pain got too much.

The procedure went smoothly. As soon as Haig had excised the bit of the bony growth he sent the sample across to the hospital's pathology laboratory and began stitching up the wound. He had just finished when from across the room the voice of the pathologist came over the intercom; unaware Ellen was still in the room, he began telling Haig what he had found—an aggressive cancer. Ellen gasped ('Oh, my God. Oh, my God. My kids.') And then passed out: the anaesthetist had pumped in a dose of propofol as soon as he heard the word cancer.

Ellen woke ten minutes later, oblivious. She never even knew she had been asleep. Haig arranged to talk with her when the pathology report arrived, and she left.

Haig was adamant that the anaesthetist had made the right decision. In removing not only Ellen's consciousness but her memory, he had made it possible for Haig to deliver the information sensitively and privately—and at a time of his choosing. This, he said, was ethics at the front line. 'Questions of withholding bad news, wiping out bad memories—plastering over wayward cracks in our minds with chemicals—are answered thousands of times every day without ever being asked,' he wrote. 'Ethics committees and experts exist in our hospitals, but what they have to say counts precious little down in the trenches, where intercoms fail and human minds treat human minds, in real time.'

But despite Haig's conviction that it was the right thing to do, he also understood that something had been breached: '...only a little and, obviously, with benevolent intent. But it hadn't been as simple as pushing a rewind button. Something there had borne the unmistakable quality of wrong.'

Ellen died six years later of cancer. Haig never told her what happened in the operating room that day. More than ten years later, he was still not sure that he had made the right decision in staying silent.

MERGING CURRENTS

Coming apart

Scene 1, foreshore, exterior: There are two of us, myself and another young woman about the same age. It is dusk. Around us are groups of malevolent men, some in cars, some just prowling. We try to stay hidden but some of the men grab my friend and drag her away. I can hear her screaming and I know they are raping her. I know I should go and help her, but there are too many of them. I am too scared. I move off quietly through the sandy scrub, staying low.

Scene 2, house, interior: I am inside a house not far from the beach where I have left my friend. There is a young woman here and her blind mother. I tell the mother what has happened and ask what to do. The mother says, do nothing. She has white hair. She seems to imply that what is happening to my friend is not unusual and will sort itself out in the end. The damage is inevitable, but my friend will not die. I feel guilty at having abandoned my friend but also relieved at not having to go back out there to save her.

Scene 3, house, interior: It dawns on me (dreamlike) that the daughter, who has so far been silent, has herself been through the same awful experience as my friend—that she may indeed be my abandoned friend—but as if she has stayed young, while time has moved on for the rest of us. So I am middle aged, and the mother is old. I turn to the daughter and ask, 'Has anything worse ever happened to you?' Even dreaming, I am aware that it is an indirect way of trying to minimise what has taken place, appease my complicity in the mother's denial. The daughter, however, seems calm. Yes, she says, worse things have happened to her. My relief brushes up alongside the knowledge of having betrayed my friend, who I know in my heart is still out there where I left her, in the dark with those circling men.

I flew into Detroit late one afternoon and took a taxi to my hotel, past dark trees and a dim watery sky, on my way to meet Ann Arbor's most over-qualified trainee anaesthetist. I had spoken by email to George Mashour and he had replied immediately. ('It would be my absolute pleasure to discuss this subject with you...I'm anxious to hear all about your project, as these subjects are near and dear to my heart!') While still technically a trainee anaesthetist, Mashour at thirty-eight was already onto his third or fourth incarnation in a precocious and eclectic academic ascension. As an undergraduate he had studied philosophy before switching track ('I regarded myself as pretty much a scientific idiot until college') and eventually doing a PhD in neuroscience, as well as a medical doctorate. For a while he studied tumours in the brain and nervous system, but soon started to focus on less tangible questions. What was the relationship between the brain and consciousness, for instance? Switching to Harvard, he did a year of psychiatry, thinking this might combine his interest in neuroscience, medicine and philosophy. Instead he got hooked by anaesthesia.

I had not originally intended to come to Ann Arbor. I rearranged my itinerary at the last moment when, during our correspondence, Mashour sent me the draft of an intriguing and, from the standard medical perspective, all but heretical paper. In it he put forward a view of anaesthesia so compellingly at odds with almost everything else I had heard that I rang my travel agent immediately and booked an overnight stopover. Mashour's paper compared two disciplines seemingly at opposite ends of the medical spectrum, anaesthesia and psychoanalysis—the latter largely concerned with talking; the former, by necessity, with silence. In his paper, Mashour pointed out the almost universally ignored fact that, despite their apparent differences, both disciplines shared a fundamental preoccupation with unconscious states, and wondered if they could share an underlying process or mechanism.

'The anesthesiologist seems to "put people to sleep",' he wrote, 'while the analyst "wakes people up". Despite these superficial disparities, however, both fields share a common focus of inquiry...'

Mashour picked me up out the front of my hotel in a yellow sports car and we drove to his apartment, a multi-levelled loft in a converted armaments factory. Fast talking, precisely spoken, his shaven head sloshing with ideas, he exuded an aura of intensity in no way offset by his casual black T-shirt, pale cotton pants and sandals. After finishing a year of post-doctoral research in Europe, he had done his anaesthesia fellowship in Boston before moving to the University of Michigan at Ann Arbor for a six-month residency in neuro-anaesthesia—anaesthesia for brain and spinal surgery—which he was one month away from finishing. At the time of our conversation he was in the process of editing a book on anaesthesia and consciousness, and was also engaged in setting up his own neuroscience laboratory.

Inside, his apartment was sparse, tasteful and devoid of detritus. His study, on the top level, was an exercise in geometry—books, laptop computer and piles of cards arranged at angles on the desk. 'You're very tidy,' I said. 'All my friends say that,' he agreed. On a shelf by the stairs was a small model of the brain, wrinkled and intestinal. He was an attentive and generous host. We sat downstairs in a lounge decorated in shades of cream and brown and Mashour opened a bottle of pinot noir.

The reason, he argued, that these two ideas, anaesthesia and psychoanalysis, had remained quarantined from each other within scientific debate, despite sharing nomenclature and at least some features, was that the conventional view of anaesthetic unconsciousness was of a state of cognitive stasis—with all higher brain function including memory and learning effectively shut down—while the Freudian unconscious was active and energetic.

Mashour believed, however, that the two states might have more in common than was comfortable to consider. He had seen the conclusions drawn by the Canadian researchers Merikle and Daneman, whose meta-analysis showed that even deeply anaesthetised patients could take in and remember information without knowing it. He had also, through his study of psychiatry, developed a knowledge of and interest in the ideas that Freud had first begun to articulate through his study of psychoanalysis.

Central to Mashour's thinking was Freud's concept of the psychoanalytic defence—the process whereby the brain is understood to effectively exile upsetting thoughts or memories into the realm of the 'unconscious' where they exist in an uneasy sort of limbo—not available to conscious thought or reason, but influencing us all the more powerfully for that.

'You don't have to believe Freud's theories of psychosexual development or whatever,' added Mashour quickly, 'but, Freud is basically saying, the unconscious mind is not this black sea of nothingness, it is active and dynamic.' Freud, he said, had coined the term 'dynamic unconscious'.

'What I was realising when I thought more about anaesthesia

was, *wait,* this is also a kind of dynamic unconscious. The brain can learn, it can register information, there is discrete cognitive activity going on. It is active.'

To help build a theoretical framework for his strange new idea, Mashour looked first to anaesthesia, drawing his focus back from the technical preoccupations with the sites and structures of anaesthetic action—the realm of lipids and proteins and brain geography—and shifting instead to tackle consciousness front-on. Given that the ultimate effect of anaesthetics was to suppress consciousness, he said, it was to this mysterious process that science must turn.

He chose as his guide the eighteenth-century German philosopher Kant, who proposed that the mind, rather than being an undifferentiated neural blob, was composed of distinct faculties that processed different sensory and other information. Here, for instance, I sit at my desk: in this moment I can see the computer screen, feel my fingers on its keys, hear the bleats of early-morning birds beyond the window. What Kant wanted to know was how all these distinct inputs were synthesised into a single unified experience: in this case me typing. He proposed that for me or anyone to make sense of these individual blips of disconnected data, the blips (he did not call them that) must be integrated through some unifying principle that he termed the 'transcendental unity of apperception'.

More than two centuries after Kant, neuroscientists have established that the brain does indeed process different types of information in discrete regions: even a single brief memory is processed in various separate areas. What they are still trying to work out is how these inputs come together into the shimmering edifice of consciousness—into me sitting at my desk in the quiet hour before the family wakes, knowing that not only do I exist but that I am writing this book.

Using terminology first coined in the 1980s, Mashour had gone on to describe this process as 'cognitive binding', and summarised various mechanisms by which such binding is now known to take place—either through chemical links between individual neurons or neural circuits, or through the synchronisation of electrical frequencies across different areas of the brain—a sort of mind music—though he stressed such binding in itself may not be necessary, or enough, for consciousness.

Mashour was not at this stage offering insights into how this all happened, simply speculating that bits of information collected by the brain are somehow (through processes known and unknown) drawn together and collated into something greater than the sum of their parts, which we call consciousness.

Yet this deceptively simple construct provides the basis for a mirror theory on how anaesthetics might work formally proposed by Mashour in 2004 and later published in the influential journal *Anesthesiology*. Rather than simply suppressing the brain's neural activity, he argued, perhaps anaesthetics dismantled it.

His thesis was elegant. If consciousness was a process of binding, then anaesthesia might be one of unbinding. If consciousness was integration, unconsciousness was disintegration. If consciousness could be depicted as a group of individual instruments making sounds that, through a process known as music, cohered into a symphony—here Mashour waved his hands like a conductor's—perhaps anaesthesia could be seen as the orchestra falling apart: 'The cello player starts getting out of sync with the violinist and the percussion section.'

Central to this is the understanding that, under anaesthesia, information (such as pain, or sounds, or perhaps speech) reaches the brain and is processed there to some degree, but does not evolve into a conscious experience. 'There's no *structural* problem—all the instruments are working, all the people are playing—there's a *functional* disruption.' This was not the same, he emphasised, as if he had gone and smashed up the cello. The cello could still play, but instead of music there was just noise.

He pointed to evidence that anaesthetics could interrupt cognitive binding—by interrupting the electrical circuitry of, and 'coherence' between, different parts of the brain; thus curbing the ability of clusters of neurons carrying fragments of information to synthesise and translate that information into a message that could be consciously processed.

Mashour's was only one of many theories that attempted to explain how anaesthetics might bring about unconsciousness, but it had the benefits of being flexible and inclusive. It allowed for the diversity of anaesthetic agents and effects on different levels of brain processing—and, satisfyingly, it provided a framework for integrating the study of anaesthesia with that of consciousness. While he was not the first to suggest that anaesthetic drugs might bring about unconsciousness through disrupting the brain's ability to process information, he was the first to propose and articulate unbinding as a formal theory.

The paper that came out under Mashour's name not long after my visit was not published in *Anesthesiology*. Nor in any anaesthesia journal. It appeared instead in the *Journal of the American Psychoanalytic Association*, where, Mashour said, he could be fairly confident that none of his colleagues would come across it. And here he took his huge and speculative leap.

This time, Mashour beamed his spotlight upon the theories of British psychoanalyst Wilfred Bion who proposed last century that conscious experience arose from the brain's synthesis of blocks of raw data into more complex arrangements. From these, thoughts and ideas could eventually be formed. In this schema, psychiatric problems might be associated with 'attacks on linking' between blocks, effectively exiling painful or unwanted information into unconsciousness, where it remained as fragments (splinters). Thoughts, he said, without a thinker. Could it be, asked Mashour, that anaesthesia was an extreme form of such censorship? That instead of simply shutting down the mind, anaesthetics *activated* a system—the same one that kept all the unwanted and unnecessary information, ideas, experiences and memories out of consciousness?

The idea, or the kernel of the idea, of a possible overlap between the anaesthetic and psychological unconscious came to Mashour early in his anaesthetic residency.

He had been anaesthetising a woman, a difficult patient, he said, in her forties, who had come into hospital to have her cancerous breast removed. 'She never smoked, she never drank,' said Mashour, 'she was an athlete, she was a high achiever, a healthy woman and she was really wrapped up tight...'

'Psychologically?'

'Yes. And employing—and I had done a year of psychiatry, so I could see that she was employing a lot of defence mechanisms: was being very controlling...trying to make me feel inadequate, but just not displaying any emotion about the process.'

Anyway, he continued, they had taken the woman to the operating theatre and he had hooked her up to an intravenous anaesthetic. Until this moment, he said, she had remained stiff and impassive—what he described in psychiatric terminology as 'still in this mode of defence'. But as the anaesthetic started going in, he said, and the woman began to lose consciousness, everything changed. 'She just started bawling; she just started crying. And the affect [*emotion*] that was released at that moment was just so striking to me—and it was so clear that on the way down under she was able to access the emotions that she was sort of controlling and defending against.

'I don't know whether that has any place in your thinking,' he added, 'but to me...that's often why people drink...'

Mashour stressed that this idea was not yet a theory, just something he had been thinking about. But one of the appealing aspects of his proposition is that it attempted to make sense of some of the anomalies routinely overlooked in most anaesthetic theories—to start with, Bernard Levinson's mock crisis. Despite its flaws, said Mashour, that study hinted that emotional material ('Just a moment! I don't like the patient's colour' etc.) laid down under chemical hypnosis and then lost to the conscious mind could be retrieved (perhaps reassembled) under psychological hypnosis. This suggested that these two very different sorts of unconsciousness might share a common cognitive structure.

Further strengthening his theory, Mashour argued, was the fact that it could also be generalised to other states such as coma and sleep. He pointed to brain scans of unconscious patients in so-called persistent vegetative states whose brains still lit up in response to spoken instructions. Something similar happened in sleep. He argued finally that not only did anaesthesia and the psychological defence mechanism share a similar structure, but a common aim— the alleviation of distress. In the end, and despite their differences, anaesthetists and analysts might both be engaged in the same business: dismantling and reconstructing consciousness. The mosaic re-imagined, restored from the scattered fragments.

Sometimes when George Mashour allows himself to drift and his mind to roam over the boundless possibilities of consciousness and unconsciousness and anaesthesia, he has strange thoughts that even he is not sure what to make of. One of these concerns how long after surgery it can take patients to 'remember' periods of awareness. To him, it doesn't add up. 'I mean, I don't know...but why should it take somebody a week to remember that they were awake and in pain during surgery? Does that make any sense to you, as a lay person? It doesn't make any sense to me. I mean, if you punch me in the face, right now, or beat the crap out of me, I should be able to tell you about that more vividly tomorrow than I should a week from now.'

So what has happened to the memory, he wonders? Or was there ever a memory? Or even an experience, at least in the way we understand experience? What if, rather than an orchestra, there was only ever a set of individual players? What if the orchestra doesn't assemble until later? 'When we think of awareness and awareness with recall, we think of somebody being awake during the procedure, at the event, and then remembering it…What if, during the surgery, they actually just acquired the tools, the parts to the experience and actually didn't really experience it quite literally until after the event, when their ability to synthesise this information returned? What if the awareness actually does happen a week later?

'I mean, it is kind of mind-boggling and I don't know if I am right about this, but do you see what I am saying?'

'So do you talk to any of your colleagues about this stuff?' I asked Mashour towards the end of our discussion.

'No. I don't,' he said. 'I mean, I don't have any colleagues to talk to about this stuff because they don't think about it this way.'

'So who do you talk to about it?'

'Nobody,' he said. And then, laughing slightly, 'I talk to you.'

o

The more I think about George Mashour's theory, the more I am reminded of the process of the writing of this book. The extraordinary slowness of synthesis. The pushing together of the opposing poles. It seemed to me that at the start of each section I would have a flash of understanding, a moment of completion in which for an instant I saw the exact shape and content of what it was I was trying to say. Then all that disappeared and I spent weeks, months, sometimes years, trying to pull or shove it all together again. It was all there, or much of it, and sometimes if I could let myself speak unguardedly, let the ideas flow out unchecked in a rush, I found that the connections were already in place, the deep shape of it, and all I was trying to do was reunite them. Or maybe that was not what I was doing at all. Maybe I was trying to keep them apart. I couldn't tell.

Lying in bed one morning, waiting for the alarm to go off, I found myself drifting in that in-between state, neither here nor there, or rather in both places, able to watch as my mind unspooled the last of the night's imagery. Suddenly I was slipping between selves. One moment 'I' was there; the next, it was as if there were three versions of myself, each floating in my mind in its own little bubble. They were visual images—pictures—not words or ideas and, although I no longer remember the content of each bubble, I understood without the need or capacity for thought that each not only represented myself in some way, but that each was, in a sense, me. Becalmed. It was a fleeting moment. Then one bubble began rising towards the surface, and I understood in that instant that the awakening part of me, the 'I' now rising from sleep towards the day, was now identifiably me. The other floating bubbles, while each representing, even containing, me, were not. I understood them to be myself, but felt no sense of ownership. And because of this, each could exist quite easily and effortlessly side by side, with neither competition nor contradiction. Boundless. Unbound. It was only in the rising towards—and more particularly the moment of entering—consciousness (and by this I mean the 'I' consciousness, the me that not only thinks but articulates these thoughts back to myself through language, the me that knows myself as 'Kate') that these other selves were lost. Left behind somewhere within me until such time, perhaps, as I merged back into selflessness.

So how many 'me's do I have, potential 'me's? And what happens to them under anaesthesia? The self who is writing this book is partial, I know; an act of creation and recreation. But I recognise her. She feels like *me*. Are there really other selves building up inside me? Pre-selves? Sometimes I feel the 'I' in this book straining at the edges, trying perhaps to absorb some other hidden part or parts of me—or to keep them from absorbing the me I know. (The feeling in my body is sludgy, resistant.)

One of these selves is, even now, folded over in the open doorway of a white Mazda Capella, Sydney 1996, trying to contain or escape a feeling that is trying equally hard to ram its way out of my mouth. My newish partner is crouched beside me, solicitous, bemused. I am maybe ten weeks into a pregnancy that will result six months or so from now in the birth of our son. But for now I have been invaded by a fear that I neither recognise nor understand. It is completely physical. It has no story attached. I have no idea what it is or why it has settled on me (for this is how it feels, that it is something that has been imposed from outside me, a terror that is not even mine). The fear moves in and stays for a month, then fades.

The hypnotist

As we walked to a friend's house one late afternoon, my daughter told me about something she had noticed. The last time she had set out to walk there on her own she had forgotten the way. She had tried hard to remember, but it wasn't until she stopped trying that she realised she knew where she was going. It was as if, she said, her thoughts were little people and if she tried too hard to think of something it was like strangling them. But if she just let them be, it was as if they were all sitting there with their books open in front of them (she gestured the holding up of a book), able to tell her everything she needed to know.

'Just let them be.' But I couldn't: I worried and niggled at my thoughts. I bullied and cajoled. I grabbed them around their necks and tried to strangle them. And the harder I tried, the more they fought me.

Waking early one morning, sleepless and tense, I realised I had been dreaming about writing a book. I could see it had possibilities but it was a bloodless process; a collating and compiling, a corralling of depleted resources. I was sick of it already.

Lying in bed, I was squashed up against a feeling of intense dislike. Dislike for self. A rancorous belittling dislike; petty and provoking. Mean and exhausted. The unconscious: I wanted to track it down. I wanted to dig it out with a metal spoon.

In pursuit of my unconscious, I went to see another hypnotherapist. I had to book a long time ahead and it cost what seemed to me an unseemly amount of money. His office was in a two-storey brick house in one of Melbourne's wealthier suburbs, with an entrance flanked by small graceful trees. After I had sat for a while in a small waiting room, the wooden door opened and the hypnotherapist, unsmiling, ushered me through.

Inside, the room was crowded with photographs and personal effects and smelled faintly of incense. The hypnotherapist sat behind a large wooden desk and asked me why I had come. I mumbled something about the book I was writing and anaesthesia and memory and then I told him about an abortion I had had under anaesthesia some years before my son's birth, when I was living in Darwin. I wondered whether this experience might be somehow related to that persistent feeling.

After I had given a brief summary to the hypnotherapist, he stared at me, still unsmiling, and recapped. 'So, you are angry at yourself for not having the courage to go ahead and have the child?' And although the truth was more complex than this, I nodded.

The hypnotherapist asked about my habits. Alcohol? (Yes.) Coffee? (Yes.) Cigarettes? (Not anymore.) He said the alcohol was probably contributing to my depression and the coffee to my anxiety. To do this sort of work, he said, the body needed to be clear. He also mentioned prayer. I tried not to look sceptical. We talked for half an hour or so, and then he gestured to an armchair alongside his desk and I lowered myself into it. The hypnotherapist sat beside me and told me to close my eyes and relax. He leaned closer and put one hand along the side of my face—almost or lightly touching, and one cool finger in the centre of my forehead. Then he asked me to roll my eyes back towards the top of my head and to feel that I was sinking. After a while he started talking in a slow, sonorous voice.

He spoke for some time, but all I can remember him talking about was drinking. I wouldn't want to drink alcohol or coffee, he said. If anyone offered, I was to say quite firmly that I didn't want to as it didn't suit me. I was also to exercise. As he spoke I was aware, once again, of the competing strains of resistance and submission. Part of me seemed to be sinking lower and lower, the other part was tight in the chest and wary. After a while he told me he would count backwards from three and that as he did so I would wake easily. Which I did, although from where I was not quite sure.

The hypnotherapist told me to come back in two or three weeks. And after I had paid, I walked away wondering if I would bother.

Two weeks later I had drunk neither alcohol or coffee. I had dieted and even swum. It was not that I no longer desired them. I missed alcohol in particular in a sad dragging way, as I once had with cigarettes. It was more that I felt resigned to their absence. In the week after I had seen the hypnotherapist I also got a crashing headache, then a snotty chest bug, then diarrhoea. I didn't know whether to feel pleased or resentful.

Despite or because of this, I returned three weeks after the first appointment. After discussing my new-found purity and talking around in circles for a while, I finally asked what I had wanted to ask the session before. Could he hypnotically regress me to the time of that previous anaesthetic? I felt foolish asking, as if I really believed that my unconscious would be sitting there waiting for me in a nice little box. Gift-wrapped. But I wanted to know. Hadn't Bernard Levinson done it forty years before in Johannesburg? Perhaps this was where I would find the key.

The hypnotherapist paused and then said slowly that he did not think this would be advisable. I didn't take it all in, but he finished by saying that even if I did come across some 'memories' under hypnosis, there was nothing to say they would be real. I appreciated his honesty, but did not go back again. I went home and had a glass of red wine.

Maybe it was a form of wish-fulfilment or confabulation, but four days after this visit my unconscious obliged by delivering me this dream.

I am to be operated upon. I am lying on my back, I am awake and unable to move. The operation has not yet started and I am trying to move my right hand to get the attention of the doctor. Throughout the dream there is an odd sense of dislocation or numbness. Oppressive. Congested. I am aware that something unpleasant is happening, but do not quite allow myself the feeling. There is, all the same, the sense that the feeling is there. The doctor seems angry. I must manage to move my hand a little because he says something like, 'You'll have to be still for this.' His voice seems hard and punitive. Then he plunges something sharp into the back of my right hand. There is a jabbing pain, then no more movement. I feel a growing dread, and the sense of his hatred, and the knowledge that I will have to endure it. The doctor is in white, very crisp, middle aged, and it is my feelings about him that are the main strand in the dream. I feel that part of him knows what is happening and doesn't care.

I cannot say what this dream represented. The plot was clear enough—almost ridiculously so. But I did not feel any great sense of attachment to the story. Not like the dream of the red dog. Maybe I was indeed re-experiencing an episode from one of my own anaesthetics; maybe this explained my interest in anaesthesia, and that strange low feeling. It was conceivable. I would have liked to believe this.

But maybe it was simply my mind doing what minds do, creating a collage out of my reading and talking and thinking, re-gifting it to me as a brand new experience. Or maybe it was my own feelings about the hypnotherapist, whose manner I had found rather aloof, finding expression as I slept. I wanted to know the truth of the dream. I still do. But I can't.

In any case, I now had more immediate concerns.

Regression

Melbourne 2009. Huddled one afternoon in a stationary car in Fitzroy with my soonish-to-be-husband Pete, I came to a terrible realisation. A couple of years before, at the prompting of a friend, I had returned to see a Melbourne orthopaedic surgeon, who had sent me for an X-ray that confirmed what I half-knew. My spine was getting worse: more bent, more twisted. In response to this news I had embarked on a belated campaign. In addition to Pilates classes, I searched out therapists who claimed to have had success treating scoliosis without surgery. Ignoring the fact that these approaches, if they worked at all, would almost certainly be too late for me, I tracked down visiting international therapists, I took up the Alexander Technique, I drove an hour across town every week for months to visit a physiotherapist who had an exercise machine that had been proven to reduce curves in younger people. I had a machine of my own imported from Italy and adjusted by an ironmonger friend. I felt fitter and better.

But now I was sitting in the car with Pete and a new set of X-rays that showed it had all been for nothing. My spine had simply used the time to add another couple of degrees to its curve. 'No!' I blurted, incredulous, appalled. 'I don't. I can't.' And then, 'I'm going to have to have the surgery.'

..

It is hard to comprehend the vulnerability of the anaesthetised patient. A newborn has more resources. An infant abandoned at birth can survive for days untended. An adult undergoing even relatively straightforward surgery might last only minutes without the doctors, nurses and the machines assembled to maintain the basic functions of life—breath, the circulation of blood, the containment of skin. Walking into a hospital to have a general anaesthetic is a profound statement of trust, or necessity.

The vulnerability starts well before surgery. To enter a hospital as a surgical patient is to experience a series of small and escalating losses: privacy, props, dignity, control and eventually, for many, consciousness. You also lose your equality. As a patient you are not equal: you are dependent. You eat what you are given; you have visitors only when you are allowed; you submit to sometimes inexplicable rules and procedures; and you are reliant always on other people's largesse—for food, painkillers, information or even company. You may or may not have given over these freedoms voluntarily, but either way, without them you are not the person who carries you through your daily life.

Sometimes this can be liberating: what a relief to stop trying, to simply relinquish. For others this letting go—this ceding of control—can be deeply disturbing. Graham Burrows (the psychiatrist who first tried, against the odds, to help me understand hypnosis) put it like this. 'So imagine the CEO of a company that's controlling billions of dollars, thousands of people, and he's got to go have an anaesthetic for his haemorrhoids, he may find it very difficult when somebody in a nice white uniform comes along and says, bend over I'm going to give you an injection.'

Either way, like it or not, your relationship with the world changes, and you become in a sense childlike. In hospital you are not the boss of you. In the presence of a doctor, even your local GP, you will tend to slip soundlessly into the patterns you learned in childhood: submission, defiance, helplessness, adulation. You are small, your doctor is big. On this level it is all the same. Even before the anaesthetic, you have entered the realm of the unconscious. In psychological terms it is known as regression: a state of vulnerability and enforced passivity in which, without realising it, you fall back on childhood ways of interpreting and dealing with frightening situations.

The slide into passivity can be alarmingly quick. New Zealand anaesthetist Alan Merry has spoken about breaking his leg badly on a skiing holiday. He knew what had happened, and even as a local medic applied a plaster cast up to his knee, Merry said, he knew she was making a mistake: he needed a full-leg cast. But instead of speaking up, Merry shut up. He didn't want to make a fuss. He eventually found his voice and told staff at the emergency department what was wrong and the leg was replastered. 'I'd never really understood before how a patient lets the wrong thing be done to them,' he later told a reporter.

In the months after my mother's diagnosis and prognosis and all that followed, I took to reading—or more often re-reading—the Regency romances of the late Georgette Heyer. Bright, witty confections filled with impatient men and irrepressible women. A slender, predictable plot (elopements, kidnappings, tangles of one sort or another) stitched together with a mass of extravagant period detail. Kid gloves, pigskin fans and so many carriages—barouches, curricles, phaetons—deftly navigating Berkeley Square or dashing from London to Bath, all drawn by high-stepping bays or Spanish greys.

I was amused and a little startled at how comforting I still found them.

It was not, of course, the horses that kept me reading late into the night; it was the yearning. An indefinite, pre-sexual ache. The longing for another skin to enclose my own, to hold me in, to keep me safe and entire and complete. A yearning that, through the ritualised choreography of Heyer's imagination, and for the duration of the book, would be satisfied. Because that is the contract. The fantasy of permanence.

Everyone is scared before surgery. 'Scared out of their minds,' one Boston anaesthetist told me. 'Very frequently people say to you, I'm more afraid of the anaesthesia than I am about the actual procedure I'm having.' Up to three-quarters of us facing surgery say we worry about the possibility of pain, paralysis and distress. The rest of us just don't admit it. US medical psychiatrist Richard Blacher pointed out thirty years ago that the patient's perception of the risk usually far outweighed the realistic dangers, although they were unlikely to share their fears with doctors. 'Indeed, some patients who seem calm and contained clinically, may reveal a level of anxiety close to psychosis when psychological tests are performed.' Blacher believed patients would often try to hide their anxieties—for fear, perhaps, of looking foolish or out of a reluctance to be seen as doubting or challenging the authority of the doctor. 'The patient wants to be admired and loved and thus treated well and cured.'

Under pressure, we stop filtering information through the rational grid of the neocortex and revert to simplistic, childlike modes of thinking. Jokes are lost on us. We become literal. Superstitious. We clutch at signs and symbols, touch wood, worry that bad things will happen in threes. We expect the worst. In a 1910 address delivered on the anniversary of Ether Day, the American surgeon George Crile likened the experience of surgery to facing a firing squad. 'If one were placed against a wall and were looking into the gun muzzles of a squad of soldiers and were told that he must not be afraid because in nine chances out of ten he would not be killed outright when the volley was fired, would it help him to be told that he must not be afraid? Such an experience would be written indelibly on his brain.'

Graham Burrows said a good anaesthetist would recognise an anxious patient. 'There's two types of behaviour commonly. They either talk like mad, and can't stop talking, because they're so nervous, or they're lying there quite quiet saying nothing and being quite petrified beneath it all.' The most anxious patients were doctors, and the most anxious doctors were probably anaesthetists and surgeons. 'The old story, the more you know, the more you know that there's a potential problem.'

If merely speaking with a doctor (or a teacher or a judge or a police officer, or even the grumpy woman from the milk bar) can be enough to spiral us backwards to our younger selves, what are the implications for someone facing a general anaesthetic? To be anaesthetised is to be about as regressed as you can get. Dairy farmers, stockbrokers, trapeze artists, all reduced to a state of infantile helplessness: immobile, voiceless, offering up their bodies and their minds for someone else to act upon. Psychiatrists describe this as regressing in the service of the ego. As a competent adult you make an informed decision to make yourself vulnerable to another human being and to trust that they will help you. In this light it is a healthy dependency.

Several of the people I met in the course of researching this book told me how much they loved general anaesthetics. Loubna Haikal, a Sydney-based, Lebanese-born doctor, novelist and playwright, said she had had quite a few anaesthetics, 'And I realised the last time I had one that it was a bit like taking a break from living. Like dying.' She did not mean this in a bad way. It was only a short anaesthetic, she said, but was in its way liberating. 'It was a very pleasurable experience to have a break from the world, in a way, and just go into total lack of consciousness. The interesting thing is that you lose the notion of time. You're free of all the boundaries, all the concepts, all the elements.'

But a general anaesthetic is still a taste of mortality. A chemical regression. At surgical levels, the eyes fix, breathing shallows, the muscles between the ribs stop working. Go deeper and the body starts to shut down. Breathing. Blood pressure. The heart. Life recedes.

Underpinning this physical dismantling is another, more primal, disintegration. Anaesthetics, it seems, switch off more recently evolved sections of the brain but leave some of the more primitive parts relatively active—at least for a while. Under their influence we travel backwards down the evolutionary ladder, losing first the brain functions that make us most particularly human—language, reasoning, analysis, impulse control—before retreating into the emotional centres of our mammalian brains, and eventually to the life-preserving realm of the oldest brain structures. Along the way, the drugs can also precipitate a more subtle regression. A dismantling of the psychic armour that defines and defends our sense of self. The habits, tics and assumptions, the postures and muscle tensions that help to maintain our day to day sense of who we are.

Even a routine anaesthetic can open unexpected doors. 'Years ago, I underwent a couple [*sic*] hernia repair surgeries in close succession'— this post from a young woman seeking advice on a medical website. 'During the first surgery, I was only on the operating room table for about twenty-five minutes, and my recovery was normal. During the second, I was under for a good two hours. Physically, I recovered well, but mentally there were problems. I was strangely depressed and didn't feel like myself at all for months afterward. In addition, I found myself lovesick over the surgeon who performed the operations and could not get him out of my head for quite some time…'

So what is it that might leave one patient lovesick, another feeling like a block of wood, and still another convinced she is going to die? It is the drugs. But not just the drugs. While some anaesthetics (ketamine in particular) can trigger delusions, today's cocktails have been designed to minimise such reactions. They remain powerful mind-altering substances, but their effect depends in part on the particular mind they are in the process of altering.

As my own surgery approached, I found myself increasingly anxious— not just about the operation, but about the people who would be involved in operating on me. Would I be paralysed? Would my anaesthetist use a BIS monitor? What drugs would they use? Could I wear headphones during the surgery? I swatted the questions about inside my head, coming up with increasingly unsatisfactory answers, but found myself unable, or unwilling, to pick up the phone and make the necessary inquiries. I felt impatient with myself, irritated. But what I felt most was powerless—a soft slippery feeling that loosened the muscles of my stomach and belly, leaving me undefended against the thoughts that drifted silkily in. Don't be difficult. Don't make a fuss. If they think you are a troublemaker they will refuse to anaesthetise you. And if they won't anaesthetise you, then your surgeon won't operate on you…and so on. I was scared of being ostracised, cast forth, abandoned, punished. I knew this was ridiculous. But I also knew that it was not as ridiculous as all that. I knew that I was in the grip of forces larger than my sensible self, forces more deeply embedded than all the knowledge and research and categories and conclusions at my disposal.

And I knew how much was at stake.

SURFACING

Pulsations and palpitations

A few months before I flew to Brisbane to have my spine reconfigured, two new papers by the Australians Kate Leslie and Paul Myles appeared in the American journal *Anesthesia & Analgesia*, both looking at how the patients in their original B-Aware study had fared over the intervening four or five years.

The first looked at the patients' long-term health. Leslie and Myles already knew from previous studies that patients whose anaesthetists used the BIS monitor generally got lower doses of hypnotic drugs and woke up quicker, feeling less sick and less likely to succumb to various serious complications. They wondered whether there might also be long-term health benefits. Their results, based on reviews of B-Aware patients' medical records and follow-up interviews, were compelling—though not in quite the way they had been imagining. As it turned out, the simple fact of using a BIS monitor did not seem to bestow any particular advantage over time. But when they looked at the patients whose BIS recordings had shown them to have been the most deeply anaesthetised, the result seemed a bit alarming. In the years following their surgery these patients turned out to be at significantly greater risk of heart attack, stroke and death.

Yet on the following page was another study by Leslie and

Myles, also following up the B-Aware patients—this time looking at the fates of those who had received not too much, but too little anaesthetic. After tracking down the seven surviving awareness patients (six having already died), the team assessed their psychological states. Five years after their surgery, '[s]evere late psychological sequelae were common and persistent', with seventy-one per cent still suffering post traumatic stress. Admittedly (and as the authors acknowledged) seventy-one per cent of only seven people is not a lot—five in fact—but it is enough to raise questions about the costs of too-light anaesthesia. Particularly if you are one of the five.

I did not want to be one of the five. Nor one of the tens, maybe hundreds, of thousands worldwide who each year are likely to remember waking during their surgeries, relaxed or otherwise. Nor on the other hand did I want to come through my surgery comfortably comatose, only to have a heart attack or a stroke five years later. Of course the chance of any of these things happening to me was remote. I didn't sit up at my computer and think, 'Oh god, I'm going to die.' The rational, analytical circuitry pinging through my frontal lobes pointed out the fact that, unlike the people who had died or had strokes or heart attacks since Myles and Leslie's original study, I wasn't actually sick to start with—just bent. But the two papers threw into unavoidable relief the central quandary confronting all anaesthetists, and by extension patients: how to know for sure, and for any given person, what is too much or too little?

It is a balance that becomes more critical as new evidence solidifies around a disturbing idea. Doctors have long known that after surgery many patients have problems thinking straight. Postoperative cognitive dysfunction, a mild but sometimes disabling mental fogginess, affects up to fifty per cent of patients in the first week after surgery, with ten to fifteen per cent, mainly elderly, still having problems three months later, sometimes forever. While some evidence suggests that the experience of surgery simply unmasks existing brain vulnerabilities, others suspect anaesthetic drugs themselves might be at least partly to blame. More dramatic—and less ambiguous—is the delirium that often affects older patients as they emerge from surgical anaesthesia, and which has been linked to dementia and even death, although again the precise causes are uncertain. Doctors wonder too about the possible long-term impact of repeated or lengthy anaesthetics on the developing brains of babies. 'From the origins of surgical anaesthesia in the 1840s through the late 1990s, the prevailing view has been that the brain emerged unscathed from the assault of surgery and the pharmacologic coma that we call general anaesthesia,' wrote Harvard Medical School anaesthetist Gregory Crosby in a 2011 editorial in *Anesthesia & Analgesia*. But in the years since, he said, the literature had been 'awash with studies suggesting that is not always the case and that sometimes, in an effort to heal the body, we might be harming the brain'.

The BIS monitor, meanwhile, despite its popularity, has a bolus of critics pointing out its failings and limitations, of which there are, as it turns out, quite a few. (It is less accurate in old people, sensitive to electronic interference and has on more than one occasion shown a wide awake but paralysed patient to be unconscious.) Myles and Leslie acknowledge the limitations but argue that the figures speak for themselves, and that, used as part of the anaesthetist's armoury, the BIS is a valuable weapon, particularly for patients with a high risk of awareness.

Other studies, meanwhile, have shown the monitor to be no more effective than traditional methods. The pointedly titled B-Unaware trial of 2008 found that BIS patients were no more or less likely than those monitored using the standard technique (measuring the concentration of gas exhaled) to wake during surgery, nor did they use less gas. The study's lead author, US anaesthetist Michael Avidan, concluded that while neither protocol was foolproof, the routine use of BIS would be expensive, unjustified and potentially dangerous in that it could lull patients and doctors into 'a false sense of security'.

There was little chance of my being lulled into a sense of security, false or otherwise. I wanted the BIS. I started fretting again about whether my anaesthetist would use it. Would he or she have even heard of it? And what was it measuring anyway?

In fact, before I finished this book, another small study from Finland would show that as we come out of anaesthesia, primitive structures deep in our brains switch on first: before the newer (in evolutionary terms) structures through which we assemble language and ideas, and which had been assumed by many to underpin consciousness. The result surprised the study's authors, who had been looking at what happened in volunteers' brains at the point at which they responded to a request to open their eyes. They had expected to see the outer brain bits (the cerebral cortex) light up first as the subjects came to. Instead, said the study leader, Harry Scheinin, they found the emergence of 'a foundational primitive conscious state' in the older brain centres including the brain stem and thalamus, which linked up with areas in the mid and front sections of the cortex. The authors speculated that this might explain the limitations of EEG-based monitors such as the BIS, which were better at measuring activity close to the skull than in the deeper structures that in fact appeared to rouse first.

Perhaps this is what Ian Russell was measuring with the help of his ludicrously simple Lyall Willis & Co. latex-free cuff—the moments we push across some threshold into another state, before we even understand what it is to be conscious, or perhaps who we are, but in which, if we hear a voice telling us to squeeze the hand holding ours, we will do so.

Or maybe it starts before that. Responding to a blog reporting on the Finnish study, one reader left this post. 'After my surgery a year ago, I remember regaining awareness before being able to see, hear, or feel anything. As the anaesthesia continued to wear off, I gradually began to hear speaking, although it was some time (I don't know how long) before I was able to identify the voices or understand their words.

'I understand that my recalled experiences aren't exactly reliable, but I only mention this because I think we need a more reliable indication of consciousness than motor responses to verbal commands,' he wrote. 'Unfortunately, as I am merely an interested layman, I have no suggestions.'

'Incidentally,' he added, 'that period of darkness, silence, and lack of sensation was probably the most peaceful experience I've ever had. =)'

I think back to Anthony Angel all those years ago at the conference in Hull, and how the professor of physiology described the effect of general anaesthetics on senses such as sight and sound and touch. *And thus, for the patients the world goes silent, black...* I wonder if this was the sort of silence and blackness he meant. Perhaps not. What has become clearer, however, in the decade and more since I heard Angel speak, is the importance of the thalamus—the sensory relay centre nesting above the brain stem, which he nominated as a central target of anaesthesia—and the role of anaesthetic drugs in hindering its ability to communicate with the cortex.

Soon after that Finnish report would come a compelling new study, this one led by American neuroscientist Patrick Purdon in collaboration with Boston anaesthetist, neuroscientist and statistician Emery Brown. I had visited Brown in 2007 at Massachusetts General Hospital where he danced me through a summary of his research into the brain science underpinning anaesthesia. Back then, Brown—beyond whose commentary I could almost glimpse the blazing trajectories of trillions of synaptic pulses—was in the early stages of a series of studies designed to establish what happens to the brain's electrical activity as people lose and then regain consciousness in the presence of anaesthetic drugs.

Six years after our meeting, his team announced they had found what they were looking for. They had slowly anaesthetised first epileptic patients and then volunteers with propofol while asking them to press a button in response to prompts. With the help of hi-tech snapshots that plotted the electrical activity inside the patients' brains, the team identified consistent patterns—what Brown calls neural signatures—they were confident could identify the moments in which subjects dipped from consciousness into unconsciousness and, finally, deep anaesthesia.

There were changes in how brainwaves organised themselves and where in the brain they did it. But in the end it all came down to communication. Soon after the propofol went in, the small choppy waves of the awake brain got bigger, slower—and very, very shouty.

> The same way a loud, long tone, like the Emergency Broad-
> cast tone, drowns out all other noise, anaesthesia drugs create
> long, large, and lasting brainwaves that make it impossible for
> new signals to be passed from one brain region to another.

Basically, said Brown, it was a neural tsunami. 'WAA-WAA-WAA.'

The particulars of the wave pattern differed in consistent ways with different drugs, and changed in consistent ways depending on a patient's age. Central in all this was the moment the enormous waves drowned out communication between the thalamus and the cortex.

Brown has pointed out that this discovery is not new. 'This

was first reported in 1937!!!' But he and his team have since set about methodically isolating the neural signatures for a range of anaesthetic drugs, investigating their mechanisms and representing them in the form of colourful visual displays called spectrograms. These, he now says, help identify in real time transitions that can be obscured by scaled monitors such as the BIS. Anaesthetists can even use the raw EEG measurements already displayed on many existing brain monitors. While he acknowledges there are other mechanisms in play, Brown believes that these neural oscillations are a primary mechanism—'most likely *the* primary mechanism'—through which anaesthetics act in the brain to create the altered states of arousal known as general anaesthesia. 'Our findings move thinking about anaesthesia away from abstract constructs to concrete neurophysiological reasoning whose consequences can be monitored in the operating room.' In a practical sense, he says, they enable him now to safely use far less anaesthetic—up to seventy-five per cent less—particularly in older and frailer patients.

That said, at this stage, Brown estimates that at best half of US anaesthetists actually use the EEG and far fewer are yet able to read the raw data and its spectrogram. 'We are teaching this now.' The technique is yet to be tested in large clinical trials.

Nor of course can this tell us anything about patients' subjective experiences as they go under or what unconscious traces may or may not be left behind. What it does tell us is that soon after receiving propofol patients stop responding first to clicking sounds and then to their names, and that shortly after that the tsunami hits.

Around which point we assume the world goes silent and black.

Before finishing this book I also spoke again with George Mashour, the trainee anaesthetist whose pristine loft I visited in Ann Arbor in 2007. A lot had happened for him in the intervening years. He had become a senior faculty member at the University of Michigan, edited major books on anaesthesia, consciousness and neuroscience, and picked up a prestigious award from the American Society of Anesthesiologists along the way. And his nascent paradigm of cognitive unbinding as an underlying principle of anaesthesia, published when he was still a clinical resident, was by now broadly accepted in the field. ('Before, I had concepts and ideas that I was giving to you; now there is a lot of data to support these hypotheses.')

His metaphors had moved on too. No longer was he describing an orchestra with musicians playing from set scores. Now he was talking about riffs rising and sparking new riffs, a supple sinuous mindscape inventing and reinventing itself as it went along ('I'm playing piano and you're playing bass'). This was jazz. And the riffs that interested him most were the ones that looped back and forth between the older brain structures, blasting notes and tones from the sensory organs (eyes, ears, big toe) into the frontal cortex where this raw data was somehow synthesised into the fluctuating music we call consciousness. And, yes, research—his own and other people's—had confirmed that while, under anaesthesia, sensory information still loops its way from the back of the brain towards the front, the second part of the process breaks down—the part where it somehow gets put together to create your awareness of lying there knowing you're being operated upon. 'In a sense you have the information that you need for experience but you don't have the tools to assemble that information.'

Mashour said a great deal more. What it meant in practical terms, he agreed, was that anaesthetists trying to gauge their patients' depth of anaesthesia may well be looking for the wrong things in the wrong places. Rather than measuring activity in a particular brain region, he argued, a monitor would need to plot the connections between those regions. These neural interactions—within the cortex and between the thalamus and cortex—are where Mashour and a bunch of other investigators from around the world are now focusing their formidable energies. But that is as much as I can tell you, and more than I let on to Mashour.

I did not, for instance, confess that despite repeated attempts I could still barely conceptualise a brainwave, let alone the mechanisms of directional connectivity between different regions of the brain. Nor multimodal association, nor global scale-free organisation. Not that Mashour wasn't patient or articulate or a dab hand (obviously) at metaphors. He was. He was terrific. And dauntingly intelligent. I just didn't understand it. Any more than I had understood Emery Brown's signature of unconsciousness or Stuart Hameroff's micro-tubules or any of the various other models and theories I have in recent years tried to stretch my head around as to what might actually happen in my brain when someone else switches it from on to off. Their research was clearly important. I was interested in the fact of it, and in the *WAA-WAA*. I was interested in the brain flaring up and down like a faulty power board. I was interested in jazz. But what I was really interested in was people. And what I could not yet see was what these discoveries might mean away from the laboratory and in the lived experience of you or me. I knew that the fact that I did not understand how the one related to the other did not mean that they did not. I knew that one day these discoveries might change the lives of millions of people for the better. And I was glad of that.

But I suspected that for all their intellectual heft and technolog-ical whizz-bangery, what these breakthroughs were on the way to solving was philosopher David Chalmers' easy problem. And what interested me much more was the hard one.

That may be why I felt more comfortable sitting one scrappy autumn day in a not-very-nice outdoor cafe on Circular Quay with my old acquaintance Michael Wang, the British psychologist. And why I perked up when he said, 'I have to say this stuff doesn't turn me on.'

Wang (stripy T-shirt, blue cap, the big open smile of a man who has just spent a week sailing the Great Barrier Reef) said the preoccupation with multi-million-dollar brain imaging machines was distorting the research agenda, imposing hi-tech solutions on a problem whose parameters had not yet been adequately defined. 'I think there's an awful lot of stuff in neuroscience literature that is totally without merit or meaning in terms of—well you found one little part of your brain lit up or didn't light up. So what?'

In the event of anyone ever giving him a great pile of money for research, Wang said, he would like to stage a large study in which he too lowered volunteers slowly under—but in which he looked not at what was happening inside their brains, but their minds. 'What mechanisms are at play? What sort of emotional meanings are there for people at different levels of consciousness? How is memory distorted during those planes of consciousness? That's the experiment I would be interested in doing.'

He called this 'the psychology of what's going on', and said these insights would be more useful than any number of neurological studies.

Wang is a psychologist, so it is unsurprising that he might say this. But he believes his approach would have practical implications for anyone going under a general anaesthetic. In the operating theatre, he argues, his experiment could help understand what you or I might experience if, during surgery, we started to rise towards consciousness. 'And how that might open doors to primitive parts of the brain and memory and processing that are really important emotionally.'

Because in the end, of course, a monitor, no matter how effective, can only ever be one part of an equation that must also include the doctors and technicians who are operating and interpreting that monitor, and, crucially, the human being it is attached to, and whose pulsations and palpitations, currents and calamities it is designed to identify and interpret.

Wang knows no one is ever going to give him that pile of money. But despite having retired from teaching he intends to continue his research. 'I just think that we're messing around with things that could be quite serious. And we just don't know what we're doing. And most anaesthetists aren't really interested.'

He is pretty sure he knows of one person who would have backed him, had he been around in the days of general anaesthetics. 'What a fabulous opportunity to really get down to studying what consciousness is all about. I think Freud would have given his right arm to do some of this stuff.'

o

At the around the time of her first diagnosis, my mother started working on some new paintings. Again, the grids. Again the high, clear eye. But now they are different. And perhaps it is also that now I can see them differently. We each have one, my sisters and I; mine is on the wall in my study. Here the lines are finer, their colours stronger. A mesh of white and red and orange resting over a flat-spread world of remnant green and dun earth. But something changes in the looking. It takes patience; this not an image to glance at. It is, I now realise, a portal. Thirty seconds. Longer. Long. And then things start to move. At first I think it is the grid, then I think it is the land beneath, then I think it must be the space between. I stand, with my back to my desk and the window and the garden beyond, and let my gaze settle on my mother's painting. Quietly, calmly. And the colours start to shimmer. It's like looking out from your window seat and seeing, far below, the shadows of the clouds above you as they break apart. Things dapple. Spread. Leap around the canvas. It is uncanny. Light appears from nowhere. *Nowhere.* It happens (I understand with my thinking brain) not in the canvas but in the relationship between the canvas and the viewer. The painting has not changed (*surely?*) but something in me has (*must* have). And now, as I gaze into my mother's marks, the grid at the centre starts to expand and throb, a steadfast beat; and the world beyond it tilts and opens; pulses <*flares*> I see.

The shallows

The day after I rang the Brisbane anaesthesia providers to confess my anxieties about my looming anaesthetic, I picked up my phone to a call from a stranger. He introduced himself as the anaesthetist who was going to put me under and hopefully keep me there for the duration of my surgery. I'll call him John.

He was lovely. Chatty, informative, reassuring. It was very important, he said at the start, that I not be anxious. He was going to do everything he could to make sure I wasn't. He started by telling me exactly what he proposed to do. He would put me to sleep with propofol and midazolam via a drip in my hand. He would then put another drip in to keep my blood pressure low. And once I was unconscious, he would keep me asleep with a potent anaesthetic gas, a modern relative of ether.

He managed to say all of this without making me feel foolish. Without my asking, he volunteered that he would be using at least one BIS monitor. He knew of Kate Leslie and Paul Myles and their B-Aware study. 'I always try and use the BIS.' Nor would he be using paralysing drugs except at the start of the procedure, to relax my muscles while he put the breathing tube down my airway. Then, he said, the assembled theatre staff would flip me, 'like a turkey', onto my belly. (This was the only moment in the conversation I felt un-soothed.) He would be monitoring me the entire time. He would not be discussing films or golf or playing Sudoku. And he was very confident that I would remember nothing. 'It's never happened in the twelve years I've been giving anaesthetics. I'd have to work hard to give someone awareness.'

But it is easy to give someone information.

Emery Brown, the Boston anaesthetist whose team have discovered what they call a neural signature for unconsciousness, would like his patients to know a bit more about the insides of their heads. Not as much as he does, obviously, but enough to have some sort of language for what is going to happen to them. Heart, lung, kidneys, the dark sump of the liver: as proprietors of these organs, we have at least some sense of what they do in our bodies, and of what might happen if they stopped doing it.

The brain less so. Our brains are mysterious not only because scientists don't know everything about them, but because we, the owners of those brains, know almost nothing about them. Yet if Emery Brown tells me there is a pulpy region inside my skull that helps me form memories, and another that tells me when I am in pain, and still others that are keeping me alert right now, and if he explains that anaesthetics temporarily 'turn down' or 'snip' the connections between these brain regions by producing large disruptive rhythms, it all starts to seem a lot less mysterious. Almost straightforward.

The fact that he doesn't understand what it is he is taking away doesn't seem to worry him. 'All we have to do is agree that there's a certain set of circuits which could, when active, allow you to have conscious processing. I may not understand how key brain areas work together to do that, but all I have to do is figure out how I can turn them off. Or on. And I'm done.' Easy.

And talk, as it turns out, is not only cheap but effective (a preoperative visit from an anaesthetist has been shown to be better than a tranquilliser at keeping patients calm). I know from experience how intensely reassuring such a conversation can be. For me it was not just the information, or even mainly the information (although I clung to it); it was the fact of the human contact, of being treated as an equal, of being included, rather than feeling an appendage to a process to which I was, after all, central. But if you were my anaesthetist, I hope you would tell me about more than just the pulpy regions inside my head; more even than my anaesthetist, John, told me in that phone call. Above all I would want you to tell me about paralysis.

Hank Bennett, the American psychologist I met in Hull, remembers a young girl whose mother brought her to see him in some time after the girl had her adenoids removed. The surgeon referred the mother to Bennett after she had returned to him anxious about her child. The surgery had been straightforward, but the mother felt that something was very wrong with her previously happy daughter: the child had withdrawn from her family and friends and had stopped working at school. She could no longer fall asleep without her mother sitting with her, and was afraid of the dark.

Bennett spoke with the girl. He told her there must be a reason she had changed her behaviour, and asked if it might have something to do with the operation.

And she said, 'Yes.' (I was very clear, she said that.) 'They said that they were going to put me to sleep, but the next thing that I know I couldn't breathe, and I felt as though I couldn't breathe anything.'

Now, she was only momentarily like that—she does not

remember the breathing tube going in—but when I asked why she was doing these things differently at school and at home, she said, 'Well, I have to concentrate and I can't be bothered by anything. I've got to make sure that I can breathe.'

Bennett referred the girl to a child psychologist and within weeks she was back to herself. Today she would be approaching middle age. 'But let's say, that was just luck,' Bennett says now. 'What if nothing had been picked up about that? Would she have been permanently changed? I think that you would say, yes, she probably would have been.'

Recently, doctors in the United Kingdom undertook a hugely ambitious project. Over three years, they audited and analysed three million general anaesthetics carried out in every public hospital in Britain and Ireland to try to establish who reports waking during general anaesthesia, what happens when they do awaken, and what might be done to stop it happening again. It was an astonishing effort. To start with, the Royal College of Anaesthetists' 5th National Audit Project on accidental awareness during general anaesthesia (NAP5 for short) gathered and scrutinised more cases of awareness than all those ever reported in all the previous literature combined. It provided some extraordinarily detailed information about the experience of anaesthetic awareness and its impact on sufferers. Among its many findings were that, despite most episodes apparently lasting less than five minutes, half those patients went on to suffer longer-term psychological problems. What the audit also confirmed beyond doubt were the potential risks in paralysing patients. Fewer than half all general anaesthetics in the UK included a muscle relaxant, but ninety-three per cent of reports to the audit involved patients who had been paralysed. Even brief experiences of paralysis could be devastating.

> The experience most strongly associated with psychological sequelae was distress at the time of the event. This in turn was strongly associated with a sensation of paralysis. The majority of patients reporting paralysis developed moderate or severe longer-term sequelae.

What was also striking was that the solution, or part of it, had been there all along. Among the many recommendations about anaesthetic regimes and training and monitoring and safety checks, the simplest and most plentiful advice to anaesthetists was to *communicate*—with each other, and particularly with their patients. To tell them beforehand that they might briefly wake and find themselves unable to move, and that this would pass; to reassure them *during* surgery if there was even a hint of them having woken; to speak to them as they emerged, explaining what was happening; and finally, to listen respectfully and sympathetically if they later complained of having been aware.

After Rachel Benmayor was wheeled, wide awake, from the operating theatre all those years ago, the first thing she did was to start trying to call for her husband, Glenn. The paralysing drugs were finally beginning to wear off, and she recalls a nurse coming across and standing over her. What happened next has stayed with her ever since.

> She started talking to me really loudly, like I was a child, in a way. I was trying to say 'Get Glenn'. And she's going 'Mrs Benmayor, you've had a lovely baby. You've had a lovely little girl.'
> And I'm like, 'I know. I know. She's fine. I know. Get Glenn!' I kept on trying but I was really blurred and she

kept on rabbiting on and just treating me like I was—it was very controlling and gross. There was no space for me there, whatsoever.

And I realised really powerfully that all over the world when people come out of general anaesthetics at that point they are very close to their own inner consciousness, and they are very vulnerable, and often have seen things or felt things that they may not have seen or felt for a long time. And when you've got staff practically bellowing at you because they think that you're unconscious—I was just so clear that it was such a wrong way to deal with people.

o

I have only ever entered a hospital as a visitor, a patient, or, from time to time, a journalist. I can only imagine the pressures of working each week in a world of limited and often contracting resources, of overarching and often competing priorities, in which every day there is a risk you might kill a client. No surprise that a patient's emotional needs will sometimes come a far second to their survival. Even then, I have heard many stories of kindness: the Italian nurses who wordlessly stroked an English-speaking friend who found herself alone and afraid in a foreign hospital; the Australian theatre nurse who reached for a violently shivering young woman about to go into surgery and held her quaking body to her own until the patient was warm and calm. I suspect the reality is that most theatre staff are professional, and many are much, much more. But some are not.

Reston, Virginia, April 2013. A man later identified in court documents only as D. B. is about to have a colonoscopy. Knowing there is a chance he will be woozy when the doctor talks to him after the anaesthetic, he pushes the record button on his mobile phone. Later, remembering nothing, he plays it back. Here is his anaesthetist: 'After five minutes of talking to you in pre-op, I wanted to punch you in the face and man you up a little bit.' She calls D. B. a 'retard'. She tells the other theatre staff he probably has syphilis and tuberculosis of the penis. She is awful.

The trial lasts three days. One of those to testify is a former president of the Academy of Anesthesiology, Kathryn McGoldrick. 'These types of conversations are not only offensive but frankly stupid,' she tells the court, 'because we can never be certain that our patients are asleep and wouldn't have recall.' D. B. describes months of anxiety and sleeplessness. The jury awards him half a million dollars.

What motivated that anaesthetist? Was this her usual bedside manner? Who knows. You can only hope that this sort of sadism is vanishingly rare. But operating theatres, like any other theatre of human endeavour, teem with the frailties that come with being human. And staff—even those who know they are being watched—sometimes say or do spectacularly inappropriate things.

Some years back, I spoke with a researcher who had sat in on an operation in which a woman was having breast implants inserted. 'The patient looked completely normal from my point of view—but she clearly was very unhappy about how she looked to want to go through that sort of procedure.' The woman was unconscious. 'And the surgeon and a male nurse were kind of juggling with these different implants and making comments about how she would look if she had one this big, or this big, or what about a massive one like this? You know, "Cor!"' The researcher, who did not want to named, had found the behaviour more stupid than offensive, but felt that the patient might have been very much more vulnerable. 'She was already prepared to have a general anaesthetic and surgery to change the way she looked, so I assumed she was pretty unhappy with how she looked at the time. So for her those might have been quite important comments, had she been able to hear them or process them.'

We'll never know.

What we do know is that while most people seem to settle back into their lives pretty easily after general anaesthesia, quite a few don't. Recently a team including George Mashour spent around two years monitoring a series of patients who had undergone elective surgery. They found that even in patients who gave no evidence of having been awake during their operations, fifteen per cent later showed signs of PTSD. There are various possible explanations—social isolation, previous medical experience, personal frailties and so on—but in the end, for whatever reasons, it seems fair to assume that a significant minority of patients will undergo their surgery at a heightened risk of emerging less psychologically healthy than they went in. This doesn't mean they are mad or bad. It just means they are vulnerable. We are vulnerable.

So if you were my anaesthetist and I your patient, there are some other things I'd hope you would do in the operating theatre. Things that Kate Leslie and Paul Myles and many others already do. Be kind. Talk to me. Nothing highbrow, just a bit of information and reassurance. Use my name. Patients who remember waking are often greatly relieved at having been told what was happening to them, and reassured that this was OK and that they would now drift back to sleep.

> The patient's interpretation of what is happening at the time of the awareness seemed central to later impact; explanation and reassurance during suspected accidental awareness during general anaesthesia or at the time of report seemed beneficial.

Most of us will remember nothing. But in keeping that small channel open, even if only in your imagination, you would be practising a form of Tonglen meditation—breathing in the difficulty: the embarrassment (yours); the terrifying vulnerability (ours); breathing out something softer. Your colleagues might think you odd, but they'd get used to it. And just to make sure, you could put a sign on the wall of the operating theatre: *The patient can hear.* Because one of the strange things about anaesthetic drugs is that they can exert their effect in each direction—not just upon the patient, but upon the doctors and theatre staff performing the procedure.

After the son of a good friend was badly burned in an accident some years ago, he had to endure weeks of intense pain culminating each week in the agonising ritual of nurses changing the dressings over his chest and arms. They did this by giving the teenager a dose of a sedative drug designed to distract him from the pain and prevent him remembering it. My friend would attempt to comfort her son as he yelled and as the nurses got on with their difficult task. What she observed was that while the drugs did give her son some distance from his pain, and certainly his memories of it, they also gave the nurses some distance from her son. It was an understandable, perhaps necessary, distance; but inherent in that tiny retreat (the lack of eye contact, the too-bright voices) was a loosening of the tiny filaments that connect us one to another, and through which we know we are connected. It is a process inevitably magnified in the operating theatre, where the patient is silent and still, to all intents absent, and where their descent into unconsciousness is routinely accompanied by the sounds of the music being cranked up (one prominent Australian surgeon is said to favour heavy metal), and the building prerogative of conversation.

It need not take a scientific study (although someone, bless them, has done one) to tell us that this deepening of respect and focus is good not only for patients but for doctors, whose neural reward centres glow when they believe they are delivering effective treatments. In the end, it might not even much matter what you say. 'To the extent that intra-operative suggestions do some good,' writes psychologist

John Kihlstrom, 'the limitations on information processing during anaesthesia may mean that any positive effects are more likely to be mediated by their prosody, and other physical features, than by their meaning: a soothing voice may be more important than what the voice says.' Kihlstrom still encourages anaesthetists to talk to their anaesthetised patients ('about what is going on, giving reassurance, things like that') but acknowledges he doesn't expect them to understand any of it—not verbally at least.

Japanese anaesthetist Jiro Kurata calls this care of the soul. In an unusual and rather lovely paper delivered at MAA9, he wondered if there might be 'part of our existence that cannot ever be shut down, which we cannot even conceive by ourselves'—a 'subconscious self' that might be resistant to even high doses of anaesthetics. He called this the hard problem of anaesthesia awareness. I have no idea what his colleagues made of it. But his conclusion seems unassailable. 'Any solution? Science? Yes and no. Monitoring? Yes and no. Respect? Yes. We must not only be aware of the inherent limitation of science and technology but, most importantly, also of the inherent dignity of each personal "self".'

Blood and blushing

A week or so after my phone conversation with John, the anaesthetist who was going to oversee my spinal surgery, I rang him back with the question I had felt too flaky to ask the first time we spoke. Would it be all right if I wore earphones during the surgery, through which to play myself music or other recordings? John was unperturbed. It was fine with him, he said, as long as my surgeon agreed. He had heard that playing music could be helpful for patients having anaesthesia. His only caution was that occasionally devices like mine could interfere with the operation of other electronic equipment such as the diathermy wands used to cut and cauterise tiny blood vessels during surgery. There had even been rare reports of players overheating or occasionally bursting into flames and burning the ears of unwitting patients. 'It's very, very rare,' he said hurriedly as I started to laugh.

'Well, take them out,' I said, 'if my ears start smoking.'

As it turned out, I did not get to wear earphones during my surgery. My surgeon told me that my iPod might interfere with the equipment with which he was monitoring my spine. But he was more than happy for me to bring music with me to be played over the operating theatre speakers while I was being put to sleep. So that is what I did. I accepted my doctor's decision: he was, after all, going to be drilling into my backbone right next to my spinal cord. If he would prefer not to have digital equipment running, then so, in the end, would I. At least I had tried. And even that, oddly, seemed to make me feel better.

The point is that it is not just what we as patients take away from the operating table that might matter, but what we bring to it in the first place. And here some doctors have been helping us to help ourselves.

Ten years ago doctors at New York City's Mount Sinai School of Medicine randomly assigned two hundred women facing surgery for breast cancer to two groups. Shortly before their operations each woman met with a psychologist for fifteen minutes. For half the women, these brief sessions were presented as a chance to chat or ask questions about their surgeries. The psychologists were very nice. They did not try to control the proceedings, but listened attentively, allowing the women to direct the conversation, and responding with a series of suitably supportive and empathic comments. This was the control group.

The second group was treated rather differently. Unlike the free-range empathising of the control group, these women were hypnotised. Beginning with relaxation and pleasant imagery, they were then given specific suggestions including that they would experience reduced pain, nausea and fatigue. They were also given instructions on how to use hypnosis for themselves.

The results were galvanising—or should have been. Not only did the hypnosis group use less drugs (during surgery and after), spend less time in surgery, and report less pain, nausea, fatigue and emotional upset upon awakening, hypnosis also saved the hospital an estimated $772.71 per patient, largely in reduced surgery time. This was whether or not the patient was even particularly hypnotisable.

Consider the more than twenty million people who each year have surgery under general anaesthesia in the US alone. As the researchers pointed out, these savings could more than compensate hospitals for the cost of hiring psychologists to spend fifteen minutes with patients before their operations. 'The present brief hypnosis intervention appears to be one of the rare clinical interventions that can simultaneously reduce both symptom burden and costs.'

As an editorial in the same edition of the *Journal of the National Cancer Institute* noted, 'If a drug were to do that, everyone would by now be using it.

'So why don't they?'

None of this, as it turns out, is new. In 2003, the year before I first visited Hull, members of the same team of doctors had analysed a bunch of similar studies and concluded that patients having hypnosis fared better than nine out of ten of those in control groups when it came to pain, anxiety and depression, as well as length of surgery and hospital stay, and stress markers including blood pressure and heart rate. This was so whether the hypnotic suggestions were made by a living, breathing person or via a (much cheaper) tape recording.

How all this actually happens remains (no surprises here) unclear. Some wonder if hypnosis might work by reducing the distress associated with surgery; others if it has more to do with changing patients' expectations. Still others suspect the magic may have nothing to do with hypnosis at all—but might simply be the result of patients getting extra attention from medical staff. And then there are the familiar question marks about study size and design. Even so, the Mount Sinai team concluded: 'This suggests that... adjunctive hypnosis is a powerful tool for addressing signs and symptoms after surgery.'

..

In the lead-up to my own looming surgery, I emailed Hank Bennett about a small study he had carried out ten years before, on ninety-two patients undergoing major spinal surgery. The procedure is one in which patients typically bleed so much that they need a blood transfusion, and Bennett wanted to know if there was anything he could do—or that patients could do—*before* the surgery that would help stem this flow. He had a hunch that instead of viewing the patient's role in surgery as completely passive, he might be able to encourage them to help themselves during their operations. During the standard pre-operative interview, he made suggestions to some of the patients, each of whom had been randomly assigned to one of three groups. The control group were simply given information about monitors that would be used during the surgery. A second group were also given some additional relaxation exercises. But those in the third group received a rather more interesting instruction: during the operation they were to shunt blood away from the site of their incision, returning it to the area after the wound had been closed.

This would almost certainly qualify as one of Kate Leslie's 'spooky little studies'. Yet the results were eye-opening. The control group lost on average a litre (about twenty per cent) of their blood. The relaxation group fared even worse, losing close to 1.2 litres. But the fifty-one people in the 'blood shunting' group had a mean estimated blood loss of only 650 millilitres—a third less than the control group.

All for an intervention that took minutes and cost nothing.

Other researchers have had varying success trying to reproduce Bennett's results. But with my own surgery drawing nearer, I thought it was worth a try.

In reply to my email, Bennett sent me a link to the audio he had made, following his experiment, for people preparing for surgery. I didn't listen to it immediately. In fact for some time I pretended it wasn't there. Then, one afternoon a few weeks before the scheduled operation, I moved the recording to my iPod and lay down on my bed to listen. Bennett's voice, slightly distorted, reassembled in my ears.

I've been working in the Department of Anesthesiology for more than fifteen years, Bennett said into my ears, *and I've talked to a lot of patients about ways of going through their surgery more comfortably, recovering more quickly and having a sense of wellbeing throughout their surgical experience.* He spoke unusually slowly and deliberately, as if pacing out each sentence in some large room (an old gymnasium, maybe) or perhaps following a cortege. *I'd like to talk to you using this tape recording about ways to go through your surgery more comfortably. As well, there will be soothing sounds and my voice present during the unconsciousness of your anaesthesia, during your surgery.* He continued at this pace, accompanied by some aimless synthesised music of the sort often played in the nineties. *In anaesthesia,* he said, *we have an old saying: the way the patient goes into anaesthesia is the way the patient will come out of anaesthesia. This has been true for over one hundred years. It is very important that as you come out of anaesthesia from your surgery that all of the muscles at the site of your operation be completely relaxed...*

Lying on my back in my bedroom, I was not completely relaxed. Instead I seemed once again to be battling the twin forces of anxiety and inertia. Part of me sinking, part of me restless, resistant. My chest was feeling tight and a long way from my stomach. What if I went into anaesthesia panicking—how would I come out then? (What if I didn't come out? What if I didn't even go in at all?)

I'm going to be talking to you about things you already know how to do, I'll be talking to you about abilities you already have— doing things that you already know about, because these are things that you can already do... He talked throughout the tape in this strange, circular manner, looping ideas over and around each other, collapsing sentences and reconstituting them slightly altered. My surgery was a way of repairing my body. He mentioned goals and exertion. Accomplishment. Then the sound of flowing water. *In order for you to have relaxed muscles at the site of your surgery and through your body as you come out of your anaesthesia it's important that you go into your anaesthesia thinking, feeling, imagining a warm relaxed place, where you have been before.* More running water. (A bath?) *Perhaps the warmth of the sun on your skin*...I was beginning to feel confused. (Bath? Beach?)... *You'll be sending signals to your body of relaxation and warmth, just the kind of signals that will take you into your anaesthesia in a way that will allow you to come out after your operation with warm and relaxed muscles throughout your body, especially under the bandages, especially at the site of your operation*...His voice plodded on...*warm relaxed place*...*site of operation*...*limp like a rag doll*...*good blood flow*...*nutrients*...*heal your body quickly*...

As he spoke, I felt I was listening carefully to everything he said, but after a while, with the repetition and the odd syntax and his deliberate, rhythmic way of speaking, his sentences started to detach and float around in the eddies of his voice.

A few years later, when I spoke with him again, Bennett had changed his mind about the need for all this rigmarole. Rather than relying on hypnotic suggestion or languorous looping tape recordings or even psychologists, Bennett now believes anaesthetists can do it themselves. All they have to do, he says, is tell people what to tell their own bodies. For an attentive and motivated patient, the rest will follow. 'You just don't need the word "hypnotic" in any of this. It is a direct instruction, it is a direct instruction to the body.' Other studies also suggest that simply giving patients information and tips on how to emerge cheerfully from an anaesthetic may sometimes do the trick. But lying on my back in bed, this was all immaterial. Bennett's circuitous tape was what I had. So I kept listening.

Now, said Bennett, *I'd like to talk about another aspect of your surgery. By way of introduction, have you ever been embarrassed, have you ever felt so embarrassed, where somebody's words said something and something happened, somebody said something and all by itself these words caused you to feel embarrassed…*On he went…*felt the warmth come up into your neck and your face…perhaps you even blushed…that warmth, that blushing, is blood moving up into your face…somebody's words caused blood to move up into your face, and what this means is that words can cause blood to move…so I want to talk you now about having very little blood loss during your surgery…*

And now he had my attention.

It's very important that during the operation the blood at the site of your surgery will move away to other parts of your body…and down deep into your body where the surgeon will be operating, the tissues will move the blood away from that site…and all you have to do is listen to my words…After the operation, as you're awakening, the blood will move back into that area, bringing the nutrients to heal your body at the site of your surgery…back into the relaxed limp tissues and muscles…

He continued in his meandering way: blood and blushing and wound sites, washing up and into, healing and warmth.

Now just allow this music to wash over you.

This suggestion came about twenty-five minutes into the forty-five-minute recording, and I took it as my cue to turn off the tape. The music annoyed me. Hank was beginning to annoy me. I was annoying me.

And yet, for all my wriggling and carping, my doubts and mental resistance, a couple of days later I listened again, and a few days after that. And I kept listening. By the time I boarded my flight to Brisbane I had probably heard the tape ten times. I kept listening because I wanted to. Because Hank Bennett's slow, repetitive voice was soothing. Because I did indeed want to be warm and relaxed as I entered my surgery. Because I wanted even more, and despite the seeming improbability of it all, to shunt the blood in my unconscious body away from the wound that would soon open in my back. And finally, and perhaps most importantly, I kept listening because I wanted to feel that there was something, anything, that I could do—some action that I, Kate, reduced by fear and passivity and circumstances, could take—that would make even a skin's depth of difference in that drear dark room towards which I felt I was hurtling. And this, it seemed, was what Hank Bennett was offering me.

Ballast

Night time. The boy is eight. He cannot stop thinking. Until a moment ago he had never thought this thought before and now it keeps rolling around inside him. One day he will die.

'I remember lying in bed in the dark trying to imagine what it would be like to be dead. Putting myself into a kind of oblivion, total darkness and just floating in nothingness, and then trying to imagine this is what eternity would be like.'

Michael Wang understands now that his logic was flawed. The death he imagined all those years ago was worse than death. 'I had this horror, this terrifying horror of being conscious and yet having absolutely no agency, and in this world of black oblivion.'

This conversation took place at the not-very-nice outdoor cafe at Circular Quay in 2015. Wang was by this stage sixty-five, newly retired, happy, healthy, although he coughed when he said the words 'black oblivion'. He had been thinking about this childhood memory quite a bit. Recently he had been involved in NAP5, the largest ever study of people who remembered waking during anaesthesia. He had helped write chapter seven, which focused on the psychological impact of accidental awareness. But this was not what we mainly talked about. Mainly we talked about death. One of the things that had struck Michael Wang most forcibly during the long and rigorous audit was hearing several vivid accounts from people who had woken under anaesthetic and concluded they had died.

Reading these reports, he thought back to his eight-year-old self, lying there in the dark trying to imagine a frozen black forever. He suspects now that this is a very common fear, one that might be most particular to cultures with a tradition of entombing or burying their dead. Then he thought about all the patients he had seen over the years who had found themselves awake under anaesthetic. It is just a theory, he says. But, 'If that is the case—think about it—even for the most trivial of surgery, if it involves a general anaesthetic, we all have the thought,'—here he lowered his voice a little—'"I might die. I might die during this operation."' Wang thinks it himself every time he goes under, even though he knows that statistically he is almost certain not to.

'I think there is something profoundly primitive, hugely frightening that surrounds becoming conscious on the operating theatre table in this state of apparent oblivion, complete lack of agency, darkness...And there you are. You've died. And this is the way you're going to be for eternity.'

In the end, the most important thing we bring to surgery is ourselves. Not just our diagnoses and prognoses, but the whole squirming bag. History, culture, psychology, stories, fears. The baggage that weighs us down and the ballast that keeps us stable. We bring them with us and afterwards they are the materials from which we reconstruct ourselves.

Lying in a Perth hospital following a car accident in 1999, his body smashed 'like a toad's' the late art critic and historian Robert Hughes had a lengthy encounter with the dead Spanish artist Goya. Hughes had for years been trying and failing to write about the great and graphic chronicler of wartime atrocity. Finally Goya, perceiving perhaps that he now had the upper hand, chose to appear. Hughes had been placed in an induced anaesthetic coma to give him a chance of surviving the impact that had wrecked much of the right side of his body. Unconscious in intensive care, his leg encased in a metal brace, he dreamed that he was in a lunatic asylum that also happened to be the Seville airport. Hughes was desperate to catch an Iberia jet to get him away from the madness. Instead, he was being tormented by a young Goya and his friends who had attached a metal implement to his right leg to prevent his escape. Each time Hughes tried to go through the security gate a buzzer would go off and he would be dragged back. The more he tried to escape the torture—and his torturers—the tighter the trap. This struggle was part of what Hughes brought to his anaesthetic. And it was what allowed him, after a slow and painful recovery of sorts, to finally write the book he had been battling for so long.

Just after Christmas 2012, Michael Wang discovered for himself some of the strange things that anaesthetic drugs can do to the mind—and the ways in which the mind tries to make sense of them. After a lifetime of good health, Wang had been admitted to hospital a month earlier for surgery to repair an errant electrical signal in the upper chambers of his heart. The procedure, known as an ablation, involved pushing a wire up through his groin and femoral vein and into the faulty organ and there burning away a fragment of tissue that had been causing the stutter. All seemed to have gone well and he had been discharged with a steadily beating heart, until four weeks later he woke up in a frozen foetal curl: rigid, fevered, delirious. ('I was basically off my head.') Back in hospital his doctors discovered that the surgeon in the previous operation had accidentally burnt a hole through the heart wall and into his oesophagus from where bacteria had migrated, then incubated. They were now in the process of killing him.

In the intensive care unit after emergency surgery, Wang became convinced he was on a hospital ship. Beyond the windows of the ICU he could see trees sliding past. 'I thought it was a riverbank. I was on a boat, and we were moving past the riverbank.' Later he was transported beneath the ICU, into a crypt—a Chinese mausoleum—where he found himself surrounded by illuminated Chinese symbols and ginger jars full of human remains. Travelling with him into the hallucinatory crypt were the two nurses from ICU, who were shouting at him.

Clearly Wang was not in a Chinese mausoleum, any more than Robert Hughes had been at Seville airport being taunted by Francisco Goya. But here in this hallucinatory melange, Wang had brought together a unique array of ingredients. There was the non-existent riverbank and the imaginary room in the basement of the hospital. Then there were props he had pulled in from the room around him: the trees, which were indeed outside the window (albeit stationary), the frantic nurses, and the lines and monitors that he was in that very moment trying to pull out. There were the metaphors: the mausoleum, the body parts. Then there was his own cultural and personal history: the Chinese vault, the ginger jars (just the sort of oriental knick-knacks Wang's father had sold in his shop when Wang was a boy). Perhaps Wang also brought with him a sanguine disposition. Certainly he brought his Christian faith. But he also brought his background as a psychologist—one with a particular interest in the strange things anaesthetic drugs can do to the mind. And instead of being alarmed by or afraid of the hallucinations, he was intrigued. 'I appreciate from the listener's point of view they sound horrific [but] I really had no significant anxiety or emotion. I didn't find them terribly traumatic experiences, and I don't have nightmares. I was very curious, to be honest...I realised that they were odd experiences, and I was curious as to what was going on.'

This is what Michael Wang would bring with him to surgery.

But it was not all that he would bring.

Three psychologists in a car. Munich, 2008. The accounts differ slightly. In one, they are driving to the airport after a conference; in another they are touring the nearby Bavarian Alps. Perhaps they are doing both. Either way, they are talking. Maybe they start by discussing the conference they have all just attended, the 7th International Symposium on Memory and Awareness in Anaesthesia. MAA7. But then they start to speculate about what might have drawn them to their professions in the first place: psychologists with a fascination in anaesthesia.

One, an American called Shelley Freeman, is pretty sure she knows. She has previously spoken about her memories of waking under ether as a six-year-old after being terribly burnt—and hearing the doctors discussing the futility of going through all this for a child who would almost certainly die. Her shock and incomprehension when her unwitting parents later sent her back for more surgery. She had flashbacks to this experience when as a young psychologist she visited a rehabilitation facility for victims of torture. She went on to attend the second MAA conference and many others, including the one in Hull where I first came across her and the two colleagues now driving with her through the German countryside.

They have met before. But today, for the first time, they realise they have something else in common. A second American, Ruth Reinsel, tells the story of reaching, as a four-year-old, for the glowing element on the electric heater. The little grey coat with red buttons she wore on the way to the hospital. And then, a year or so later, crying alone at night in a different hospital where she had been taken for a skin graft, her arm tied to the bedrail to prevent her from thrashing or lying on it.

Now the third speaks. When he was ten months old, the high chair into which he was strapped fell over, tipping him into an open coal fire. He avoided landing face first in the flames by thrusting his left arm into the coals. He remembers none of this, nor the three years of operations and anaesthetics that followed as doctors grafted new skin over his tiny, damaged hand.

'I have one memory,' he wrote to me recently, 'of standing in a hospital cot-bed (with barred sides) feeling emotionally abandoned by my parents who had been visiting me and had had to leave. I think I would be about two years old at the time.'

A little later he wrote again: 'I don't recall ever wondering before this conversation in the car why I had become a psychologist with an interest in anaesthesia. I always thought it fairly straightforward.'

In the year or so before I met Michael Wang in Sydney, both my parents were admitted unexpectedly to hospital. My father's problem was a mysteriously blocked bowel which, without modern medicine, would have killed him. The doctors, however, were reluctant to operate unless or until they had no choice, partly because my father has other ailments that would make anaesthetising him risky. For a week he waited without complaint in ICU, hooked up to a tangle of tubes that pumped nutrients in and green bile out, keeping him alive, though not comfortable. The doctors kept trying and failing to open the blockage. No one knew what it was.

Eventually he had an MRI scan, which involved lying perfectly still in a cylindrical echo chamber while radio waves translated the soft tissue of his body. When I saw him the next day he mentioned in passing that the experience had been 'rather painful'. My father is claustrophobic; he coped in the tube, he said, by reciting Shakespeare.

He was curled on his side as we spoke, in his meagre hospital gown, smaller and frailer than I had seen him before. His voice was thinner too, but the cadences were all there. 'To-morrow, and to-morrow, and to-morrow,' he muttered, 'creeps in this petty pace...

'Rather gloomy, I'm afraid,' he added apologetically.

I wanted to tell him that it was fine. That this is what stories are for. To say the things that our social habits prevent us from saying. To talk about death and loss and fear. And I mumbled something to this effect. My father shrugged, a gesture at once helpless and resigned. He knew the score.

Eighteen months later, in the home he had shared with my mother for thirty years, he would pull from the glass-fronted bookshelf in the hallway a tattered green volume—his father's complete works of Shakespeare—and open it to reveal on the inside cover an inscription in blurred blue.

Bernard Randall Cole-Adams took this volume (which has since been rebound) with him into internment with the Japanese in January 1942, along with 'In the King's Presence' (a book of prayers), 'Intimation of Christ,' and a book of daily texts from the Bible. During three years and eight months of internment these books must have been a great solace to him. B. R. Cole-Adams, who was born on 5th of July 1897, died on 15th September 1945 of meningitis and malnutrition on the day that the internees and prisoners of war in [?] Kuching were liberated by the Australian Forces.

The note was marked with the stamp of my grandfather's friend and superior officer Charles Macaskie, who would later marry my grandmother and become a benevolent father figure to her children.

This too is what my father brings to anaesthesia.

..

Face down at the pool, I watch the sliding blue of the tiles, and populate each oblong interval with a series of connected, sequential thoughts. This one leading from this, arising in turn from this, and then this. I must remember, I tell myself. I build a mnemonic—the spreading grid of the submerged tiles overlaid, for a reason I can't fathom and don't question, with the face of a colleague from work—and within this grid I feel the line of my thoughts is implanted. But when I come to the surface, I bring only the shapes, the stringiness of the connections, not the fullness of the vision. What was it? Absences? The way they are passed from generation to generation. The mechanics of silence, and how it translates, each tiny retreat, into eddies or whorls against which the next generation must kick or gain traction, or into which they must dive or be pulled.

I remember, as I dry my hair in the tiled change room, a moment that the psychiatrist Bernard Levinson described during his 1965 experiment. Later I rummage in my desk for the unpublished experimental results he faxed me after one of our phone conversations. There on page forty is his typed account of the last patient to have been operated on that day, a forty-seven-year-old accountant, whom he calls Mrs M. S.

It begins, 'The EEG is unusual in this patient's case.'

Once the surgery had begun and Mrs M. S. appeared to be deeply anaesthetised, Levinson had signalled to the anaesthetist Dr Viljoen that the patient was ready. At this point, and before Viljoen had said a word, the theatre staff fell silent.

'The EEG changed markedly,' Levinson wrote in his notes. 'The sudden silence seemed to startle the patient.'

He reported a change in the woman's brainwave patterns, an increase in activity that continued for many minutes after Dr Viljoen had said he was satisfied. It was as if, Levinson said later, the patient was responding not to the clatter and hum of the operating theatre, but to the sudden lack of it.

When he hypnotised her a month later, the woman remembered details of the surgery but not of the mock drama. When he tried to guide her back there, asking if she had heard anything disturbing, the woman became agitated and woke.

The report is appended to a note handwritten by Levinson in what appears to be dark chiselled fountain pen, a bygone architecture of tilting italics and generous rounded curves. Levinson writes: 'I love this quote by Hughlings Jackson (1931): "There is no such entity as consciousness: we are from moment to moment differently conscious."'

o

Waking after her second surgery, in a fitful morphine swell, my mother murmured in dismay, 'Oh, I'm just like Peter.' Peter, my father, whom she had calmly watched thrashing his ungainly way towards consciousness one surgery after another. But she was not like him, or anyone else. Soon after, when my sister asked how she was feeling now, Mum delivered a wry, one-word summation: 'Disgruntled.' A not-quite smile. Herself again. The self we knew.

o

I find in the cardboard box sent by my uncle my maternal grandfather's photocopied obituary from the *Medical Journal of Australia*:

> Approaching the peak of his career and with a great future before him in his profession, ill health beset his path before he was fifty. He continued to work, however, as hard as ever, until he died, quite suddenly on April 17, 1956, while he was quietly preparing a paper, and with a book which he was writing still only half finished.

Not long after leaving hospital the second time, my mother told me again about that day in April 1956 when she found him in his room. She was seventeen. (What did she *do*, I asked her, appalled, when I was about the same age. What did she *feel*?) In revisiting that day, decades later, my mother would describe not the room where she found him, or what she found there, but the moments afterwards, her adolescent self standing alone on the landing outside, the way the house was organised around her; the doors, the stairway, the light entering from the opposite window. She told me now what she had told me back then, which was simply what she knew: that from then on she would have to make her own life. Her mother would live for several more years but, standing outside the room where her dead father lay, what my mother understood was that, in some essential way, she was now on her own. And that she would have to get on.

This is what my mother brought with her to the operating theatre. It is what she brought with her all her life. A clear-eyed appraisal of her situation and options. A willingness to act. And, with it, a calm acceptance, a refusal to dwell.

It is part of what she brought.

All those typewritten notes. Those words and phrases and links. (*Nothing to think with / nothing to love and link with*). My grandfather's manuscript runs to maybe two hundred pages, many of them unnumbered. Some are repeated or revised. Some are in seemingly random order. Throughout, he keeps circling the subconscious mind, outlining its mechanistic, physiological underpinnings, enclosing it in its neural mesh. 'The human animal is then a reflex machine...' But it is a struggle for him, I sense, to think like this all the time. He tries to contain us—mankind, all those wounded men, himself—within the confines of the nervous system, the bounds of science, but then he keeps seeping or leaping out. The human animal may be a reflex machine. 'The machine however is sensitive to and modified by its experience. Within his structure he carries his past and his future, his past extending back to the beginning of all things and his future envisaging the kingdom the power and the glory of which in his more lucid moments he dreams.'

He pulls himself back then with a matter-of-fact list cataloguing the 'primary instinctive reactions of man', which are, he notes, relatively few and simple. We are on the third from last page now, at the bottom of my cardboard box, a page that may have been intended for elsewhere in the book, or that might eventually have finished up as another of my grandfather's emphatic crossings out. But which feels for now like an ending.

> He seeks, in short, food, drink, shelter, and a mate. He is impelled to care for his young. He is interested in environmental threats and promises and curious as to novelties. He avoids pain, discomfort, nausea and excessive cold and heat. Lacking other outlet he laughs when his behaviour is biologically successful and weeps when he is thwarted. He projects his experience as a world, and endows the objects and even events of that world with natures pleasing and unpleasing, good or evil, moral and immoral. In the presence of threat or promise he fears or rages and attacks or flies. He dreams and dances and thinks and sings. He grows up, lives his life, grows old and dies. He speaks. He draws pictures.

My mother.

o

And what about Rachel Benmayor, what did she bring to that surgery all those years ago? One of the more surreal moments in the devastating saga that was the birth of Rachel's second child came not on the operating table, but in the kitchen of her Blue Mountains home a week or so before the birth. Rachel had been feeling, she said, not quite at peace with her life. The birth of her son some years before had been difficult, and he had been taken from her almost immediately for treatment, leaving her bereft. Now she was about to have another child. She knew she should be feeling excited, but she also felt empty, as if something was lacking. Rachel is not religious in any conventional sense, although she is open to the idea of mystery. She is unsurprised by coincidences. She speaks in a casual, familiar way about 'the universe'. She sees herself as engaged in a search for some sort of spiritual meaning. All of which was true that day more than two decades ago as she looked out the window and across the valley beyond.

'I'd never done this before but I had a really strong feeling to ask—and I'm an agnostic—but I put out, to the universe basically, to have an experience that was of a spiritual nature—that would wake me up, or provide some sort of learning, powerful learning, for me.' Her voice trailed off. 'But I was not at all sophisticated, I just asked for that...'

Later she told me that she had asked for one other thing as she sat at her kitchen table that day. Please, she had said to the universe, let me be present for the birth of my child.

More than a decade after that conversation I still don't know what to make of this revelation, except that, if this were a novel, I might enlist such a moment as a visceral illustration of how powerfully we think ourselves towards our lives; how the stories we tell ourselves become the lives that we lead. Rachel has never found out quite what happened during her surgery—whether, as seems most likely, the hypnotic gas or drug that was supposed to keep her unconscious was somehow disconnected and failed to ever reach her; or whether the anaesthetic simply didn't do its job. (Her anaesthetist's entry in the hospital record is largely illegible.) And this in turn flowers into other questions, such as whether Rachel might be one of those people who, due to their physiology, require more anaesthetic than most, or whether (and this thought leaves me teetering at the outer edge of my own world view) somehow the force of her desire for consciousness, or perhaps her fear of unconsciousness, helped bring about its own end. She had always, she told me later, had a corrosive fear of death.

That younger me

And now it was my turn. What was I about to bring to my now inevitable surgery?

Well, much of what is in this book. Too much thinking, too much drinking, a submerged, possibly self-inflicted melancholy, a certain stubborn stoicism. Fear, of course. Of death, of extinction, of separation—most particularly of separation from myself.

Resistance? Less so, by the time I got there. I thank the psychologist I was seeing for that. Yes, she said, you might die or end up paralysed or wake up in the middle of the operation, although you probably won't. But it is you who has to weigh up the odds, acknowledge the risks, and make the choice. Seek advice, of course: but you alone take responsibility for your decision. And to make that choice you need to be fully conscious, fully present in this moment, this accounting. This, at any rate, is what I took from our discussions.

I brought information. Far too much information, but information that in the end I found very helpful. An understanding of what my surgeon proposed to do, and of the drugs and monitors my anaesthetist would use to make that possible. The instruction to relax. The idea of drawing blood away from my spine.

The idea of myself as an active participant in my own surgery—

and by extension in my own life, conscious and otherwise.

And of course I brought the enormous, invisible sack of my unconscious self. A sack that I cannot open at will, or often at all, but through whose bulging outline I can feel the shapes of the habits and hurts and hopes I carry with me, and sometimes even the hint of a body part (an elbow, a brow, a tiny foot); an imprint that might at any moment connect me to a two-year-old who has been left behind for a short period by her young parents, or even to a thirty-two-year-old who has flown down from Darwin for her appointment and is now lying semi-conscious on a trolley in a suburban clinic in Melbourne.

A funny thing can happen under a light anaesthetic. You lose yourself even when you are still there. You can see it on those YouTube videos of people waking in dentists chairs. Staring, fascinated, at the fingers waving vaguely in front of them, but with no idea that the hands are theirs. Doctors call it dissociation. In itself it is not bad—it can be fun—but it can do strange things to your mind. Sometimes the swoopy, disconnected feeling you get under low levels of anaesthetic drugs can mimic other previous dissociative states—hypnosis, fever, extreme stress, even a previous anaesthetic—and you become a time traveller. A man half-waking from an anaesthetic and finding himself, arms tied down, in intensive care, is catapulted back into traumatic wartime experiences buried for forty years. A woman wakes to flash-backs of her childhood sexual abuse. These stories keep repeating. In my publisher's office, a senior editor sets aside my contract and talks instead about her parents, both Holocaust survivors, and her mother who, each time she goes under, returns in Yiddish, a tongue her children neither speak nor understand. Poet Jean Kent writes of her husband's father emerging from heart surgery: *Post-operative, pethidine-high, plucking his language/ of youth*

..

And so, the youngish woman. What did she bring to that brief anaesthetic all those years ago? A jumble of feelings. Truncated. Half-felt. A history of preemptive departures; a habit of leaving but not letting go. Most evidently, at least to herself, a blank resolve to simply get on, get it over with. Be done. The grieving, if that is what it was (for it never came in the daylight, this feeling) came later and in that strangely attenuated undertow. A dragging malaise that was not, I now understand, just to do with the death of a foetus, and with it the potential for a child. She was also grieving the relationship with the man, which she knew in her deep self, though refused to acknowledge for some time, had also been terminated—as had the self, or the version of herself, she had been diligently and wilfully propagating since falling for him and by which she had set such store.

What I am pretty sure I did not bring into that abortion was the word 'Gadget', the name of the red dog who would visit me in a dream all those years later in the yellow house in the Blue Mountains.

In the emotional unmasking of that dream (the grief, the awful regret) the word sits uneasily, like something that has been inserted from outside. An implement I have been passed by someone else and am still holding. I wonder if there were other uninvited gifts.

The first patient Bernard Levinson hypnotised in his rooms in 1965 after the fake crisis was an eighteen-year-old dental nurse, Miss A. According to Levinson's notes, during her dental surgery the woman's EEG changed markedly when the anaesthetist Viljoen stopped the operation to deliver his prepared script. There was a sudden change in her brainwaves that took some minutes to settle down.

'The hypnotic session a month later was traumatic,' wrote Levinson. 'Miss A. entered a trance easily, and was regressed to the morning of the operation. As she began to relive the operation she suddenly blocked. Said she couldn't speak. She began to cry and burst out of the trance state weeping.'

Levinson made another appointment to see the woman and try to take her back to the operation. Again without success. 'She resisted going into a deep trance, and became anxious. After many minutes of gentle persuasion she began to relive the operation.' Instead of the dental surgery, though, she was reliving a different operation altogether. 'This proved to be an earlier operation that she had had for an abortion. I could not get her to relive the operation at the Dental Hospital…Her previous experience seemed to have given her a mental set against operations and accounted for her anxiety reaction.'

I have been thinking lately about that younger me all those years ago in the counselling room in Darwin. That great murky torrent, and the non-memory of that small moment in my small life when I was for ten days without parents. For a long time I have felt embarrassed to talk about it. *A little thing*. But it persists. Like that small dog yapping behind me. I doubt I will ever remember why I made the appointment to see the young counsellor in the first place, or know what it was that pitched me back into those childhood fears. But I believe the visit probably happened after the abortion. What I think now is that just because something is a non-memory does not make it a non-event. And while I do not recall my second birthday or the days leading up to and away from it (any more than I recall my fourth), I do have one clear memory that belongs to that time, though it didn't happen until some years later.

A sleepover. I was to spend the night with the same family I had stayed with during my parents' brief absence when I was two. Now I was perhaps six or seven. I do not remember the circumstances. What I do remember is evening—the other girls, and now a young boy as well, already in bed—and me in the lounge room pacing. No particulars. Just the soothing entreaties of the mother trying to talk me gently into bed, and me unable, utterly unable, to oblige, caught up in a feeling so powerful that all I could do was prowl from room to room: the sense of my feet on the floor, the necessity of motion. (It is a feeling that balloons even now, in the process of writing, into my chest; rhythmic bursts that billow and clump at the base of my throat.) Later, after they had called my parents, I think I remember sitting or standing in a window alcove, face reflecting back from the darkness outside as I watched through the glass for headlights. Perhaps I accepted a mug of milk. I did not want to upset the mother and father whose hospitality I was supposed to be enjoying but it was impossible for me to stay. I knew that, though not why.

In all of this I am aware of the constant tension of trying to push together things that do not want to go.

In the weeks after I separated from my son's father—this was not the Darwin man, nor the man to whom I am now married—I began to dismantle. Cycling home from work the day before the removalists were due, I experienced myself in a momentary flash as a series of rectangular boxes, four small wooden coffins, lined up side by side. I understood that the function of the boxes was to simultaneously hold and separate my feelings—like body parts: left arm, right arm, torso, legs (where was my head?) And that the reason for this was that if all the fragmented feeling parts were to come together, they would engulf me.

In the end it was my son who forced me to stay present, anchored me, even as I dismembered the creature that had been our small and briefly perfect family. Long before the final breakdown of our relationship we had booked a beach holiday with my parents, my sister and her family. I went down early with our son, and his father followed a little later. I went back to town soon after, to work a late shift at the paper where I was sub-editing. I left my no-longer-partner in the beach house glowering in pain and barely suppressed resentment. My chest was a tight brick of tension. Our son was anxious. When I tried to leave the house, he clung and hugged, called me back for more, struggled to make it all right. I watched the wave of feelings rise and spill in him. Felt the pitch and yaw of my own appalled, appalling heart. I did not go until he told me I could. I did not leave him crying. I held one hand across my stomach, and one across his. I told him that my love was in his stomach, and his in mine. And that if he was finding it hard, he could put his hand on his tummy at any time and feel me there. I told him to go upstairs and wave to me.

'I don't want you to go,' he said.

'I know you don't darling, but I have to. I'll be back in the morning.'

At last, quietly, he said, 'What would you do if you were me, Mummy?'

I held him then with my hands, each palm cradling a shoulder, moved him back enough that I could see his face. 'If I were you, I'd say "I love you, Mummy, I'll see you later," and I'd go upstairs and wave.'

'Is that what you'd do?'

'Yes. Even though it's hard, that's what I'd do.'

And he did. Stepped away. Looked at the ground, said in a tight little voice, 'I love you Mummy. I'll see you later,' and headed upstairs on his small muscled legs.

How does a subject come so completely loose from its moorings? I am writing about anaesthesia / I am in Darwin / I am in Sydney / I am in Melbourne / I am abandoning my partner / dividing my son / my self. My mother is dying.

Everything separating, detaching. Falling apart.

..

Sometimes I wonder too about that tiny accumulation of life that was once inside me, the wordless clutch of cells, divided, dividing; and what it might have been to exist for that brief time, to expand and accrue; an assemblage that might eventually have cohered into consciousness, but that may even in that early unfolding have constituted—perhaps not experience, but *something*.

At my wedding many years later, my husband, Pete, surprised even himself by quoting Woody Allen. One of the things he loved about me, he told our merged and extended family and friends, was that, like Alvy Singer in *Annie Hall*, I believed that a relationship was like a shark: it moved forward constantly or died. And it is true that these days I interrogate myself and other people. 'You think *way* too much,' my son tells me. Certainly I leave less to chance. But back then—before my son, my husband, my daughter, myself as I know myself now—I didn't think at all; that's how it feels from here. It probably isn't true; perhaps I just thought about things I now think of as futile. An obsessive forensic analysis of the details of a life contingent on a belief that any one relationship could save me from the self I did not want to know. So, yes, these days I think a lot. I just think about different things.

What do I wish I had brought in with me to that Melbourne clinic? More information, to start with. What to expect during the short procedure; the fact that the anaesthetic would be very light, not general anaesthesia at all, more a sedative to settle me on the table; the fact that I might still be able to hear during the procedure. The fact that forgetting something was not the same as it never having happened. What I also wish is that I had made my decision in a different way. Indeed, that I had made a decision at all, rather than letting myself be borne along on the competing currents of a mutinous refusal to take responsibility for my own life or the one forming inside me: that, and a desire for a child that was stronger than I knew, or had allowed myself to know. Because, in truth, whatever happened or didn't happen on that metal trolley, I had anaesthetised myself well before I walked into the clinic.

Maybe I have simply imagined the rest. Or made it up. It doesn't matter.

Most of all I wish I had brought myself.

Sky

One of the most moving moments in Jesse Watkins' ten-day voyage—the epic visionary delirium that enveloped him following a 1940 anaesthetic, and which he later described to R. D. Laing—was its ending. Watkins, exhausted and overwhelmed by the intensity of his vision ('It shivered me up'), terrified he would 'go under', determined to find his way back. Refusing further sedation, he sat on the bed in his padded cell and held his own hands, said his own name, over and over. Until, suddenly, 'just like that', it was over. He was back.

My own journey back to self (one that began for real with the birth of my son twenty-one years ago) has been far less dramatic. It is a journey many of us make at various times and in various guises, and which in my case has involved more plodding than poetry. Exercise, meditation, counselling, writing; the simple passing of time. As part of the process, I have taken to watching the sky. It is almost as if I have suddenly realised it is there. At first, when I started looking up, dutifully, from the back porch, I saw just that—sky, in its various familiar guises: blue sky, grey sky, pale sky with wispy clouds, Simpsons sky, etcetera. A series of statements. Lacking conviction. But now I find myself gazing into the blue and once I start it is hard to stop. It sounds so obvious, but I am amazed. Up there nothing is as it seems; it just is. Lying beneath a distance I would once have called flat, I am utterly absorbed in the intricacy of it: the swells and billows, the subtle irrevocable shifts; purple softness yielding to membranes of tensile white, and now an impossible arctic blue; one sky opening incessantly into another. And if I can just stay with it, something starts to happen in my body, my mind. I cannot see it or name it or know what it is, but I can feel the deep interior articulation of it, the click and release. And, above it all, high up, a fluid pulse, the heaving striations of some great ribcage.

All I have to do is wait.

On a crystalline winter's afternoon in the mountains I went to visit Rachel Benmayor. She looked older, as did I, but familiar now; slightly dishevelled as if she had been racing from place to place all morning. We hugged comfortably before she suggested we drive up and buy takeaway for lunch and then eat it at her house, the one she and her husband Glenn had built together, and which, she explained in the car, they were now renting out for weekends and holidays while they lived for a time with friends. Twenty minutes later we pulled up in front of a stylish mud-brick and corrugated-iron building with whimsical adobe-style garden beds and a veggie patch out the front. But it wasn't until we had entered through a side door and taken off our shoes in the small entrance foyer that the house unfolded itself in two or three levels (I couldn't quite tell), richly and strikingly decorated in strong earth colours against the textured walls. From each room, or rather within each room, great teetering views across a eucalyptus valley and humped mountains in the distance pulsed outwards and inwards at once.

We ate on a wide verandah. Two magpies, a grey-chested adolescent and an adult in binary black and white, flung droplets of sound back and forth in a nearby tree, and everything—the sky, the valley, the massive gums, even our brightly coloured salads in their plastic containers—was plumped and raucous with light. It was glorious. And although, as we talked, I put my voice recorder on the table between us and turned it on, I felt for the first time that we were no longer simply interviewer and subject, but women who might in the right circumstances be something closer to friends. She pointed to the place in the sky where the full moon rose. I asked if there had ever been fires and she described twice having stood on this same verandah as flames twisted along the ridge and towards the house. The sound, she said, 'was like roaring'. After a while I asked about her anaesthetic experience—if she had changed the way she viewed it over time.

No,' she said straight away. 'Not at all. The memory of it is as acute as it was.'

She said it wasn't something she thought would ever go away. 'I think it's very powerfully become part of who I am.' Small, unexpected things could trigger it. A sound. Not being able to breathe. 'I got the flu two or three weeks ago, and I couldn't breathe. And it was just the same...It's so physical.'

She spoke about her daughter, Allegra, the child who was cut from her womb without anaesthetic and into whose dark eyes she later gazed and gazed to try to keep herself on the planet. They had talked a lot about what had happened, she said. 'She knows. She's read what I wrote about it. And she knows that I don't have any regrets about her birth. That's not something I'd wish on anybody, it was absolutely horrendous, but having gone through it I wouldn't change it—I know that sounds strange—because there have been a lot of gifts from that.' She talked then about the 'messages' she had received while paralysed on the operating table, which, she said, had been 'so very pertinent' in her life since then and had given her, among other things, 'the opportunity to learn, whether I liked it or not, of that very deep surrender. I'll never forget that.'

These days she uses that lesson whenever she goes to the dentist. 'For obvious reasons I don't like anaesthesia. I don't like injections. I prefer to stay very awake. But then of course I have to deal with the pain.' She tries to remember not to resist or fight the pain, but to let herself go into it. She tries to do the same with emotions. 'I guess I know that even if I'm in a horrible situation and I'm finding it really difficult to cope, I say to myself, "You have experienced your own strength. It's there. Just trust that you know that incredible pain will pass. It will pass."'

The other lesson Rachel keeps coming back to is that powerful conviction that hospital workers need to be more attuned to the intense vulnerability of their patients as they come out of anaesthesia. Some time after her daughter's birth, she was invited back to the hospital to talk to the nurses who worked in the recovery ward. 'The thing that really upset me a lot was the fact that I absolutely knew, I absolutely *knew*—it was really important that the nurses get told how to behave with people when they're in recovery, because I reckon there are a lot of people who feel things.'

I was about to comment on the fact that during the birth she had *not* in fact been anaesthetised at all. But before I had formed the words, she started talking about an anaesthetic she had been given some years before Allegra was born. Her doctor, concerned that she might have cervical cancer, had given her a sedative anaesthetic and a curette. 'When I came out from that, in recovery, I was…flooded with feelings and memories that were very real and truthful. I think this is something I experienced again with Allegra, that when I was in recovery it was like being in the presence of the truth. And I *wanted* to be heard, and I was very scared that I wasn't going to be heard.'

Years afterwards, when she spoke to the group of nurses she

asked them a question. 'I said, "Look, do you experience people coming out of anaesthesia and saying strange things?"

'"Oh yeah, it happens all the time. They're just mumbling."

'And I said, "I want you to know that...what they may be experiencing may be incredibly important for them, and it may be very important that they integrate that into their consciousness. So my advice to you is, don't just placate them. If they want to talk, if you've got time, sit down and listen"...Because it can be a gift—that kind of vulnerability is very rare in most people's lives. And I think if it can just be treated a little differently it can be a hugely different experience, and powerful, and can bring good things.'

Then she told me a story about a friend of hers, a woman whose mother had never held her. When the mother was in her seventies she was diagnosed with cancer and went to hospital for an operation. Her daughter, said Rachel, sat beside her as she came out of the anaesthetic. 'And her mother, as she came round, took her hand and told her how much she had loved her. For the first time in her life. Took her hand, stroked it, told her how grateful she was and that she's a good daughter and that she loved her.'

We sat a while longer in the sun and the light, and the magpies flew off and we gathered our forks and glasses, our plastic containers.

'So,' said Rachel, 'I would encourage anybody these days if having a major operation to ask if they could have a loved one present when they come around, I think it would just make all the difference.

'Someone who can just be there and speak to them gently, and if there's things that they need to say, to listen...Because her mother's never going to say that again. But, boy, did it make a difference to my friend.'

Letting go

July 7, 2010. In my whitish hospital room in Brisbane I lay out my totems. I have brought with me a spell bag from my daughter containing three lucky stones and a wishing angel, and the Buddhist prayer beads a friend pressed into my hand before I left Melbourne. I have a card showing a small, brightly coloured bird straddling two massive tree trunks. Taped inside is a strip with two gold stars with arrows leading to them:

1) For getting to this point in time.

2) For waking up after the operation.

Finally, there is a small leprechaun doll given to me by a friend when I left England thirty-five years ago, and whose name I later passed on to my son.

I lay them all out on the tray table over the bed and I crouch down and take a photo of them and another of me crouched on the bed behind them. Then I turn off the main switch and stand for a while at the window looking out at all the tiny glittering lights.

They come just after seven the next morning. I have already showered and scrubbed myself with disinfectant wipes, folded my clothes away in my suitcase with my lucky charms, donned the white starched gown. My mother is here, with my Uncle Jim, to see me off. Nine hours from now, as I emerge in a splintering of pain and delirium, I will try to tell her about a dream I have just had; then I will forget. For now, however, they stand side by side before the window and chat in a soothing sing-song, as if this is normal. Beyond them, beneath a pale clear sky, a road darts up and away between concrete cubes towards the hills that edge the city. It is too soon. I am not ready. I climb as instructed back onto my bed, now a trolley, and we set off in slow procession. 'Mum,' I say. 'You have to do something for me. As soon as I wake up after the operation, you have to ask me if I remember anything.' When we reach the lifts, I grasp her hand and consider, for a moment, not letting go. Her eyes look grey, uncertain. The doors slide open; the doors slide closed. My mother disappears. Someone in the lift says something cheerful. I try to smile.

I am parked now in a curtained anteroom staring up at the mottled ceiling tiles. Someone, it occurs to me, has become rich making such tiles. These ones have seen better days; they are misaligned and cracked in places, with black marks around some of the edges. Lined up next to me, through a filmy nylon curtain I can hear somebody else, a man, breathing too loudly; and beyond him, low voices. I lie here, it seems, for ages. From time to time people dressed in surgical scrubs approach and ask me the same set of questions. What is your full name? Date of birth? Any allergies? What are you here for? Consent form?

My anaesthetist, John, arrives in a gust of cheerful certainty. In the flesh, he is young (but not too young, I tell myself) and chatty, with oblong glasses and a cropped beard. He tells me again how he will put me to sleep (we both know it is not sleep, but now is not the time for that conversation), the drugs he will use to keep me there, the monitors he will attach to help measure my descent. He too asks about the consent form before moving off. He will see me soon, he says. Perhaps he gives me a sedative—I can't recall. There is more rustling and quiet chatting from the other bays. The man beside me coughs. Two theatre staff appear silently at my feet. What is my name? Consent form? As they wheel me out (ceiling tiles accelerating), I turn my face to the right, glance first at the coughing man and then into the next cubicle where an older man is lying on another trolley, a woman sitting next to him, holding his hand. As I pass, she holds my gaze and mouths to me, *Good luck.* In the isolation of that moment (suspended, unreal) the gesture feels intensely, penetratingly human, and I hold it to me—even now, as I write—a small vital connection to myself and my life: I am here, she can see me; she wishes me well.

A clatter of white light. Theatre. My surgeon is here, a blue cap, a preoccupied smile. Someone hands me a new consent form, which I sign lying down. John attaches a needle to the back of my right hand. He tells me that over the next ten minutes, as he fits and adjusts my monitors, I will be awake but that I will not remember this later. There is a muffled pause, which could be seconds or minutes, and which may or may not include further conversation, and I am suddenly aware of something against my face, a puffy, pushed-up-upon feeling, a smell of plastic and decay, as if my face is being held against someone's ageing shower cap (an insistent buffeting) and I cannot escape. There is a sense not so much of falling as of being pushed, a moment of tumultuous, belated outrage, then—

o

It is odd where the mind goes, when it is off the leash. I think about all the researchers who have made it into this book, and many who haven't, day in, day out, harnessing their quick, clever brains to the study of consciousness and the borderlands where it bleeds into something else. Each operating within the rigorous constraints of science, each with his or her own fascinations, preoccupations.

When he is not researching the subjective experiences people have as they are lowered towards anaesthesia, Lithuanian neuroscientist Valdas Noreika (whose sedated volunteers in Finland in 2011 reported visions of playing football and coming out of their bodies) studies dreaming, including lucid dreams, in which you not only know you are in a dream but may even get to direct what happens.

In Plymouth, Jackie Andrade's attention drifted some years ago to our habit of doodling while on the phone, or in the lecture theatre or any time we have a pen and paper and are supposed to be focusing on something else (it turns out it actually improves our memory for boring information).

A while ago, in between investigating consciousness and the neural correlates of unconsciousness, George Mashour contributed to a small but mind-bending paper on what happens as rats die. He had been approached by a colleague at the University of Michigan, Jimo Borjigin, who had been monitoring rats' brain activity as part of a different project. One night two of her animals died suddenly. When she later looked at the readings she found something unexpected: a surge in their brain chemistry around the time of their deaths. Weird.

A small team of researchers decided to explore. This time they monitored the brainwaves of rats as they anaesthetised them, then killed them by inducing cardiac arrest or asphyxiation. What they found was that shortly after the animals' hearts had stopped beating and blood had stopped flowing to their brains—the markers of clinical death—their brains went briefly into overdrive, displaying patterns consistent not just with conscious perception, but with *heightened* conscious perception.

The team had expected their study to yield something, but not this. '[W]e were surprised by the high levels of activity,' said

Mashour, 'In fact, at near-death, many known electrical signatures of consciousness exceeded levels found in the waking state, suggesting that the brain is capable of well-organised electrical activity during the early stage of clinical death...' While agreeing that the practical implications are unclear, the authors say the results might tell us something not only about the dying human brain—but also about the brains of the two in every ten survivors of cardiac arrest who later report strange visions; that this provides the first scientific framework for these so called near-death experiences; these impossible moments, unfettered, unforgettable, 'realer than real'.

It is strange to think that the self could stay present even for a moment after the conditions for life, as we conceive of it, have passed. Especially given how *hard* it is to be present, even on a regular day, a not-dying day. To simply be. So hard not to slip or glide or dive into the alternative: into blankness, or stupor, or the multitude of grappling grasping thoughts waiting in every instant to be thought (*choose me, choose me*), most of which are not relevant or helpful or even interesting, but which might, even so, serve their purpose of keeping at bay other thoughts, other presences—

Oh, and here she comes. Our mother. Swinging smoothly across the room in her pneumatic hoist. Up and out of the padded day bed, gliding over the visitors chair, the night table laden with notebooks and lists, tubs of green jelly. The nurses raise their arms to steady her as she sways between them in her sling, calico legs dangling thinly, the bulging pad, trailing tubes. That look. A look that knows exactly what is going on: the pathos, the incongruity, the sheer slapstick of it all. A look that says, here we are then. Here am I—flying. Her dignity is sublime.

o

On the last day my youngest sister rang early. She was doing the first shift at the hospice. Two days before, Mum had developed an infection. Maybe she would pull through, maybe she wouldn't; it would announce itself in time. This was the world we had entered. Now, my sister said, Mum was unconscious. Maybe a good idea to head in soonish. No rush. Then a while later, as I was preparing to leave, another call. Come now. Get Dad.

Come now. The trip across town, first to pick up my father and his wheelchair then straight down Johnston Street to Kew, had the elastic contagion of dreams. Everything sticky and altered and unendurably slow. Lights clanged red as we approached. Cars streamed around and ahead of us, while we (my father beside me, gracious, resigned) were sucked down and down, under and back.

In my mother's room were my sisters and the sound of breathing. Mum had spoken once that morning—briefly, to a nurse—and now she laboured steadily. We felt the cold moving up her body, a blue tide that began at her feet and over the coming hours slowly occupied her calves, thighs, belly. She kept breathing. Or the breathing kept coming, uneven at times, but still engrossed somehow with the apparatus of my mother's chest and lungs, throat and lips, as if uncertain or unready yet to separate. There was no sign of pain. Just the halting corrugation of breath. We talked to her or through her or about her and occasionally about other small things. The nurses left us to it, materialising to offer help, or as time went on to wonder at how long it was all taking, while we, the four of us, rotated slowly around her, stroking or whispering or urging or weeping or completely silent.

Eventually we decided we would leave the room for a spell, to let her go without us, if that was what she wanted. Stepping into the hallway was almost shocking, as if the air beyond the room was already cold, the space stark and flat and empty. Outside the men's toilet I wanted to scream and scream at my invalid father to hurry up. Hurry up! We returned as a group in a sort of suppressed panic, almost running, this was how it felt to me, appalled suddenly at the idea that we had abandoned her, or that she might have left of her own accord.

Back inside, breathing; less breathing now than breath. A slow and slowing shunt (mother/wife/child). We did whatever we did, stroked, said, sat, attending each minuscule momentous shift. Then a final flutter or flurry, an exhalation so sweet I still have no idea what to make of it. Except that in that tiny opening—that moment before the next part, the afterwards, began—what I felt in the room was not a nothing, it was a something. A wriggle, a twist. Release. When I think of it now, I can trace in my mind the joyful zig-zag of my mother's final breath hanging for a moment slightly above her face and to the left, and then I don't know.

A little later, as we sat or stood or stroked or said; as our own bodies shaped themselves around their new habits of resistance and knowledge and loss, a magpie called outside the window, and a shaft of light shredded the glass and landed *bam* upon her face, like in a painting.

o

One of my mother's earliest memories was of herself in a cot in a dark room in a house far from home. An orphanage, she called it. Wartime. She told me the story a number of times, perhaps because after the first time I kept on asking. She was not an orphan but her father had been relocated to Melbourne, where he was working long hours at a hospital for returning soldiers, and her mother, who had brought the children (my mother, three, and her older brother) down from Brisbane to be with him, had fallen ill with pneumonia. And so for a short period, I don't know how long, the children were in care. In the memory it is dark and my mother is standing up in the cot.

Outside the room, coming down the corridor, are footsteps, which she knows are for her. She has been making a noise. My mother tells this story quite cheerfully. She has no memory of alarm. But what she knows, or remembers knowing, is that she should not be awake, and she certainly should not be standing at the railings of her cot making a racket. So she lies down quietly and pretends to sleep. When the owner of the footsteps arrives my mother keeps her eyes closed. She knows the woman is looking at her, and knows too that the woman knows she is not asleep at all—so she stays quite still. Now the woman turns and leaves the room and the child who will nineteen years later become my mother rolls onto her back, or curls on her side, and does whatever it is she does within the small hot hub of her head, her chest, the quick and canny circuitry of her nerves and notions and feelings. Was she scared? Satisfied? Simply curious? What did she see through the struts of the cot? What would she make of it all? I don't know. But years later she tells me this story, and I take it and I make it mine. One day she will look across at me from the padded chair near the window at the hospice: that quick clear gaze; the drifts of falling hair. She will say: I am not at all afraid.

Wings

Brisbane, July 7, 2010. I do not wake, so much as emerge, wings of neon pain sprouting from my shoulder blades.

I am aware of the sound before I am aware of myself—a melodic wailing, almost satisfying, and then: language. *Owwww* (a series of these, drawn out). And eventually: 'My shoulders. *Owwww.*' Something like this.

I am being pushed on a trolley (I am convinced) from Brisbane airport along the endless outdoor walkway to the temporary short-term car park. And each time the metal wheels hit the cracks in the paving, the pain streams upwards into the livid apparatus that has erupted from within me, and through which I am now being transmitted, a hallucinatory signal, fractured and distorted; so that the pain exists alongside but independent of my mother, now walking with my uncle at the end of my trolley (why are they pushing me? where is the car park?) and another self, all synthesised laughter, a reckless hilarity still zinging through my bloodstream. Falling together and apart; my shoulders high as kites.

Of the past seven-and-a-half hours I remember nothing, not even the conversation I have just had with Mum. Nor obviously do I have a clue what is to come: the weeks and then months of morphine, the halting reassembly of the self. I certainly don't know yet that tomorrow or the next day, my anaesthetist, John, will stand beside me and confess sadly that despite his best efforts, once the operation was underway and I had been turned over (like a turkey, I keep thinking), he had been unable to reattach *either* of the precious BIS monitors for fear of obstructing the surgeon working at the base of my neck—so I would never know how far down I went, or up, none of which would by then seem relevant. Nor do I know what my surgeon will say when I finally find the energy some days hence to ask how much blood I lost during the operation. (I did not mention to him the patients in Hank Bennett's study who, like me, had listened beforehand to his instruction to shunt the blood away from their wounds, and who lost on average 650 millilitres of blood—a third less than the control group.)

'Oh,' the surgeon will tell my future self cheerfully. 'Surprisingly little! Only about four hundred mils.'

'So did I say anything?' I will ask my mother casually at last, and she will look at me a little quizzically (as if to say, don't go reading too much into this) and say, 'Yes, though I couldn't make most of it out.'

'And?'

'All I could hear was mumble mumble mumble, and then—'

'Yes?'

'All I could make out was, "bad playground".'

Bad playground.

I like that.

For now, though, I am in a different kind of playground. Surging along the corridor on a wave of synthetic morphine, my mother and uncle contracting and expanding in my wake, and beyond it all—the bulb-bright pain, the wings, the streaming walls—is the extraordinary good fortune of my continued existence.

In intensive care the nurse (sitting in an illuminated cubicle near the end of my bed, dissected by tubes and cables) tells me to stop pushing the button in my right hand—my 'patient controlled analgesia'.

'Why?' I ask, surprised.

'Because you're hallucinating,' she says.

'No, I'm not.' (Puzzled.)

'Yes you are. You're talking to yourself.'

'No I'm not!' (Indignant.) 'I'm talking to my friends.'

They are very convincing, my friends, though I cannot quite remember their names. ('Is she awake?' asks someone.) Each time I close my eyes, they are there, in ones and twos, and I move down the line, chatting as I go, filling them in on all that has happened. I am very intent and thorough, imparting information; deeply engrossed.

'You'll make yourself vomit,' says the nurse. But I won't.

My wings are pulsing, glorious—I *am*.

Acknowledgments

This book has had a long gestation. So many people have contributed their time, insights, specialist knowledge, personal stories, patience, good will and support that it is hard to know where to begin.

I am greatly indebted to the scientists, medical practitioners, historians, philosophers and other experts who gave me access to their minds, writings, work spaces and sometimes much more. Some appear in the book, others don't. Either way, their forbearance and generosity were indispensible in navigating material that was at times complex, nuanced and technical.

I am equally and deeply thankful to the people who shared with me their own experiences of anaesthesia and beyond, many of whom allowed me to include their accounts here. In particular, Rachel Benmayor's extraordinary story provided an emotional and philosophical pivot around which I have circled for nearly two decades; her courage and dignity are inspiring. There are many others who don't appear in these pages but whose accounts have informed and enriched the book. They include Harriet Davis and Deborah Shaw.

Underpinning the research are countless conversations—with friends, colleagues, strangers—that have helped me plot a path through a topic as slippery, layered and entirely fascinating as anaesthesia.

The extraordinary community of staff and writers at the Varuna writers' centre provided intellectual, creative and physical sustenance (in Sheila Atkinson's case, magical comfort food), and crucial feedback, as well as a surprising number of odd stories about anaesthetics. This book benefited greatly from a three-week fellowship at the centre as well as regular sojourns. My particular thanks again to former creative director Peter Bishop whose insights and expansive, permissive curiosity helped keep me open and honest.

My agent, Jenny Darling, backed the book from the start, commented wisely on early drafts and then waited patiently for nearly a decade until a workable version finally lobbed.

Once again, the team at Text Publishing have been everything I could hope for: supportive, enthusiastic and rigorous. Particular thanks to Michael Heyward for championing the book; to Khadija Caffoor, Anne Beilby and Jane Finemore for working to get it out into the world; to Danielle Bagnato for help with social media, and to Sandy Cull for the beautiful cover design. Above all to my editor Mandy Brett for her fierce advocacy, fine ear and shrewd, perceptive guidance.

Readers who offered valuable perspectives on drafts of the manuscript include Peter Kenneally, Sophie Cunningham, Karen Kissane, Margaret Simons, Peter Cole-Adams, Jennet Cole-Adams and Kate Leslie. Others who read and commented on sections include Penelope Trevor, Kim Langley, Anne Crawford, Mary Anne Butler and Brigid Cole-Adams. I am grateful for their insights and candour.

Practical support came from Sally Ruljancich who transcribed many interviews and did some additional early research. James Button, May Lam, Shane Higgs, Penny Gibson, Kerry Proctor and Clive Meltzer offered peaceful working spaces at crucial points; Siegi Edward designed me one of my own. Bobbi Mahlab asked the right questions and offered strategic advice. Angie Paton provided psychological support and existential theories. And the staff of the Australian and New Zealand College of Anaesthetists were unfailingly friendly and helpful as I wandered in and out of their library over a decade or more.

Much of the research and related travel was made possible with an Australia Council grant. My thanks also to the estates of Philip Larkin, for use of the poem 'Aubade', and R. D. Laing, for kind permission to quote sections of *The Politics of Experience*.

In all this, my husband, Peter Kenneally, has been an astute and enabling presence, managing by and large not to glaze over during sundry impromptu tutorials on anaesthesia, amnesia, memory and forgetting. My children, Finn and Francesca, have spent most of their lives sharing me with this project. Despite this—and along with my sisters, Sarah Boyd and Jennet Cole-Adams, and father, Peter Cole-Adams—they submitted graciously to being co-opted as characters in a drama not of their own making. I am deeply grateful for their support.

My thanks also to my uncle and aunt Jim and Aldyth Love who shared with me their medical knowledge and, in the weeks after my surgery, their home. And to my late grandfather Harold Russell Love, whom I never met, but sections of whose unfinished manuscript found their way into this book. I don't know what he would have made of the result.

And, finally, to my mother, Brigid, who died before I had finished writing or she reading, but whose faith in me was constant and whose clarity and spirit have informed and imbued the book.

NOTES

Into the blue

This chapter draws on books including: Eger et al., *The wondrous story of anesthesia*; Keys, *The history of surgical anesthesia*; Davies et al., *All about anaesthesia*; Dormandy, *The worst of evils*.

Sections of this chapter first appeared in the articles 'Switching off brain and pain', *Age*, 4 September 2010: http://www.smh.com.au/national/switching-off-brain-and-pain-20100903-14uhr.html; and 'Eyes wide shut', *Good Weekend Magazine*, 10 February 2001.

'Suffering so great as I underwent cannot be expressed in words'—Eger, *The wondrous story of anesthesia*, p. 13.

Until the mid-1800s, surgery was almost always an agonising last resort—There had been intermittent reports of other doctors using ether or other drugs to operate on their own patients, but none that had been widely broadcast or publicly demonstrated: Izuo, 2004; Hammonds et al., 1993.

A Napoleonic surgeon called Langeback claimed—Melanie Thernstrom, *The pain chronicles*, p. 143.

'To avoid pain, in surgical operations, is a chimera'—This is one of various translations from the French, which you can read here: http://www.histanestrea-france.org/Velpeau.html (accessed 3 December 2016).

Levinson, then thirty-nine, persuaded a professor of surgery—Levinson, 1965 and 1989.

Awake

Sections of this chapter first appeared in the article 'Eyes wide shut', *Good Weekend Magazine*, 10 February 2001.

Many years ago in the Blue Mountains—It was 1999, in a weatherboard house in Lawson.

...one to two patients in a thousand report waking under anaesthesia—Avidan and Mashour, 2013; Bischoff and Rundshagen, 2011; Mashour and Avidan, 2015; Sandin et al., 2000; Sebel et al., 2004.

More, it seems, in China—Xu et al., 2009; Shi, 2013.

More again in Spain—Errando et al., 2008.

...twenty thousand to forty thousand people are estimated to remember waking each year in the US alone—Avidan et al., 2008; Sebel et al., 2004.

Last time I searched, the paper had been adjusted slightly—http://sydney.edu.au/medicine/anaesthesia/resources/lectures/anaesthesia_basics.html (accessed 28 November 2016).

One study in the 1980s found that close to half—forty-three per cent: Bogetz and Katz, 1984.

Children wake far more often than adults—Davidson et al., 2005.

Some people might simply have a genetic predisposition to awareness—Kate Leslie has been investigating this possibility.

All of this training helps explain why the death rate from general anaesthesia has dropped—Li et al., 2009; Gibbs and Borton, 2000.

'If you have an inclination to travel take the ether—https://www.general-anaesthesia.com/people/henry-thoreau.html (accessed 3 December 2016).

Jeffrey Mifflin—has since retired, but when I met him he was the Massachusetts General Hospital archivist.

It was here, on Friday October 16, 1846—The history of the discovery of surgical anaesthesia is well documented, though the knives are still out over who gets recognised as the founder of modern anaesthesia. Some of the historic material in this chapter is based on accounts in Fenster, Julie M. *Ether Day* and Snow, Stephanie J. *Blessed Days of Anaesthesia.*

For most of them it ended very badly—It really did: Fenster, Julie *Ether day.*

'Why cannot a man have a tooth extracted and not feel it under the effects of the gas?'—http://www.americanheritage.com/content/%E2%80%9Cgentlemen-no-humbug%E2%80%9D?page=3 (accessed 28 November 2016).

...at a rented hall in Boston—The popular version of this story has Wells' demonstration also taking place in the Ether Dome, but medical historian Rajesh Haridas' research suggests otherwise. Haridas, 2013.

'a glorious conquest for humanity'—https://www.lib.uchicago.edu/ead/pdf/ofcpreshjb-0048-009.pdf (p. 7).

'During the operation the patient muttered—Bigelow, 1846.

It took until 1942 for Canadian anaesthetists to act on what Sir Walter Raleigh had known in 1596—Feldman, *Poison Arrows*; http://www.med.uottawa.ca/historyofmedicine/hetenyi/milner.html.

About half the people who wake unexpectedly during surgery are apparently OK with it—Cook et al., 2014.

One Italian woman who woke peacefully—Bonke, Fitch and Millar (eds) *Memory and awareness in anaesthesia,* p. 246.

To compensate, anaesthetists still routinely overestimate the amount of anaesthetic—Short et al., 2015.

Denial

Sections of this chapter first appeared in the article 'Eyes wide shut', *Good Weekend Magazine*, 10 February 2001.

In the early 1990s, *New Idea* **invited readers to write in**—Cobcroft and Forsdick, 1993.
… anaesthetists greatly underestimate the chances of patients—particularly their patients—waking up under the knife—Myles et al., 2003.
The authors of a 2014 British study wondered—Pandit et al., 2014.
A recent report from a North American registry of awareness patients—Kent et al., 2015.
I had been struck by a 2005 interview in which Frank Guerra—http://www.washingtonpost.com/wp-dyn/articles/A4207-2004Nov22.html (accessed 23 November 2016).
And I refused all elective surgery as an adult—'I had a benign testicular tumor that I refused to have surgically removed due to my fear of having anesthesia. The tumor grew over a 5 year period until it was so big that the heat sensing devices used at airports triggered an alarm. I had to be physically examined by the security to ensure it was not some sort of explosive device. Soon after that I had the tumour removed under epidural anesthesia. I distrusted anesthesiologists to the extent that I returned to the department that I was a resident and had one of my teachers give me the epidural. In 2011 I was 57 years of age. This was approximately 50 years after my awareness experience.' (email to Kate Cole-Adams, 24 October 2016).
America's Joint Commission on Accreditation of Healthcare Organizations finally issued an alert—https://www.ahcmedia.com/articles/4393-jcaho-awareness-during-anesthesia-is-a-problem (accessed 2 December 2016).
The American Society of Anesthesiologists subsequently acknowledged—in its 2006 Practice Advisory for Intraoperative Awareness and Brain Function Monitoring: http://anesthesiology.pubs.asahq.org/article.aspx?articleid=1923386 (accessed 2 December 2016).
Before that, however, then ASA president Roger Litwiller made a small but telling observation—This was during a JCAHO teleconference marking the release of its sentinel alert on 6 October, 2004.
More than half of all patients worry about pain, paralysis and distress—Sandin et al., 2000.
'You cannot stare straight into the face of the sun or death.'—Yalom, Irvin D. *Staring at the sun.*
In the early nineties a Dutch team tracked down—Moerman et al., 1993.
'It is difficult to imagine a more exquisite form of torture'—Wang, 1998.
In a 2005 interview, Wang—https://www.theguardian.com/lifeandstyle/2005/

feb/19/weekend.iansample (accessed 28 November 2016).
In a study published in *The Lancet* in 2000—Sandin et al., 2000.

Paralysis

'The apparent corpse before us hears and distinguishes all that is done'—Fishkin, *Mark Twain's book of animals,* p. 139.

…harrowing early references to doctors operating on paralysed patients who were awake—Winterbottom, 1950.

Take that Swedish study—Sandin et al., 2000.

… the Swedish team decided to follow up the same group of eighteen awareness patients—Lennmarken et al., 2002.

…similar stories I had heard, one from a dear school friend—Harriet Davis woke from an anaesthetic paralysed after the birth of her second son. She thinks it was close to an hour before she could move. These days she says she will do anything to avoid going under. 'I don't care how much blood or whatever. I want to be there. I want to be able to see what's going on . I know it's crazy—it's like I don't feel safe in a plane but I do feel safe in a car because I can see the road, it's nonsense, I know that, but, God, it makes a difference. It's that blank that's terrifying to me. Absolutely terrifying.'

It turns out that about two-thirds of awareness cases happen like this—Cook et al., 2014.

American psychologist Peter Levine has written a lot about paralysis—Levine, *Waking the tiger.*

Two hearts

Sections of this chapter first appeared in the article 'Eyes wide shut', *Good Weekend Magazine*, 10 February 2001.

'When voluntary movement ceases, with the eyes fixed in an upward gaze'—Power et al., 1998.

The first case of awareness involving muscle relaxants was officially reported in 1950—Winterbottom, 1950.

Ten years later a study put the incidence at an alarming 1.2 per cent—Hutchinson, 1961.

Then in January 1998 an American musician called Carol Weihrer underwent anaesthesia for eye surgery—https://www.theguardian.com/lifeandstyle/2005/feb/19/weekend.iansample (accessed 8 October 2016); http://news.bbc.co.uk/2/hi/health/3769245.stm (accessed 28 November 2016).

'Nothing gets much darker than those seconds'—speaking at the 6th International Symposium on Memory and Awareness in Anaesthesia and Intensive Care, Hull, England.

Weihrer's website—http://www.anesthesiaawareness.com/ (accessed 28 November 2016).

Questions without answers

His team…had just published the results of their three-year B-Aware trial—Myles et al., 2004.

Apply an electric shock to the side of a giant sea slug—This information is from Carr's presentation to the annual scientific meeting of the Australia New Zealand College of Anaesthetists in 2000.

…Clifford Woolf, who had established that pain, even unconscious pain, could trigger chronic responses in the spinal cord—Woolf and Chong, 1993.

… a paper published in the early 1960s by a doctor who had reported operating on paralysed patients without anaesthesia—Burn, 1963.

Much later I would come to understand other things about pain—This is a very compressed version of a long and fascinating conversation with Melbourne pain doctor and anaesthetist Malcolm Hogg.

Brainless amoeboid cells have been shown to not only learn but pass that information onto other cells – Vogel and Dussutour, 2016.

What is worth considering, however, is this possibility—Pryor et al., 2014.

Things you don't know you know

Sections of this chapter first appeared in the article 'Eyes wide shut', *Good Weekend Magazine*, 10 February 2001.

'Hillary has just climbed Mount Everest and I had made the astounding discovery'—Levinson, 1989.

Among Levinson's patients at this time was a young woman, Peggy—Levinson, 1989. This is the text of a lecture given by Levinson at the First International Symposium on Memory and Awareness in Anaesthesia in Glasgow, 1989.

'I remember Louie,' wrote Cheek of one patient. 'He was an asthmatic'—Levinson, 1989.

Cheek, who published a series of papers on the subject, argued that such unconscious learning, if allowed to remain unconscious—Levinson, 1989.

…a decade in which American scientists studied inter-species communication with horny dolphins—http://mentalfloss.com/article/26483/4-bizarre-experiments-should-never-be-repeated (accessed 10 October 2016).

…a Yale professor set out to control the mind of a charging bull with an electrical implant—http://mentalfloss.com/article/26483/4-bizarre-experiments-should-never-be-repeated (accessed 10 October 2016).

…the CIA tried to control the minds of unwitting US citizens through the secret application of LSD and other brain-frying drugs—U.S. Senate Report on CIA MKULTRA Behavioral Modification Program 1977 | Public Intelligence. https://publicintelligence.net/ssci-mkultra-1977/ (accessed 10 October 2016).

When I last googled 'unconsciousness' I found a link to the textbook *Adams and Victor's Principles of Neurology*—Ropper et al., 2014.

There was the strange case reported in the mid-1980s by Australian psychologist Julius Howard—Howard, 1987.

Adams and his team had taken twenty-five unconscious heart surgery patients and played them audiotapes of paired words: boy/girl, bitter/sweet, ocean/water—Adams et al., 1998.

'[T]he subjects often complained that they could not see anything at all'—Sidis, 1898. Or online at http://www.sidis.net/psychologyofsugg.pdf (accessed 11 October 2016).

…a team led by US psychologist Henry Bennett—Bennett et al., 1985.

Weird science

This chapter draws on interviews with Graham Burrows and Graham Wicks.

Hypnosis is a curiously liquid phenomenon—Wobst, 2007; Burrows and Dennerstein, *Handbook of hypnosis and psychosomatic medicine.*

A decade later, Scottish physician James Esdaile reported having carried out around three hundred such operations in India—Esdaile, *Mesmerism in India.* (https://www.rickcollingwood.com/sites/default/files/resources/pdf/free/Mesmerism-in-India-and-its-practical-application-in-surgery-and-medicine-by-James-Esdaile-MD.pdf).

By the 1950s, the British Medical Association had recognised a place for hypnotism—Wobst, 2007.

Some years ago I collected from this office a videotape—The video, *Entranced: hypnosis health and healing,* featured South Australian doctor and hypnotherapist Graham Wicks.

…your capacity to be hypnotised remains stable throughout life—http://www.nhne.com/misc/hypnosis.html (accessed 27 November 2016).

One study found there were differences between the corpus callosums—Wobst, 2007.

Moonless nights

It may also be that surgery by its nature imprints itself into her brain's more primitive emotional memory centres—Deeprose et al., 2004.

Neurobiologist James McGaugh writes that in medieval times…a young child might be—McGaugh, 2013.

One theory is that, under anaesthesia, the stress hormones that surge into the

bloodstream—Deeprose et al., 2004; Ghoneim, *Awareness During Anaesthesia*, preface xiii.

At least one study has shown that anaesthetised patients are more likely to learn words during 'surgical stimulation' than before the knife goes in—Deeprose et al., 2004.

But it is also true that some fields…are simply much harder to investigate—as biostatistical whizz Roger Peng explains in his Simply Statistics blog: http://simplystatistics.org/2016/08/24/replication-crisis/ (accessed 12 October 2016).

Some researchers have speculated that one reason patients tested soon after an operation show the most evidence of memories—Merikle and Daneman, 1996.

Some suggest this may also explain reports of patients heading home after surgery, minds soothingly marinated in nothing-muchness—Moerman et al., 1993; Osterman et al., 1998.

One of my favourite studies, mainly because they actually went to the trouble of doing it—Godden et al., 1975.

…I came across a written account by US anaesthetist Anthony Messina—Messina, 1996.

He recently completed a high-level review of data—Messina et al., 2016.

'I am walking across a suspension bridge…'—Levinson, Quo Vadis, in Sebel et al., 'Memory and awareness in anesthesia'. *International Symposium on Memory and Awareness in Anesthesia*.

The most famous anaesthetist in the world

…Eger had set out to solve a problem so basic it seems astonishing that nobody had done it before—Eger, 2002.

The replication study was driven by Ted Eger—Chortkoff et al., 1995.

The island

Their 1996 review, which analysed the data for more than forty experiments—Merikle and Daneman, 1996.

…it may, in the end, be impossible to 'prove' once and for all the existence of unconscious perception—Merikle and Daneman 1998.

Consider the work of American researchers Sheila Murphy and Robert Zajonc—Murphy and Zajonc, 1993.

The ideograph experiment was one of a number of studies that Merikle and Daneman went on to examine in a paper—Merikle and Daneman, 1998.

Scientists at Columbia University Medical Centre did this in 2004—http://newsroom.cumc.columbia.edu/blog/2004/12/17/fleeting-images-of-fearful-faces-show-where-the-brain-processes-unconscious-anxiety-new-cumc-research-3/ (accessed 27 November 2016).

…a study by New York psychologist John Bargh—Bargh et al., 1996.

But a 2016 meta-analysis of the literature in the prestigious *Psychological Bulletin*
—Weingarten et al., 2016; http://www.sciencedirect.com/science/article/pii/
S2352250X16300392 (accessed 4 February 2017).

We know that the brain's auditory pathways can continue to process sound after
we are unconscious—There's plenty of evidence for this (and also in people
who are asleep or in comas). Here are a few anaesthesia papers that discuss it:
Veselis, 2015; Mashour and Avidan, 2015; Deeprose et al., 2005.

We know that implicit memory or priming can continue in anaesthetised surgical
patients—Iselin-Chaves et al., 2005; Andrade, 2005.

We know too that, at light doses of some anaesthetic drugs…the threat-detecting
amygdala can keep pinging away—Pryor et al., 2015.

…an odd and inventive German study from more than twenty years back—
Schwender et al., 1994.

…Wang would attempt a replication of the Man Friday study—Wang et al.,
2015.

After a preliminary study led by one of her PhD students, Catherine Deeprose—
Deeprose et al., 2004.

…they mounted a painstaking study designed to confirm whether memories could
really be awakened and reactivated during deep anaesthesia—Andrade and
Deeprose, 2007.

Dreams

Patients often wake from surgery and report having dreamed—Leslie et al., 2007.

…the exhilaration has been quite as great, though perhaps less pleasurable, than
that of this gas [nitrous oxide], or of the Egyptian haschish—Bigelow, 1846.

…reports had started appearing in journals of patients, mainly women, waking
from anaesthesia in a state of high arousal—Most of the historic material in
this section comes from a fascinating article by Strickland and Butterworth
(2007). The cases of Stille and Dubois are sourced from this article, as well as
that of the Parisian dentist, and the reference to cases reported in *The Lancet*
and *Boston Medical and Surgical Journal*.

'[t]he authors have encountered the problem of sexual ideations or dreams'—
Strickland and Butterworth, 2007.

In July 2009, amid emotional courtroom scenes, a Pittsburgh dentist was
acquitted—http://www.post-gazette.com/local/west/2009/07/09/Oral-surgeon-
acquitted-of-assaults-on-patients/stories/200907090373 (accessed 30 October
2016).

…a Canadian anaesthetist who was convicted of sexually assaulting twenty-one
sedated women—http://www.dailymail.co.uk/news/article-2567632/Canadian-
doctor-sentenced-sexual-assault.html#ixzz44wJbu5kI (accessed 28 November
2016).

'The dream which I had during anaesthesia came to mind'—Aceto et al., 2003.
Either way, various researchers have pointed out that dreaming is in itself a form
of consciousness—Sanders et al., April 2012.
...she and Myles had asked surgical patients if they remembered dreaming during
the anaesthetic—Leslie et al., 2005.
In a new study she and her colleagues monitored the BIS values of three hundred
patients undergoing elective surgery—Leslie et al., 2007.
His name was Stuart Hameroff and he was a respected anaesthetist—Hameroff
conceded in an email that much of *What the Bleep* was pretty silly, but stood by
all that he had said in the film, which, he said, brought the connection between
quantum physics and consciousness to a broad public audience.
He believed that consciousness was a quantum process—There's plenty of material
around if you want to try to wrap your head around this stuff. You could try
Hameroff 1998 or 2006 or Craddock, Hameroff et al., 2015.
...what Bernard Levinson has described as the 'flamboyant charade' of dreams—
Gurman et al., 2005.

Altered states

Australian philosopher David Chalmers has argued—Chalmers, 1995.
'Truth lies open to the view in depth beneath depth of almost blinding evidence,'
wrote William James—'The subjective effects of nitrous oxide', 1882: https://
ebooks.adelaide.edu.au/j/james/william/nitrous/ (accessed 13 October 2016).
It sounds oddly like the experiences described by Jesse Watkins—Laing, *The
Politics of Experience*, pp. 120–37. With thanks to the R. D. Laing Estate for
kind permission to use these extracts.
It was the same for a J. A. Symonds whose own experience following an operation
under ether he recounted to William James—William James. *The Varieties
of Religious Experience*. In http://www.gutenberg.org/files/621/621-h/621-h.
html (citation 10. Accessed 29 November 2016).
'One conclusion was forced upon my mind at that time, and my impression of
its truth has ever since remained unshaken—William James. *The Varieties
of Religious Experience*. In http://www.gutenberg.org/files/621/621-h/621-h.
html (p. 388).

General amnesia

In 1993, as a little known anaesthetist from the recursive Hull, Russell published
a startling study—Russell, 1993.
US anaesthetist Peter Sebel has described a disconcerting plane flight—Sebel, 1995.
On an anaesthesia discussion site I came across the following exchange—the
GASNet site is no longer active.

A working hypothesis

Nine years after that encounter, in an arresting and provocative paper—Kihlstrom and Schacter. 'Anesthesia, amnesia, and the cognitive unconscious' in Bonke et al., *Memory and awareness in anaesthesia*.

The pair did go on to publish a study that showed implicit memory in surgical patients—Kihlstrom et al., 1990.

Neuroscientist Antonio Damasio thinks about this question a lot—*Self comes to mind*.

Britain's Jaideep Pandit posits a state he calls 'dysanaesthesia'—Pandit, 2014. (Others talk about 'disconnected consciousness'.)

In mid-2006, to prove his point, he published a new study using the IFT in conjunction with a commercial depth of anaesthesia monitor, the Narcotrend—Russell, 2006.

While the number of women who responded dropped to closer to one-third when using an inhalation anaesthestic (Russell, October 2013), another study using an intravenous drug showed that during BIS-guided surgery nearly three quarters of patients still responded to command (Russell, May 2013).

Debate ricochets back and forth over the IFT's alleged technical limitations—Pandit, 2013; Russell, 2013; Sleigh, 2013; Sneyd, 2015.

The manufacturers of the Narcotrend sent me a long and cordial defence of the monitor—Barbara Schultz, a member of the working group that developed the classification algorithm, made various points including:

- The monitor pauses its numeric readout when the data include potentially misleading electronic or other artefacts.
- The intermittent readout in the 2006 study may have been partly the result of artefacts due to patients moving in response to Russell's questions—or even to Russell himself lifting the headphones to speak to them.
- Russell's study could have done with some additional data and details.
- Other studies have shown the monitor to reflect changing levels of anaesthesia. (Russell counters that this doesn't mean the patients were unconscious.).
- The monitor's hard and software have in any case evolved a lot in the past decade.

...concerns that Russell has fiercely disputed but which were also raised about the studies using the BIS—Andrzejowski and Wiles, 2013; Brigue and Lanigan, 2013; Russell, August 2013.

A 2012 literature review by a fellow Brit, Robert Sanders, showed thirty-seven per cent of anaesthetised patients responding to the IFT—in Sanders et al., April 2012.

The memory keepers

Whether this would have been preferable to the practice...of treating post-operative delirium with a laudanum enema—Dupuytren, 1834.

The next time I came across him was in this editorial, 'The remarkable memory effects of propofol'—Veselis, 2006.

The article drew a swift response from Bristol anaesthetists Khaled Girgirah and Stephen Kinsella—Girgirah et al., 2006.

In an eloquent response to his Bristol counterparts in *BJA*— Girgirah et al., 2006.

None of which would be news to Rolf Sandin—Sandin et al., 2000.

A new international study—the biggest so far—suggests that things may be quite a lot better—Sanders et al., 2016; Pryor and Veselis, 2016.

This is a lot less than the previous estimate of thirty-seven per cent—Sanders et al., 2012.

In Hull in 2004, on the second day of that perplexing memory and awareness conference, psychologist Michael Wang delivered a brief verbal report—Wang et al., 2004 (pp. 492–3).

On the same day in Hull, Wang and Russell presented another brief 'poster session'—Wang 2004 (p. 493).

Here is US medical psychiatrist Richard Blacher—Blacher, 1984.

New York psychiatrist David Forrest has a novel theory—Forrest, 2008.

The perfect anaesthetic

...in an article subtitled What Sound Does a Tree Make in the Forest When it Falls on Your Head? —Mehlman et al., 1994.

Mehlman mentioned a practice in which medical trainees in the US used to use newly dead patients to practise intubation—Rakatansky et al., 2002.

Years later a big British audit would confirm that Robin's experience was far from unique—Cook et al., 2014. Full report: http://www.nationalauditprojects.org.uk/NAP5report (accessed 2 December 2016).

...anaesthetists Michael Avidan and Jamie Sleigh would praise the project for its insights into patients' subjective experiences—Avidan and Sleigh, 2014.

In a 2011 Finnish study sedated volunteers later reported a kaleidoscope of thoughts, sensations and experiences—Noreika et al., 2011.

Shortly after I interviewed Chortkoff in April 2010, he emailed me with a link to a radio program—http://www.npr.org/templates/story/story.php?storyId=125869707 (accessed 15 Oct 2016); Feinstein et al., 2010.

In 2007, shortly after I returned from my research trip, New York surgeon Scott Haig published an eloquent and disturbing article in *Time* magazine—http://content.time.com/time/health/article/0,8599,1671492,00.html (accessed 15 Oct 2016).

Coming apart

...a mirror theory on how anaesthetics might work formally proposed by Mashour—Mashour, 2004.

The paper that came out under Mashour's name not long after my visit—Mashour, 2008.

Regression

Sections of this chapter first appeared in the article 'Eyes wide shut', *Good Weekend Magazine*, 10 February 2001.

New Zealand anaesthetist Alan Merry has spoken about breaking his leg badly on a skiing holiday—Adam Dudding, 'When doctors become patients', *Sunday Star Times*, 13 August 2006.

Up to three-quarters of us facing surgery say we worry about the possibility of pain, paralysis and distress—Mitchell, 2010. See also: http://www.sciencedaily.com/releases/2010/05/100520093032.htm (accessed 2 December 2016).

US medical psychiatrist Richard Blacher pointed out thirty years ago that the patient's perception of the risk usually far outweighed the realistic dangers—Blacher, *The psychological experience of surgery*.

In a 1910 address delivered on the anniversary of Ether Day, the American surgeon George Crile likened the experience of surgery to facing a firing squad—Crile, 2010. http://www.fullbooks.com/The-Origin-and-Nature-of-Emotions1.html (accessed 3 February 2017).

Anaesthetics, it seems, switch off more recently evolved sections of the brain but can leave some of the more primitive parts relatively active—Veselis, 2015.

'...I found myself lovesick over the surgeon who performed the operations and could not get him out of my head for quite some time...'—http://en.allexperts.com/q/Anesthesiology-962/anesthesia-psychological-side-effects.htm (accessed 2 December 2016).

Pulsations and palpitations

The first looked at the patients' long-term health—Leslie et al., 2010.

Yet on the following page was another study by Leslie and Myles also following up the B-Aware patients—Leslie et al., 2010.

Post-operative cognitive dysfunction, a mild but sometimes disabling mental fogginess, affects up to half of patients in the first week after surgery—Crosby and Culley, 2011; Fines and Severn, 2006.

More dramatic—and less ambiguous—is the delirium that often affects older patients as they emerge from surgical anaesthesia—Robinson et al., 2009. See also: http://www.nytimes.com/2010/06/21/science/21delirium.html (accessed 2 December 2016).

Doctors wonder too about the possible long-term impact of repeated or lengthy anaesthetics on the developing brains of babies—a big study in 2015 found that single, shortish anaesthetics did not seem to pose much of a problem: Sun et al., 2016. See also: https://www.scientificamerican.com/article/general-anesthesia-causes-no-cognitive-deficit-in-infants/.

…the literature had been 'awash with studies suggesting that is not always the case and that sometimes, in an effort to heal the body, we might be harming the brain'—Crosby and Culley, 2011.

…and has on more than one occasion shown a wide awake but paralysed patient to be unconscious—Messner et al., 2003; Schuller et al., 2015.

The pointedly titled B-Unaware Trial of 2008—Avidan et al., 2008.

…another small study from Finland would show that as we come out of anaesthesia, primitive structures deep in our brains switch on first—Långsjö et al., 2012.

Instead, said the study leader, Harry Scheinin, they found the emergence of 'a foundational primitive conscious state'—http://www.aka.fi/en/about-us/media/press-releases/2012/SCIENTISTS-solving-the-mystery-of-human-consciousness/ (accessed 12 February 2016).

Responding to a blog reporting on the Finnish study, one reader left this post—http://mindblog.dericbownds.net/2012/10/brain-correlates-of-switching.html?utm_source=feedburner&utm_medium=feed&utm_campaign=Feed:+Mindblog+%28MindBlog%29&m=1]%E2%80%9D (accessed 2 December 2016).

I wonder if this was the sort of silence and blackness he meant. Perhaps not—When I later put this question to him, Angel responded thus: 'If I were to be a pedantic Limey twit it's a touch simplistic but I'm not a Limey twerp and you have beautifully caught the essence of what I said. Best wishes, Tony.' Thanks Tony.

'…I only mention this because I think we need a more reliable indication of consciousness than motor responses to verbal commands'—some anaesthetists feel the same: Sanders et al., 2012; Williams and Sleigh, 1999.

Six years after our meeting, his team announced they had found what they were looking for—Purdon et al., 2013; Lewis et al., 2012.

'This was first reported in 1937!!!'—other researchers also involved in this line of research include Germany's Eberhart Koch (Koch et al., 1994) and New Zealander Jamie Sleigh (Bennett et al., 2009).

The same way a loud, long tone, like the Emergency Broadcast tone, drowns out all other noise—http://news.mit.edu/2015/new-strategies-anesthesia-emery-brown-0223 (accessed 2 December 2016).

We are teaching this now—In addition to national lectures, Brown and Purdon have an online teaching program: anesthesiaeeg.com or eeganesthesia.com.

...his nascent paradigm of cognitive unbinding as an underlying principle of anaesthesia—Mashour, 2004.

... while, under anaesthesia, sensory information still loops its way from the back of the brain towards the front, the second part of the process breaks down—Mashour, June 2014.

These neural interactions...are where Mashour and a bunch of other investigators... are now focusing their formidable energies—Mashour, June 2014.

The Shallows

...a preoperative visit from an anaesthetist has been shown to be better than a tranquilliser at keeping patients calm—Egbert et al., 1963.

Recently, doctors in the United Kingdom undertook a hugely ambitious project—Cook et al., 2014; Pandit et al., Oct 2014. Full report: http://www. nationalauditprojects.org.uk/NAP5report (accessed 3 December 2016). It's worth noting too that this audit also found a greatly reduced incidence of anaesthesia awareness—but given a methodology relying on patients' unsolicited recollections, sometimes many years after the event, this was not all that surprising. US-based Australian anaesthetist Kane Pryor noted: 'The greatest contribution of NAP5 may not the story of the AAGA cases that were detected, but the uncomfortable knowledge that in routine practice, the vast majority of occurrences are never revealed.' Pryor and Hemmings, 2014.

Among its many findings—On a slightly different tack, Research Implication 7.3: 'Building upon existing work, research is needed to establish if implicit memories for anaesthesia have consequences for patients' wellbeing on recovery.' Pandit et al., Oct 2014.

The experience most strongly associated with psychological sequelae was distress at the time of the event—http://www.nationalauditprojects.org.uk/NAP5report (full report, p. 15).

Reston, Virginia, April 2013. A man later identified in court documents only as D.B. is about to have a colonoscopy—https://www.washingtonpost. com/local/anesthesiologist-trashes-sedated-patient-jury-orders-her-to-pay-500000/2015/06/23/cae05c00-18f3-11e5-ab92-c75ae6ab94b5_story.html (accessed 30 October 2016).

And staff—even those who know they are being watched—sometimes say or do spectacularly inappropriate things—Dutch psychologist Benno Bonke emailed me recently with his memories of working in surgery in the 1970s: 'Having worked in the OR myself, for my PhD in the late seventies, I got intrigued by the phenomenon of awareness. Most notably because I attended so many operations where the conversation of the surgeons (mainly) was sometimes so appalling and degrading towards the supposedly unaware patient that I felt so sorry for them.'

What we do know is that while most people seem to settle back into their lives pretty easily after general anaesthesia, quite a few don't—Whitlock et al., 2015.

'The patient's interpretation of what is happening at the time of the awareness seemed central to later impact'—Cook et al., 2014.

It need not take a scientific study (although someone, bless them, has done one) —'Brain Scans Show Doctors Feel Their Patients' Pain—and Their Relief.' *Medical News Today* http://www.medicalnewstoday.com/releases/255566.php (accessed 2 December 2016).

'To the extent that intra-operative suggestions do some good,' writes psychologist John Kihlstrom—http://socrates.berkeley.edu/~kihlstrm//Blackwell Anesthesia_2015_Long.html (accessed 2 December 2016).

Japanese anaesthetist Jiro Kurata calls this care of the soul—Kurata, 2015.

Blood and blushing

Not only did the hypnosis group use less drugs (during surgery and after)—Montgomery et al., 2007.

Consider the more than twenty million people who each year have surgery under general anaesthesia in the US alone—Purdon et al., 2013.

As an editorial in the same edition of the *Journal of the National Cancer Institute* noted—Spiegel, 2007.

In 2003, the year before I first visited Hull, members of the same team of doctors had analysed a bunch of similar studies —Montgomery et al., 2007.

In the lead-up to my own looming surgery, I emailed Hank Bennett about a small study he had carried out ten years before—Bennett et al., 1986.

Other studies also suggest that simply giving patients information and tips on how to emerge cheerfully from an anaesthetic may sometimes do the trick—Lang et al., 2000; Watcha and White, 1992.

Ballast

Lying in a Perth hospital following a car accident in 1999, his body smashed 'like a toad's'—Hughes R., *Goya*, pp. 8–10.

I find in the cardboard box sent by my uncle—Fraser K., 1956.

That younger me

A man half-waking from an anaesthetic and finding himself, arms tied down, in intensive care—Moerman et al., 1993.

Sometimes the swoopy, disconnected feeling you get under low levels of anaesthetic drugs can mimic other previous dissociative states—Umholtz et al., 2016.

Poet Jean Kent writes of her husband's father waking from heart surgery—'After Heart Surgery' in *The satin bowerbird*.

Sky

One of the most moving moments in Jesse Watkins' ten-day voyage—Laing, *The politics of experience*, p. 131.

Letting go

…a small but mind-bending paper on what happens as rats die—Borjigin et al., 2013.
'[W]e were surprised by the high levels of activity,' said Mashour—http://www. uofmhealth.org/news/archive/201308/electrical-signatures-consciousness-dying-brain (accessed 2 December 2016).

SOURCES

Books

Archer, William Harry. *Life and letters of Horace Wells, discoverer of anesthesia: chronologically arranged with an appendix.* American College of Dentists, 1944.

Blacher, R. S. *The psychological experience of surgery.* John Wiley & Sons, 1987.

Blackmore, Susan. *Consciousness: an introduction.* Hodder and Stoughton, 2003.

Bonke, Benno, William Fitch and Keith Millar (eds). 'Memory and awareness in anaesthesia.' *International Symposium on Memory and Awareness in Anaesthesia, 1st, April 1989, Glasgow.* Swets & Zeitlinger Publishers, 1990.

Burrows, Graham D. and Lorraine Dennerstein. *Handbook of hypnosis and psychosomatic medicine.* Elsevier-North-Holland Biomedical Press, 1980.

Crile, G. W. *Phylogenetic association in relation to certain medical problems.* Barta Press, 1910.

Damasio, Antonio. *Self comes to mind: Constructing the conscious brain.* Vintage, 2012.

Davies, Jan and Rod Westhorpe. *All about anaesthesia.* Oxford University Press, USA, 2000.

Dormandy, Thomas. *The worst of evils: The fight against pain.* Yale University Press, 2006.

Eger II, Edmond I. *The wondrous story of anesthesia.* Eds: Lawrence J. Saidman and Rod N. Westhorpe. Springer New York, 2014.

Esdaile, James. *Mesmerism in India, and its practical application in surgery and medicine.* Silas Andrus and Sons, 1847.

Feldman, Stanley A. *Poison arrows.* Metro Books, 2005.

Fenster, Julie M. *Ether day: the strange tale of America's greatest medical discovery and the haunted men who made it.* Harper Collins, 2002.

Fishkin, Shelley Fisher (ed.) *Mark Twain's book of animals.* University of California Press, 2010.

Ghoneim, Mohamed (ed.) *Awareness during anesthesia.* Butterworth-Heinemann, Oxford, UK, 2001.

Hughes, Robert. *Goya.* The Harvill Press, 2003.

Kent, Jean. *The satin bowerbird.* Hale & Iremonger, 1998.

Keys, Thomas Edward. *The history of surgical anesthesia.* Dover Publications, 1963.

Laing, Ronald David. *The politics of experience and the bird of paradise.* Penguin UK, 1990.

Larkin, Philip. *The complete poems of Philip Larkin.* Faber & Faber, 2012.

Levine, Peter A. *Waking the tiger: Healing trauma: The innate capacity to transform overwhelming experiences.* Vol. 17. North Atlantic Books, 1997.

Mashour, George A., ed. *Consciousness, awareness, and anesthesia.* Cambridge University Press, 2010.

Ropper, Allan H., Samuels, Martin A. and Klein, Joshua P. *Adams and Victor's principles of neurology.* McGraw-Hill Education, New York, 2014.

Sebel, Peter S., Benno Bonke and Eugene Winograd. *Memory and awareness in anesthesia, International Symposium on Memory and Awareness in Anesthesia, 2nd, April 1992, Atlanta, GA, US.* Prentice-Hall, Inc, 1993.

Sidis, Boris. *The psychology of suggestion.* D. Appleton & Company, 1898.

Snow, Stephanie J. *Blessed days of anaesthesia: How anaesthetics changed the world.* Oxford University Press, 2009.

Thernstrom, Melanie. *The pain chronicles.* Farrar, Straus and Giroux, New York, 2010.

U. S. Senate, joint hearing before the Select Committee on Intelligence and the Subcommittee on Health and Scientific Research of the Committee on Human Resources. *Project MKULTRA, the CIA's program of research in behavioral modification.* 95th Congress, 1st session. US Government Printing Office 1977.

Yalom, Irvin D. *Staring at the sun: Overcoming the dread of death.* Scribe Publications, 2008.

Journal papers and articles

Aceto P., Valente A., Gorgoglione M., Adducci E., De Cosmo G. Relationship between awareness and middle latency auditory evoked responses during surgical anaesthesia. *British Journal of Anaesthesia.* 2003 May 1;90(5):630–5.

Adams D. C., Hilton H. J., Madigan J. D., Szerlip N. J., Cooper L. A., Emerson R. G., Smith C. R., Rose E. A., Oz M. C. Evidence for unconscious memory processing during elective cardiac surgery. *Circulation.* 1998 Nov;98(19 Suppl):II289-92.

American Society of Anesthesiologists Task Force on Intraoperative Awareness. Practice advisory for intraoperative awareness and brain function monitoring: a report by the American Society of Anesthesiologists task force on intraoperative awareness. *Anesthesiology.* 2006 Apr;104(4):847.

Andrade J., Jones J. G. Is amnesia for intraoperative events good enough? *British Journal of Anaesthesia.* 1998 May 1;80(5):575–6.

Andrade J. Does memory priming during anesthesia matter? *Journal of the American Society of Anesthesiologists.* 2005 Nov 1;103(5):919–20.

Andrade J., Deeprose C. Unconscious memory formation during anaesthesia. *Best Practice & Research Clinical Anaesthesiology.* 2007 Sep 30;21(3):385–401.

Andrzejowski J., Wiles M. Bispectral index compared with the isolated forearm technique. *Anaesthesia.* 2013 Aug 1;68(8):871–2.

Avidan M.S., Zhang L., Burnside B. A., Finkel K. J., Searleman A. C., Selvidge J. A., Saager L., Turner M. S., Rao S., Bottros M, Hantler C. Anesthesia awareness and the bispectral index. *New England Journal of Medicine.* 2008 Mar 13;358(11):1097–108.

Avidan M. S., Mashour G. A. Prevention of intraoperative awareness with explicit recall making sense of the evidence. *Journal of the American Society of Anesthesiologists.* 2013 Feb 1;118(2):449–56.

Avidan M. S., Sleigh J. W. Beware the Boojum: the NAP5 audit of accidental awareness during intended general anaesthesia. *Anaesthesia.* 2014 Oct 1;69(10):1065–8.

Bargh J. A., Chen M., Burrows L. Automaticity of social behavior: Direct effects of trait construct and stereotype activation on action. *Journal of Personality and Social Psychology.* 1996 Aug;71(2):230.

Beecher H. K. Anesthesia's Second Power. *Science.* 1947 Feb 14;105(2720):164–6.

Bennett C., Voss L. J., Barnard J. P., Sleigh J. W. Practical use of the raw electroencephalogram waveform during general anesthesia: the art and science. *Anesthesia & Analgesia.* 2009 Aug 1;109(2):539–50.

Bennett H. L., Davis H. S., Giannini J. A. Non-verbal response to intraoperative conversation. *British Journal of Anaesthesia.* 1985 Feb 1;57(2):174–9.

Bennett H.L., Benson D.R., Kuiken D. A. Preoperative instructions for decreased bleeding during spine surgery. *Anesthesiology.* 1986 Sep 1;65(3A):A245.

Bennett H. L. The mind during surgery: The uncertain effects of anesthesia. *Advances.* 1993.

Bigelow H. J. Insensibility during surgical operations produced by inhalation. *Boston Medical and Surgical Journal.* 1846 Nov 18;35(16):309–17.

Bischoff P., Rundshagen I. Awareness under general anesthesia. *Prevalence.* 2011 Jan 10;85(100):27–46. (Germany).

Blacher R. S. Awareness during surgery. *Anesthesiology.* 1984 Jul;61(1):1–2.

Blankfield R. P. Suggestion, relaxation, and hypnosis as adjuncts in the care of surgery patients: a review of the literature. *American Journal of Clinical Hypnosis.* 1991 Jan 1;33(3):172–86.

Bogetz M. S., Katz J. A. Recall of surgery for major trauma. *Anesthesiology.* 1984 Jul;61(1):6–9.

Borjigin J., Lee U., Liu T., Pal D., Huff S., Klarr D., Sloboda J., Hernandez J., Wang M. M., Mashour G. A. Surge of neurophysiological coherence and connectivity in the dying brain. *Proceedings of the National Academy of Sciences.* 2013 Aug 27;110(35):14432–7.

Brigue U., Lanigan C. Bispectral index compared with the isolated forearm technique. *Anaesthesia.* 2013 Aug 1;68(8):872–3.

Burn J. M. Relaxant anaesthesia for abdominal operations using hyperventilation with air. *Anaesthesia.* 1963 Jan 1;18(1):84-7.

Chalmers D. J. Facing up to the problem of consciousness. *Journal of Consciousness Studies.* 1995 Mar 1;2(3):200–19.

Chortkoff B. S., Gonsowski C. T., Bennett H. L., Levinson B., Crankshaw D. P., Dutton R. C., Ionescu P., Block R. I., Eger II E. I. Subanesthetic concentrations of desflurane and propofol suppress recall of emotionally charged information. *Anesthesia & Analgesia*. 1995 Oct 1;81(4):728–36.

Cobcroft MD, Forsdick C. Awareness under anaesthesia: the patients' point of view. *Anaesthesia and Intensive Care*. 1993 Dec;21(6):837–43.

Cook T. M., Andrade J., Bogod D. G., Hitchman J. M., Jonker W. R., Lucas N., Mackay J. H., Nimmo A. F., O'Connor K., O'Sullivan E. P., Paul R. G. The 5th National Audit Project (NAP5) on accidental awareness during general anaesthesia: patient experiences, human factors, sedation, consent and medicolegal issues. *Anaesthesia*. 2014 Oct 1;69(10):1102–16.

Cork R. C., Heaton J. F., Campbell C. E., Kihlstrom J. F. Is there implicit memory after propofol sedation?. *British Journal of Anaesthesia*. 1996 Apr 1;76(4):492–8.

Craddock T. J. A., Hameroff S. R., Ayoub T. A., Klobukowski M., Tuszynski J. A. Anesthetics act in quantum channels in brain microtubules to prevent consciousness. *Current Topics in Medicinal Chemistry*. 2015 Mar 1;15(6):523–33.

Crosby G., Culley D. J. Surgery and anesthesia: healing the body but harming the brain? *Anesthesia and analgesia*. 2011 May;112(5):999.

Custers R., Aarts H. The unconscious will: How the pursuit of goals operates outside of conscious awareness. *Science*. 2010 Jul 2;329(5987):47–50.

Cyna A. M., McAuliffe G. L., Andrew M. I. Hypnosis for pain relief in labour and childbirth: a systematic review. *British Journal of Anaesthesia*. 2004 Oct 1;93(4):505–11.

Cyna A. M., Andrew M. I., McAuliffe G. L. Antenatal self-hypnosis for labour and childbirth: a pilot study. *Anaesthesia and Intensive Care*. 2006 Aug 1;34(4):464.

Davidson A. J., Huang G. H., Czarnecki C., Gibson M. A., Stewart S. A., Jamsen K., Stargatt R. Awareness during anesthesia in children: a prospective cohort study. *Anesthesia & Analgesia*. 2005 Mar 1;100(3):653–61.

Deeprose C., Andrade J., Harrison D., Edwards N. Unconscious auditory priming during surgery with propofol and nitrous oxide anaesthesia: a replication. *British Journal of Anaesthesia*. 2005 Jan 1;94(1):57–62.

Deeprose C., Andrade J., Varma S., Edwards N. Unconscious learning during surgery with propofol anaesthesia. *British Journal of Anaesthesia*. 2004 Feb 1;92(2):171–7.

Dupuytren B. D. On nervous delirium. *The Lancet*. 1834;1:919–23.

Editorial. On being aware. *British Journal of Anaesthesia*. 1979 August; 51: 711–12.

Egbert L. D., Battit G. E., Turndorf H., Beecher H. K. The value of the preoperative visit by an anesthetist: A study of doctor-patient rapport. *JAMA*. 1963 Aug 17;185(7):553–5.

Eger E. I. A brief history of the origin of minimum alveolar concentration (MAC). *Journal of the American Society of Anesthesiologists*. 2002 Jan 1;96(1):238–9.

Eger E., Bowdle T. A., Sebel P. S., Ghoneim M. M., Rampil I. J., Padilla R. E., Gan T. J., Domino K. B. How likely is awareness during anesthesia? *Anesthesia & Analgesia*. 2005 May 1;100(5):1544–6.

Errando C. L., Sigl J. C., Robles M., Calabuig E., Garcia J., Arocas F., Higueras R., Del Rosario E., López D., Peiró C. M., Soriano J. L. Awareness with recall during general anaesthesia: a prospective observational evaluation of 4001 patients. *British Journal of Anaesthesia*. 2008 Aug 1;101(2):178–85.

Esaki R. K., Mashour G. A. Levels of consciousness during regional anesthesia and monitored anesthesia care: patient expectations and experiences. *Anesthesia & Analgesia*. 2009 May 1;108(5):1560–3.

Feinstein J. S., Duff M. C., Tranel D. Sustained experience of emotion after loss of memory in patients with amnesia. *Proceedings of the National Academy of Sciences*. 2010 Apr 27;107(17):7674–9.

Fines D. P., Severn A. M. Anaesthesia and cognitive disturbance in the elderly. *Continuing Education in Anaesthesia, Critical Care & Pain*. 2006 Feb 1;6(1):37–40.

Forrest D. V. Alien abduction: A medical hypothesis. *Psychodynamic Psychiatry*. 2008 Oct 1;36(3):431.

Fraser, K. Harold Russell Love. *Medical Journal of Australia*. 1956 September 1; 361–2.

Freeman S. Unconscious synaesthesia: a layered perspective. *British Journal of Anaesthesia* 2012 Feb 1 (vol. 108, no. 2, pp. 339P–340P).

Ghoneim M. M., Block R. I., Haffarnan M., Mathews M. J. Awareness during anesthesia: risk factors, causes and sequelae: a review of reported cases in the literature. *Anesthesia & Analgesia*. 2009 Feb 1;108(2):527–35.

Gibbs N., Borton C. Safety of anaesthesia in Australia. A review of anaesthesia-related mortality. 2000;2002:1–33.

Ginandes C., Brooks P., Sando W., Jones C., Aker J. Can medical hypnosis accelerate post-surgical wound healing? Results of a clinical trial. *American Journal of Clinical Hypnosis*. 2003 Apr 1;45(4):333–51.

Girgirah K., Kinsella S. M., Veselis R. A. Propofol and memory. *British Journal of Anaesthesia*. 2006 Nov 1;97(5):746–8.

Glannon W. Anaesthesia, amnesia and harm. *Journal of Medical Ethics*. 2014 Oct 1;40(10):651–7.

Godden D. R., Baddeley A. D. Context-dependent memory in two natural environments: On land and underwater. *British Journal of Psychology*. 1975 Aug 1;66(3):325–31.

Gurman G. M., Levinson B., Weksler N., Lottan M. Freud and anesthesia—an essay. *Israel Medical Association Journal*. 2005 Sep 1;7(9):554.

Hameroff S. Quantum computation in brain microtubules? The Penrose–Hameroff 'Orch OR' model of consciousness. *Philosophical Transactions* (Royal Society of London Series A Mathematical Physical and Engineering Sciences). 1998 Aug 25:1869–95.

Hameroff S. R. The entwined mysteries of anesthesia and consciousness: is there a common underlying mechanism? *Journal of the American Society of Anesthesiologists*. 2006 Aug 1;105(2):400–12.

Hammonds W. D., Steinhaus J. E. Crawford W. Long: Pioneer physician in anesthesia. *Journal of Clinical Anesthesia*. 1993 Mar 1;5(2):163–7.

Haridas R. P. Horace Wells' demonstration of nitrous oxide in Boston. *Journal of the American Society of Anesthesiologists*. 2013 Nov 1;119(5):1014–22.

Howard J. F. Incidents of auditory perception during anaesthesia with traumatic sequelae. *Medical Journal of Australia*. 1987 Jan;146(1):44–6.

Hutchinson R. Awareness during surgery: A study of its incidence. *British Journal of Anaesthesia*. 1961 Sep 1;33(9):463–9.

Iselin-Chaves I. A., Willems S. J., Jermann F. C., Forster A., Adam S. R., Van der Linden M. Investigation of implicit memory during isoflurane anesthesia for elective surgery using the process dissociation procedure. *Journal of the American Society of Anesthesiologists*. 2005 Nov 1;103(5):925–33.

Izuo M. Medical history: Seishu Hanaoka and his success in breast cancer surgery under general anesthesia two hundred years ago. *Breast Cancer*. 2004 Nov 1;11(4):319–24.

Joint Commission. Sentinel event alert: preventing, and managing the impact of, anesthesia awareness. Issue 32. October 6, 2004.

Kent C. D., Posner K. L., Mashour G. A., Mincer S. L., Bruchas R. R., Harvey A. E., Domino K. B. Patient perspectives on intraoperative awareness with explicit recall: report from a North American anaesthesia awareness registry. *British Journal of Anaesthesia*. 2015 Jul 1;115(suppl 1):i114–21.

Kerssens C., Lubke G. H., Klein J., van der Woerd A., Bonke B. Memory function during propofol and alfentanil anesthesia: predictive value of individual differences. *Journal of the American Society of Anesthesiologists*. 2002 Aug 1;97(2):382–9.

Kerssens C., Klein J., Bonke B. Awareness: monitoring versus remembering what happened. *Journal of the American Society of Anesthesiologists*. 2003 Sep 1;99(3):570–5.

Kerssens C., Ouchi T., Sebel P. S. No evidence of memory function during anesthesia with propofol or isoflurane with close control of hypnotic state. *Journal of the American Society of Anesthesiologists*. 2005 Jan 1;102(1):57–62.

Kerssens C., Hadzidiakos D. A., Buchner A., Rehberg B. Implicit memory phenomena under anesthesia are not spurious. *Journal of the American Society of Anesthesiologists*. 2010 Mar 1;112(3):764–6.

Kihlstrom J. F., Schacter D. L., Cork R. C., Hurt C. A., Behr S. E. Implicit and explicit memory following surgical anesthesia. *Psychological Science*. 1990 Sep 1;1(5):303–6.

Kihlstrom J. F., Cork R. C. Consciousness and anesthesia. In Max Velmans & Susan Schneider (eds) *The Blackwell Companion to Consciousness*. Blackwell, 2007, pp. 628–39.

Kochs E., Bischoff P., Pichlmeier U., Schulte A. E. Surgical stimulation induces changes in brain electrical activity during isoflurane/nitrous oxide anesthesia. A topographic electroencephalographic analysis. *Anesthesiology*. 1994 May;80(5):1026–34.

Kurata J. Minding the mind of subconscious self. *British Journal of Anaesthesia* 2015 Jul 1 (Vol. 115, pp. 122–3). (In: Kurata J., Pandit J. J., Messina A. G., Wang M., Ward M. J., Wilker C. C., Smith B. B., Vezina D. P., Pace N. L., Morimoto Y., Domino K. B. The 9th International Symposium on Memory and Awareness in Anesthesia (MAA9). *British*

Journal of Anaesthesia. 2015 Jul 1;115(suppl 1):i122–44.).

Lang E. V., Benotsch E. G., Fick L. J., Lutgendorf S., Berbaum M. L., Berbaum K. S., Logan H., Spiegel D. Adjunctive non-pharmacological analgesia for invasive medical procedures: a randomised trial. *The Lancet.* 2000 Apr 29;355(9214):1486–90.

Lang E. V., Hatsiopoulou O., Koch T., Berbaum K., Lutgendorf S., Kettenmann E., Logan H., Kaptchuk T. J. Can words hurt? Patient–provider interactions during invasive procedures. *Pain.* 2005 Mar 31;114(1):303–9.

Långsjö J. W., Alkire M. T., Kaskinoro K., Hayama H., Maksimow A., Kaisti K. K., Aalto S., Aantaa R., Jääskeläinen S. K., Revonsuo A., Scheinin H. Returning from oblivion: imaging the neural core of consciousness. *Journal of Neuroscience.* 2012 Apr 4;32(14):4935–43.

Lennmarken C., Bildfors K., Enlund G., Samuelsson P., Sandin R. Victims of awareness. *Acta Anaesthesiologica Scandinavica.* 2002; 46: 229–31.

Lennmarken C., Sydsjo G. Psychological consequences of awareness and their treatment. *Best Practice & Research Clinical Anaesthesiology.* 2007 Sep 30;21(3):357–67.

Leslie K., Myles P. S., Forbes A., Chan M. T., Swallow S. K., Short T. G. Dreaming during anaesthesia in patients at high risk of awareness. *Anaesthesia.* 2005 Mar 1;60(3):239–44.

Leslie K., Skrzypek H., Paech M. J., Kurowski I., Whybrow T. Dreaming during anesthesia and anesthetic depth in elective surgery patients: a prospective cohort study. *Journal of the American Society of Anesthesiologists.* 2007 Jan 1;106(1):33–42.

Leslie K., Myles P. S., Forbes A., Chan M. T. The effect of bispectral index monitoring on long-term survival in the B-aware trial. *Anesthesia & Analgesia.* 2010 Mar 1;110(3):816–22.

Leslie K., Chan M. T., Myles P. S., Forbes A., McCulloch T. J. Posttraumatic stress disorder in aware patients from the B-aware trial. *Anesthesia & Analgesia.* 2010 Mar 1;110(3):823–8.

Levinson, B. W. 'Quo Vadis', in P. S. Sebel, B. Bonke & E. Winograd (eds), *Memory and Awareness in Anesthesia.* Prentice-Hall, 1993.

Levinson B. W. States of awareness during general anaesthesia. Preliminary communication. *British Journal of Anaesthesia.* 1965 Jul 1;37(7):544–6.

Levinson B. The states of awareness in anaesthesia in 1965. *SA Family Practice.* 1989 Oct: 517–521.

Lewis L. D., Weiner V. S., Mukamel E. A., Donoghue J. A., Eskandar E. N., Madsen J. R., Anderson W. S., Hochberg L. R., Cash S. S., Brown E. N., Purdon P. L. Rapid fragmentation of neuronal networks at the onset of propofol-induced unconsciousness. *Proceedings of the National Academy of Sciences.* 2012 Dec 4;109(49):E3377–86.

Li G., Warner M., Lang B. H., Huang L., Sun L. S. Epidemiology of anesthesia-related mortality in the United States, 1999–2005. *Journal of the American Society of Anesthesiologists.* 2009 Apr 1;110(4):759–65.

Lubke G. H., Kerssens C., Phaf H., Sebel P. S. Dependence of explicit and implicit memory on hypnotic state in trauma patients. *Journal of the American Society of Anesthesiologists.* 1999 Mar 1;90(3):670–80.

Lubke G. H., Sebel P. S. Awareness and different forms of memory in trauma anaesthesia. *Current Opinion in Anesthesiology.* 2000 Apr 1;13(2):161–5.

Lubke G. H., Kerssens C., Gershon R. Y., Sebel P. S. Memory formation during general anesthesia for emergency cesarean sections. *Journal of the American Society of Anesthesiologists.* 2000 Apr 1;92(4):1029–34.

McGaugh J. L. Making lasting memories: Remembering the significant. *Proceedings of the National Academy of Sciences.* 2013 Jun 18;110 (Supplement 2):10402–7.

Mashour G. A. Consciousness unbound. Toward a paradigm of general anesthesia. *Journal of the American Society of Anesthesiologists.* 2004 Feb 1;100(2):428–33.

Mashour G. A. Integrating the science of consciousness and anesthesia. *Anesthesia & Analgesia.* 2006 Oct 1;103(4):975–82.

Mashour G. A. Toward a general theory of unconscious processes in psychoanalysis and anesthesiology. *Journal of the American Psychoanalytic Association.* 2008 Mar 1;56(1):203–22.

Mashour G. A. Posttraumatic stress disorder after intraoperative awareness and high-risk surgery. *Anesthesia & Analgesia.* 2010 Mar 1;110(3):668–70.

Mashour G. A. Dreaming during anesthesia and sedation. *Anesthesia & Analgesia.* 2011 May 1;112(5):1008–10.

Mashour G. A. Fragmenting consciousness. *Proceedings of the National Academy of Sciences.* 2012 Dec 4;109(49):19876–7.

Mashour G. A. Top-down mechanisms of anesthetic-induced unconsciousness. *Frontiers in Systems Neuroscience.* 2014 Jun 23;8:115.

Mashour G. A., Avidan M. S. Psychological trajectories after intraoperative awareness with explicit recall. *Anesthesia & Analgesia.* 2014 Jul 1;119(1):1–3.

Mashour G. A., Avidan M. S. Intraoperative awareness: controversies and non-controversies. *British Journal of Anaesthesia.* 2015 Jul 1;115(suppl 1):i20–6.

Mehlman M. J., Kanoti G. A., Orlowski J. P. Informed consent to amnestics, or: what sound does a tree make in the forest when it falls on your head?. *Journal of Clinical Ethics.* 1994;5(2):105.

Merikle P. M., Daneman M. Memory for unconsciously perceived events: evidence from anesthetized patients. *Consciousness and Cognition.* 1996 Dec 31;5(4):525–41.

Merikle P. M., Daneman M. Psychological investigations of unconscious perception. *Journal of Consciousness Studies.* 1998 Jan 1;5(1):5–18.

Messina A. G., Paranicas M., Yao F. S., Illner P., Roman M. J., Saba P. S., Devereux R. B. The effect of midazolam on left ventricular pump performance and contractility in anesthetized patients with coronary artery disease: Effect of preoperative ejection fraction. *Anesthesia & Analgesia.* 1995 Oct 1;81(4):793–9.

Messina A. G. Awareness in anaesthesia: a personal view. *Memory and Awareness in Anaesthesia.* Assen: Van Gorcum & Comp. BV. 1996:134–36.

Messina A. G., Wang M., Ward M. J., Wilker C. C., Smith B. B., Vezina D. P., Pace N. L. Anaesthetic interventions for prevention of awareness during surgery. The Cochrane Library. 2016.

Messner M., Beese U., Romstöck J., Dinkel M., Tschaikowsky K. The bispectral index declines during neuromuscular block in fully awake persons. *Anesthesia & Analgesia.* 2003 Aug 1;97(2):488–91.

Mitchell M. General anaesthesia and day-case patient anxiety. *Journal of Advanced Nursing.* 2010 May 1;66(5):1059–71.

Moerman N., Bonke B., Oosting J. Awareness and recall during general anesthesia: facts and feelings. *Anesthesiology—Philadelphia then Hagerstown.* 1993 Sep 1;79:454.

Montgomery G. H., David D, Winkel G., Silverstein J. H., Bovbjerg D. H. The effectiveness of adjunctive hypnosis with surgical patients: a meta-analysis. *Anesthesia & Analgesia.* 2002 Jun 1;94(6):1639–45.

Montgomery G. H., Bovbjerg D. H., Schnur J. B., David D., Goldfarb A., Weltz C. R., Schechter C., Graff-Zivin J., Tatrow K., Price D. D., Silverstein J. H. A randomized clinical trial of a brief hypnosis intervention to control side effects in breast surgery patients. *Journal of the National Cancer Institute.* 2007 Sep 5;99(17):1304–12.

Münte S., Münte T. F., Grotkamp J., Haeseler G., Raymondos K., Piepenbrock S., Kraus G. Implicit memory varies as a function of hypnotic electroencephalogram stage in surgical patients. *Anesthesia & Analgesia.* 2003 Jul 1;97(1):132–8.

Münte S. Strategies to avoid awareness during anaesthesia. *British Journal of Anaesthesia.* 2012 Feb 1 (Vol. 108, No. 2, pp. 352P–353P).

Murphy S. T., Zajonc R. B. Affect, cognition, and awareness: affective priming with optimal and suboptimal stimulus exposures. *Journal of Personality and Social Psychology.* 1993 May;64(5):723.

Myles P. S., Symons J. A., Leslie K. Anaesthetists' attitudes towards awareness and depth-of-anaesthesia monitoring. *Anaesthesia.* 2003 Jan 1;58(1):11–6.

Myles P. S., Leslie K., McNeil J., Forbes A., Chan M. T., B-Aware Trial Group. Bispectral index monitoring to prevent awareness during anaesthesia: The B-Aware randomised controlled trial. *The Lancet.* 2004 May 29;363(9423):1757–63.

Myles P. S. Generalizability of anaesthesia study populations. *British Journal of Anaesthesia.* 2014 Oct 1;113(4):535–6.

Noreika V., Jylhänkangas L., Móró L., Valli K., Kaskinoro K., Aantaa R., Scheinin H., Revonsuo A. Consciousness lost and found: subjective experiences in an unresponsive state. *Brain and Cognition.* 2011 Dec 31;77(3):327–34.

Osterman J. E., van der Kolk B. A. Awareness during anesthesia and posttraumatic stress disorder. *General Hospital Psychiatry.* 1998 Sep 30;20(5):274–81.

Osterman J. E., Hopper J., Heran W. J., Keane T. M., van der Kolk B. A. Awareness under anesthesia and the development of posttraumatic stress disorder. *General Hospital Psychiatry.* 2001 Aug 31;23(4):198–204.

Pandit J. J. Isolated forearm—or isolated brain? Interpreting responses during anaesthesia—or 'dysanaesthesia'. *Anaesthesia*. 2013 Oct 1;68(10):995–1000.

Pandit J. J. Acceptably aware during general anaesthesia:'dysanaesthesia'—the uncoupling of perception from sensory inputs. *Consciousness and Cognition*. 2014 Jul 31;27:194–212.

Pandit J. J., Andrade J., Bogod D. G., Hitchman J. M., Jonker W. R., Lucas N., Mackay J. H., Nimmo A. F., O'Connor K., O'Sullivan E. P., Paul R. G. The 5th National Audit Project (NAP5) on accidental awareness during general anaesthesia: Summary of main findings and risk factors. *Anaesthesia*. 2014 Oct 1;69(10):1089–101.

Pollard R. J., Coyle J. P., Gilbert R. L., Beck J. E. Intraoperative awareness in a regional medical system: A review of 3 years' data. *Journal of the American Society of Anesthesiologists*. 2007 Feb 1;106(2):269–74.

Power C., Crowe C., Higgins P., Moriarty D. C. Anaesthetic depth at induction. An evaluation using clinical eye signs and EEG polysomnography. *Anaesthesia*. 1998 Aug 1;53(8):736–43.

Proceedings of the 6th International Symposium Memory and Awareness in Anaesthesia and Intensive Care. *British Journal of Anaesthesia*. 2004; 93 (3): 482–94.

Proceedings of the 7th International Symposium Memory and Awareness in Anaesthesia. *British Journal of Anaesthesia*. 2008; 100(6): 868–80.

Proceedings of the 9th International Symposium Memory and Awareness in Anaesthesia. *British Journal of Anaesthesia*. 2015; 115 (suppl 1): i122–i144.

Pryor K. O., Hemmings H. C. NAP5: intraoperative awareness detected, and undetected. *British Journal of Anaesthesia*. 2014 Oct 1;113(4):530–3.

Pryor K. O., Root J. C. Chasing the shadows of implicit memory under anesthesia. *Anesthesia & Analgesia*. 2014 Nov. 1;119(5):1026–8.

Pryor K. O., Root J. C., Mehta M., Stern E., Pan H., Veselis R. A., Silbersweig D. A. Effect of propofol on the medial temporal lobe emotional memory system: a functional magnetic resonance imaging study in human subjects. *British Journal of Anaesthesia*. 2015 Jul 1;115(suppl 1):i104–13.

Pryor K. O., Veselis R. A. Isolated forearm test: replicated, relevant, and unexplained. *Anesthesiology*. 2016 Dec 15.

Pullman M., Andrzejowski J. Comfortably numb. *Anaesthesia*. 2013 Sep 1;68(9):896–8.

Purdon P. L., Pierce E. T., Mukamel E. A., Prerau M. J., Walsh J. L., Wong K. F., Salazar-Gomez A. F., Harrell P. G., Sampson A. L., Cimenser A., Ching S. Electroencephalogram signatures of loss and recovery of consciousness from propofol. Proceedings of the National Academy of Sciences. 2013 Mar 19;110(12):E1142–51.

Rakatansky H., Riddick F. A., Morse L. J., O'Bannon J. M., Goldrich M. S., Ray P., Weiss M., Sade R. M., Spillman M. A., Morin K., Kao A. Performing procedures on the newly deceased. *Academic Medicine*. 2002 Dec 1;77(12):1212–16.

Robinson T. N., Raeburn C. D., Tran Z. V., Angles E. M., Brenner L. A., Moss M. Postoperative delirium in the elderly: risk factors and outcomes. *Annals of Surgery*. 2009 Jan 1;249(1):173–8.

Rowan K. J. Awareness under TIVA: a doctor's personal experience. *Anaesthesia and Intensive Care.* 2002 Aug 1;30(4):505.

Russell I. F. Midazolam–alfentanil: an anaesthetic? An investigation using the isolated forearm technique. *British Journal of Anaesthesia.* 1993 Jan 1;70(1):42–6.

Russell I. F. The Narcotrend 'depth of anaesthesia'monitor cannot reliably detect consciousness during general anaesthesia: an investigation using the isolated forearm technique. *British Journal of Anaesthesia.* 2006 Mar 1;96(3):346–52.

Russell I. F. The ability of bispectral index to detect intra-operative wakefulness during total intravenous anaesthesia compared with the isolated forearm technique. *Anaesthesia.* 2013 May 1;68(5):502–11.

Russell I. F. Fourteen fallacies about the isolated forearm technique, and its place in modern anaesthesia. *Anaesthesia.* 2013 Jul 1;68(7):677–81.

Russell I. F. A reply. *Anaesthesia.* 2013 Aug 1;68(8):872–3.

Russell I. F. The ability of bispectral index to detect intra-operative wakefulness during isoflurane/air anaesthesia, compared with the isolated forearm technique. *Anaesthesia.* 2013 Oct 1;68(10):1010–20.

Sanders R. D., Tononi G., Laureys S., Sleigh J. External awareness under general anaesthesia: data from the isolated forearm technique. *British Journal of Anaesthesia.* 2012 Feb 1 (Vol. 108, No. 2, pp. 358P–359P).

Sanders R. D., Tononi G., Laureys S., Sleigh J. W. Unresponsiveness ≠ unconsciousness. *Journal of the American Society of Anesthesiologists.* 2012 Apr 1;116(4):946–59.

Sanders R. D., Absalom A., Sleigh J. W. V. 'For now we see through a glass, darkly': the anaesthesia syndrome. *British Journal of Anaesthesia.* 2014 May 1;112(5):790–3.

Sanders R. D., Gaskell A., Raz A., Winders J., Stevanovic A., Rossaint R., Boncyk C., Defresne A., Tran G., Tasbihgou S., Meier S. Incidence of connected consciousness after tracheal intubation: a prospective, international, multicenter cohort study of the isolated forearm technique. *Journal of the American Society of Anesthesiologists.* 2016 Dec 15.

Sandin R. H., Enlund G., Samuelsson P., Lennmarken C. Awareness during anaesthesia: a prospective case study. *The Lancet.* 2000 Feb 26;355(9205):707–11.

Schuller P. J., Newell S., Strickland P. A., Barry J. J. Response of bispectral index to neuromuscular block in awake volunteers. *British Journal of Anaesthesia.* 2015 Jul 1;115(suppl 1):i95–103.

Schwender D., Kaiser A., Klasing S., Peter K., Pöppel E. Midlatency auditory evoked potentials and explicit and implicit memory in patients undergoing cardiac surgery. *Anesthesiology.* 1994 Mar;80(3):493–501.

Schwender D., Kunze-Kronawitter H., Dietrich P., Klasing S., Forst H., Madler C. Conscious awareness during general anaesthesia: patients' perceptions, emotions, cognition and reactions. *British Journal of Anaesthesia.* 1998 Feb 1;80(2):133–9.

Sebel P. S. Memory during anesthesia: Gone but not forgotten? *Anesthesia & Analgesia.* 1995 Oct 1;81(4):668–70.

Sebel P. S., Bowdle T. A., Ghoneim M. M., Rampil I. J., Padilla R. E., Gan T. J., Domino K. B. The incidence of awareness during anesthesia: a multicenter United States study. *Anesthesia & Analgesia.* 2004 Sep 1;99(3):833–9.

Sebel P. S. Are indirect memory studies in anaesthesia subject to the decline effect?. *British Journal of Anaesthesia.* 2012 Feb 1 (Vol. 108, No. 2, pp. 361P–361P).

Shi X., Wang D. X. The incidence of awareness with recall during general anesthesia has been lowered: a historical controlled trial. *Zhonghua Yi Xue Za Zhi.* 2013; 93: 3272–5.

Short T. G., Leslie K., Chan M. T., Campbell D., Frampton C., Myles P. Rationale and design of the balanced anesthesia study: a prospective randomized clinical trial of two levels of anesthetic depth on patient outcome after major surgery. *Anesthesia & Analgesia.* 2015 Aug 1;121(2):357–65.

Sleigh J. The place of the isolated forearm technique in modern anaesthesia: yet to be defined. *Anaesthesia.* 2013 Jul 1;68(7):681–3.

Sleigh J. No monitor is an island: Depth of anesthesia involves the whole patient. *Journal of the American Society of Anesthesiologists.* 2014 Apr 1;120(4):799–800.

Sneyd J. R. NAP5 and the isolated forearm technique. *British Journal of Anaesthesia.* 2015 Jul 1;115(1):138–9.

Spiegel D. The mind prepared: Hypnosis in surgery. *Journal of the National Cancer Institute.* 2007 Sep 5;99(17):1280–1.

Strickland R. A., Butterworth J. F. Sexual dreaming during anesthesia: Early case histories (1849–88) of the phenomenon. *Journal of the American Society of Anesthesiologists.* 2007 Jun 1;106(6):1232–6.

Sun L. S., Li G., Miller T. L., Salorio C., Byrne M. W., Bellinger D. C., Ing C., Park R., Radcliffe J., Hays S. R., DiMaggio C. J. Association between a single general anesthesia exposure before age 36 months and neurocognitive outcomes in later childhood. *JAMA.* 2016 Jun 7;315(21):2312–20.

Tinnin L. Conscious forgetting and subconscious remembering of pain. *Journal of Clinical Ethics.* 1994 5(2):151–2.

Tunstall M. E. On being aware by request: A mother's unplanned request during the course of a Caesarean section under general anaesthesia. *British Journal of Anaesthesia.* 1980 Oct 1;52(10):1049–54.

Umholtz M., Cilnyk J., Wang C. K., Porhomayon J., Pourafkari L., Nader N. D. Postanesthesia emergence in patients with posttraumatic stress disorder. *Journal of Clinical Anesthesia.* 2016 Nov 30;34:3–10.

Veselis R. A. The remarkable memory effects of propofol. *British Journal of Anaesthesia.* 2006 Mar 1;96(3):289–91.

Veselis R. A. Memory: A guide for anaesthetists. *Best Practice & Research Clinical Anaesthesiology.* 2007 Sep 30;21(3):297–312.

Veselis R. A. Anaesthetic amnesia: Where is a memory to hide? *British Journal of Anaesthesia.* 2012 Feb 1 (Vol. 108, No. 2, pp. 365P–365P).

Veselis R. A. Memory formation during anaesthesia: plausibility of a neurophysiological basis. *British Journal of Anaesthesia*. 2015 Mar 3:aev035.

Vogel D., Dussutour A. Direct transfer of learned behaviour via cell fusion in non-neural organisms. *Proceedings of the Royal Society B* (Vol. 283, No. 1845, 2016.2382).

Voss L., Sleigh J. Monitoring consciousness: the current status of EEG-based depth of anaesthesia monitors. *Best Practice & Research Clinical Anaesthesiology*. 2007 Sep 30;21(3):313–25.

Wang M. Inadequate anesthesia as a cause of psychopathology. *Royal College of Anaesthetists Newsletter*. 1998 May;40.

Wang M., Russell I. F., Nicholson J. A 10-year retrospective follow-up of alfentanil–midazolam patients who indicated intraoperative pain without explicit recall. *British Journal of Anaesthesia*. 2004 Sep 1 (Vol. 93, No. 3, pp. 493P–493P).

Wang M., Russell I. F., Logan C. D. Light anaesthesia without explicit recall during hysterectomy is associated with increased postoperative anxiety over a 3-month follow-up period. *British Journal of Anaesthesia*. 2004 Sep 1 (Vol. 93, No. 3, pp. 492P–493P).

Wang M. Implicit–explicit dissociation after conscious sedation: implications for inadequate general anaesthesia. *British Journal of Anaesthesia*. 2012 Feb 1 (Vol. 108, No. 2, pp. 366P–366P).

Wang M., Rich N., Trubshaw E., Thompson J. Implicit emotional memory in intensive care unit patients: Replication of the Robinson Crusoe study. *British Journal of Anaesthesia*. 2015 Jul 1;115(suppl 1):i125–126).

Watcha M. F., White P. F. Postoperative nausea and vomiting. Its etiology, treatment, and prevention. *Anesthesiology*. 1992 Jul;77(1):162–84.

Weingarten E., Chen Q., McAdams M., Yi J., Hepler J., Albarracín D. From primed concepts to action: a meta-analysis of the behavioral effects of incidentally presented words. *Psychological Bulletin*, Vol 142(5), May 2016, 472–97.

Whitlock E. L., Rodebaugh T. L., Hassett A. L., Shanks A. M., Kolarik E., Houghtby J., West H. M., Burnside B. A., Shumaker E., Villafranca A., Edwards W. A. Psychological sequelae of surgery in a prospective cohort of patients from three intraoperative awareness prevention trials. *Anesthesia and analgesia*. 2015 Jan;120(1):87–95.

Williams M. L., Sleigh J. W. Auditory recall and response to command during recovery from propofol anaesthesia. *Anaesthesia and Intensive Care*. 1999 Jun 1;27(3):265.

Winterbottom E. H. Insufficient anaesthesia. *British Medical Journal*. 1950 Jan 28;1(4647):247.

Wobst A. H. Hypnosis and surgery: Past, present, and future. *Anesthesia & Analgesia*. 2007 May 1;104(5):1199–208.

Woolf C. J., Chong M. S. Preemptive analgesia—treating postoperative pain by preventing the establishment of central sensitization. *Anesthesia & Analgesia*. 1993 Aug 1;77(2):362–79.

Xu L., Wu A. S., Yue Y. The incidence of intra-operative awareness during general anesthesia in China: a multi-center observational study. *Acta Anaesthesiologica Scandinavica*. 2009 Aug 1;53(7):873–82.

INDEX